Schizophrenia FOR DUMMIES®

Schizophrenia FOR DUMMIES®

by Jerome Levine, MD, and
Irene S. Levine, PhD

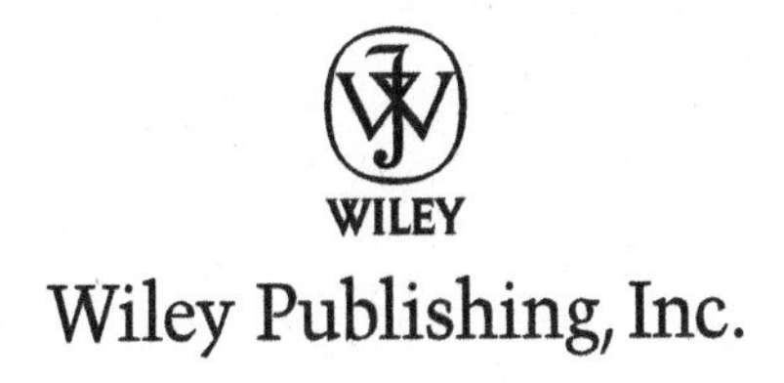

Wiley Publishing, Inc.

Schizophrenia For Dummies®

Published by
Wiley Publishing, Inc.
111 River St.
Hoboken, NJ 07030-5774
`www.wiley.com`

For general information on our other products and services, please contact our Customer Care Department within the U.S. at 877-762-2974, outside the U.S. at 317-572-3993, or fax 317-572-4002.

For technical support, please visit `www.wiley.com/techsupport`.

Wiley also publishes its books in a variety of electronic formats. Some content that appears in print may not be available in electronic books.

Library of Congress Control Number: 2008936638

ISBN: 978-0-470-25927-6

Manufactured in the United States of America

10 9 8 7 6 5

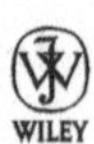

About the Authors

Jerome Levine, MD: Jerome Levine is a board-certified psychiatrist whose research and clinical career has spanned almost 50 years. For a major portion of that time, Dr. Levine served as chief of psychopharmacology at the National Institute of Mental Health. There, he worked both nationally and internationally to help design, manage, and conduct much of the federally supported research that serves as the foundation for current approaches to the pharmacologic treatment of schizophrenia and other serious mental disorders.

After leaving the federal government, Dr. Levine joined the faculty of the University of Maryland Department of Psychiatry and the Maryland Psychiatric Research Center. Both settings treat and carry out treatment studies of hospitalized and community-based individuals diagnosed with schizophrenia. In Maryland, he also directed a program training early-career psychiatrists to become research psychiatrists.

In 1994, Dr. Levine moved to New York State, where he joined the faculty of the Department of Psychiatry of the New York University School of Medicine as a professor of psychiatry, and was appointed deputy director of the NYS Nathan S. Kline Institute for Psychiatric Research. He oversees research studying the causes, pathophysiology, and treatment of schizophrenia at basic, translational, and applied clinical levels.

Dr. Levine's residency training was at the State University of New York at Buffalo Department of Psychiatry and at St. Elizabeth's Hospital in Washington, D.C. In addition, he has served on the faculty at the U.S. Public Health Service Narcotic Hospital in Lexington, Kentucky; at the Johns Hopkins Department of Psychiatry in Baltimore, Maryland; and at the University of Pisa Department of Psychiatry in Italy.

He has published numerous papers and books in the scientific literature and is a life fellow of the prestigious American College of Neuropsychopharmacology. In addition to being listed in *Who's Who in America,* Dr. Levine was awarded the American Psychiatric Association Hofheimer Research Prize and the Distinguished Leader in Research Award from the National Alliance on Mental Illness of New York State.

Irene S. Levine, PhD: Irene Levine has a doctoral degree in clinical psychology as well as extensive experience working in the public mental health system at local, state, and national levels. She began her career as a staff psychologist and treatment team leader at Creedmoor Psychiatric Center and left to develop and direct two nonprofit psychosocial rehabilitation programs in Queens and Suffolk counties in New York.

For a period of more than 15 years, Dr. Levine held senior management roles at the National Institute of Mental Health (NIMH) and the Substance Abuse and Mental Health Services Administration (SAMHSA) in Rockville, Maryland. She was one of the architects of the NIMH Community Support Program, created and directed the NIMH Program for the Homeless Mentally Ill, and served as the first deputy director of the SAMHSA Center for Mental Health Services.

In 1994, Dr. Levine joined the Nathan S. Kline Institute for Psychiatric Research in Orangeburg, New York, where she directs communications and serves as the institute's liaison to families. She holds a faculty appointment as a professor of psychiatry at the New York University School of Medicine. She has lectured locally, nationally and internationally about the needs of families of individuals with severe mental illnesses, such as schizophrenia and major mood disorders.

For the past ten years, Dr. Levine has also been a prolific, award-winning freelance journalist and author, whose credits include some of the nation's top magazines and newspapers. She writes on mental health as well as a wide range of other health and lifestyle topics, and is currently completing a book on female friendships for Overlook Press (2009). She is a member of the American Psychological Association, the National Alliance on Mental Illness, the National Association of Science Writers, the Association of Healthcare Journalists, the American Medical Writers Association, the Authors Guild, and the American Society of Journalists and Authors.

Dedication

We dedicate this book to all the courageous individuals with serious mental illness and their families that we have met through the years, who have taught us invaluable lessons that we never learned in school. We also dedicate this book to the individuals who volunteer as research participants in the interest of helping others learn about the causes of and treatments for schizophrenia.

This book is also dedicated to our own families who have enriched our lives in ways too numerous to mention, and especially to our son, Andrew, who has been an ongoing source of pride as well as 24/7 technical computer support.

Finally, this book is dedicated to the memory of Max Schneier, one of the earliest pioneers of the family advocacy movement, who taught us about the importance of listening to the wisdom of family members.

Authors' Acknowledgments

We would like to acknowledge some of our professional colleagues, many of them our personal friends, who have dedicated their lives to improving treatment and care for individuals with schizophrenia. The knowledge upon which this book is based is derived, in no small measure, from their contributions. They include: MaryJane Alexander, MD; Thomas Ban, MD; Robert Cancro, MD; William T. Carpenter, MD; Giovanni B. Cassano, MD; Leslie Citrome, MD, MPH; Jonathan O. Cole, MD; Areta Crowell, PhD; Lynn DeLisi, MD; Joel Elkes, MD; Laurie Flynn; Risa Fox, MSW; Alan Gelenberg, MD; Howard Goldman, MD; Michael Hogan, PhD; Ron Honberg, JD; Samuel Keith, MD; Daniel Javitt, MD, PhD; John Kane, MD; Harold Koplewicz, MD; Alan Leshner, PhD; Robert P. Liberman, MD; Jeffrey Lieberman, MD; Linda Ligenza, MSW; Arnold M. Ludwig, MD; Dolores Malaspina, MD; Herbert Meltzer, MD; Stuart Moss, MLS; Fred Osher, MD; Herbert Pardes, MD; Nadine Revheim, PhD; Linda Rosenberg, MSW; Nina R. Schooler, PhD; Steven S. Sharfstein, MD; John Talbott, MD; Fuller Torrey, MD; Judith Turner-Crowson; and Peter Weiden, MD. Although these individuals have influenced our writing and our careers, such an eclectic group would not necessarily agree with everything we've written.

We are profoundly indebted to the members of the National Alliance on Mental Illness, especially Rena Finkelstein, Helen Klein, and other members of NAMI-FAMILYA of Rockland County, New York, for their inspiration and collaboration over the years.

Lastly, we appreciate the support of Michael Lewis, of Wiley Publishing, and Elizabeth Kuball and Sharon Perkins, who shepherded us through this project. Thanks also to our agent, Marilyn Allen, who served as a matchmaker and cheerleader.

Publisher's Acknowledgments

We're proud of this book; please send us your comments through our Dummies online registration form located at www.dummies.com/register/.

Some of the people who helped bring this book to market include the following:

Acquisitions, Editorial, and Media Development

Project Editor: Elizabeth Kuball

Acquisitions Editor: Michael Lewis

Copy Editor: Elizabeth Kuball

Assistant Editor: Erin Calligan Mooney

Technical Editor: Wendy Koebel, LMSW, ACSW

Senior Editorial Manager: Jennifer Ehrlich

Editorial Supervisor and Reprint Editor: Carmen Krikorian

Editorial Assistants: Joe Niesen, Jennette ElNaggar, and David Lutton

Cover Photos: © Image Source Black/Alamy

Cartoons: Rich Tennant (www.the5thwave.com)

Composition Services

Project Coordinator: Erin Smith

Layout and Graphics: Reuben W. Davis, Christin Swinford, Christine Williams

Special Art: Kathryn Born

Proofreaders: John Greenough, Caitie Kelly, Toni Settle

Indexer: Potomac Indexing, LLC

Special Help: Sharon Perkins, Alicia South

Publishing and Editorial for Consumer Dummies

Diane Graves Steele, Vice President and Publisher, Consumer Dummies

Joyce Pepple, Acquisitions Director, Consumer Dummies

Kristin Ferguson-Wagstaffe, Product Development Director, Consumer Dummies

Ensley Eikenburg, Associate Publisher, Travel

Kelly Regan, Editorial Director, Travel

Publishing for Technology Dummies

Andy Cummings, Vice President and Publisher, Dummies Technology/General User

Composition Services

Gerry Fahey, Vice President of Production Services

Debbie Stailey, Director of Composition Services

Contents at a Glance

Table of Contents

Introduction

Schizophrenia affects as many as 1 in 100 Americans over their lifetime and is twice as common as HIV/AIDS. Yet few other diseases are shrouded in quite as much misinformation, lack of information, and secrecy as schizophrenia is. On average, it takes more than eight years between the time symptoms first appear and the time a person is diagnosed and treated for the disorder. Pervasive stigma keeps most people in the dark until the disorder becomes up close and personal. As a result, when someone you love is diagnosed with schizophrenia — a no-fault, equal-opportunity brain disorder — you're not sure where to turn or who to tell. Initially, most people feel ashamed, bewildered, and alone.

During our careers working in various research, policy, and clinical roles at federal, state, and local levels, people with schizophrenia and their loved ones often asked us questions. We always tried to provide simple, straightforward answers, but we never have enough time to present the big picture — to answer their questions in a larger, more understandable context.

So we decided to write this book. This book distills what we've learned and read over our combined 85+ years in the field of mental health — and just as important, the valuable lessons we've been taught by patients and families during that time. In these pages, we give you immediate access to tools and information that otherwise might take you a much longer time to acquire.

We strongly believe that only through improved public awareness and enhanced mental-health literacy can society reverse the stigma and discrimination that stands in the way of finding cures and helping people with schizophrenia lead the full lives they deserve.

About This Book

Our goal in writing this book is to help demystify a long-misunderstood illness. We want this book to be your go-to primer to better understand:

- What schizophrenia is and what it is not
- What causes schizophrenia and what does not
- Why and how diagnoses are made
- How schizophrenia can be treated

- What barriers exist to treatment and care, and how you and your loved one can overcome them
- How consumers, families, friends, and professionals can work together to enhance the chances for recovery and quality of life for people with schizophrenia
- What other resources are available to help patients and their loved ones cope with the disorder

Conventions Used in This Book

We don't use many conventions in this book, but to help you access the information you need we do use the following:

- **Whenever we introduce a new technical term, we *italicize* it and then define it.**
- **Web addresses and e-mail addresses appear in `monofont` to help them stand out.** When this book was printed, some Web addresses may have needed to break across two lines of text. If that happened, rest assured that we haven't put in any extra characters (such as hyphens) to indicate the break. So, when using one of these Web addresses, just type in exactly what you see in this book, pretending as though the line break doesn't exist.
- **We try to avoid language that is in any way demeaning or stigmatizing to people living with schizophrenia.** In recent years, the person affected with schizophrenia has been variously called a *patient, consumer, service recipient,* or *survivor* — and the term that's preferred changes over time, and can vary from one person to the next. We tend to think of people with schizophrenia as *people,* but those in the helping professions (psychiatry, psychology, social work, nursing, rehabilitation, and so on) have a long tradition of calling the people they work with *patients.* Accepting the old adage that you can't please everyone all the time, we used the terms that flowed most comfortably for us as we wrote — although we tried to vary our language. We hope that our words don't offend or interfere with our message.
- **We try to vary the pronouns we used based on gender** — for example, not always referring to doctors as *he* and not always referring to people with schizophrenia as *she.* We didn't keep a running tally of the gender pronouns we used, but we hope you'll find it a fair balance.
- **We often refer to the person with schizophrenia as *your loved one,*** because this book is primarily geared toward people who are caring for, or closely connected to, someone with the disorder — and because we recognize that you may not be family, but your love is just as strong.

- **We generally preferred to use the term *medications* as opposed to *drugs,*** because many people confuse the latter term with street drugs or drugs of abuse (like heroin, cocaine, and marijuana). That said, we do alternate use of the terms in this book — rest assured, when we use the term *drugs,* we're referring to prescribed medications.

  Also, every medication has both a *generic name* and a *trade name* (also called a *brand name*). The trade, or brand name, is the one you hear advertised on commercials (for example, Lipitor is the trade name of a medication used to treat high cholesterol, and the generic name is atorvastatin calcium). We give you both the generic and trade names when referring to medications.

What You're Not to Read

You don't have to read everything in this book to get the information you need. Here are some pieces of the puzzle you can safely skip:

- **Anything marked by a Technical Stuff icon:** Check out the "Icons Used in This Book" section, later in this Introduction, for more on this and other icons.
- **Sidebars:** Sidebars are boxes of gray text that appear throughout this book. You'll find interesting information in sidebars, but nothing essential to understanding the topic at hand.
- **The copyright page:** If you like reading fine print, have at it. Otherwise, trust us: You don't need to know what's there.

Foolish Assumptions

In writing this book, we assumed the following about you:

- You may be caring for someone who has symptoms associated with schizophrenia or has been diagnosed with schizophrenia.
- You may be a parent, family member, friend, or colleague of someone who has schizophrenia, and you want to understand more about the disorder and what you can do to help.
- You may be a mental-health or medical professional reading the book so that you can recommend it to loved ones seeking more information about schizophrenia.

Although we haven't written this book specifically for the person with schizophrenia, if you have schizophrenia and want more information on the disorder, you'll find this book useful as well.

How This Book Is Organized

We've divided this book into five parts. Here's what you'll find in each.

Part I: Understanding Schizophrenia

In this part, we give you a broad overview of schizophrenia, separating what's real from the myths and misperceptions. We describe the symptoms and unusual (and sometime disturbing) behaviors commonly associated with the disorder and explain how clinicians distinguish the symptoms of schizophrenia from those of other serious mental disorders. We describe the onset of the disorder, which can come on suddenly, seemingly out of the blue, or may make its appearance so gradually that it's barely noticed.

Part II: Finding Out What's Wrong and Getting Help

Getting a diagnosis is the first step in getting help. In this part, we explain how the diagnosis of schizophrenia is made and identify the different types of schizophrenia. We also give you tips on how to assemble a healthcare team for diagnosis and treatment, and what to do if things don't seem to be functioning as smoothly as you would hope them to. Finally, we provide advice on starting treatment, including navigating the financial hurdles you'll likely face in paying for care and dealing with your loved one's potential lack of insight into the illness.

Part III: Treating Schizophrenia

Antipsychotic medications are the cornerstone of treatment for schizophrenia. This part explains how psychiatrists select a first medication, and how and why they make adjustments. We also provide advice about how your loved one can cope with common side effects and offer tips for encouraging your loved one to stick to her medication schedule. We explain the range of treatments for schizophrenia and fill you in on what's known and unknown about complementary and alternative treatments. Finally, we identify new and promising directions in research and explain the benefits and risks of participating in clinical trials.

Part IV: Living with Schizophrenia

Schizophrenia presents challenges not only to the individual with the illness, but also to the people around them. Families need to stay positive and optimistic, and avoid blaming each other for the illness. In this part, we tell you how families can avoid burnout, work collaboratively with professionals, and acquire the coping skills they need in order to handle their loved one's not-so-pleasant behaviors. This part also provides suggestions for finding decent affordable housing and for learning how to handle psychiatric crises to minimize their adverse impact. Finally, we define and explain the importance of recovery and meeting the needs of the whole person, which transcend treatment alone.

Part V: The Part of Tens

Every book in the *For Dummies* series includes a part called The Part of Tens, which offers helpful hints to empower readers. In *Schizophrenia For Dummies,* we debunk ten myths about mental illness, offer up ten tips for coping with your loved one's disorder, and ten ways your loved one can avoid relapse.

Icons Used in This Book

Throughout the book, we use icons — little pictures in the margin — to highlight certain kinds of information. Here's what the icons mean:

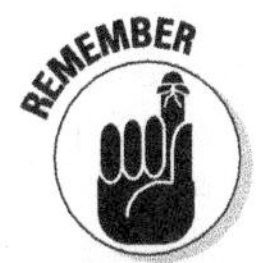

When we use the Remember icon, it means that we're highlighting essential information that's worth remembering.

Schizophrenia, like many other illnesses and disorders, is complex. When we get into the details that you don't absolutely need to understand, we mark it with a Technical Stuff icon. You can safely skip these paragraphs without missing the point — or you can read them and find even more information.

The Tip icon highlights advice or pointers to help you cope with the symptoms and behavior associated with schizophrenia and to deal with the complexities of treatment. We've worked in mental health for years — think of these paragraphs as our insider tips on dealing with schizophrenia.

The Warning icon signals potential risks and dangers. You won't see it used often, but when you do see it, be sure to heed the warning.

Where to Go from Here

If you're the kind of person who reads the morning newspaper from front to back, you'll probably want to start with Chapter 1 of this book and read straight through to the index — in fact, you've probably already read the title page, copyright information, table of contents, and everything else that comes before this Introduction. However, you don't need to read this book in sequence to get a lot out of it. If you're coping with a particular issue or problem, use the table of contents and the index to guide you to the specific portion of the book that addresses your questions. For example, if you think your loved one may have schizophrenia, but he hasn't yet been diagnosed, turn to Chapter 3. If you're looking for doctors for your loved one, Chapter 5 is the place to start. If you're looking for a place for your loved one to live, Chapter 13 has the information you need. Use this book in whatever way works best for you.

Part I
Understanding Schizophrenia

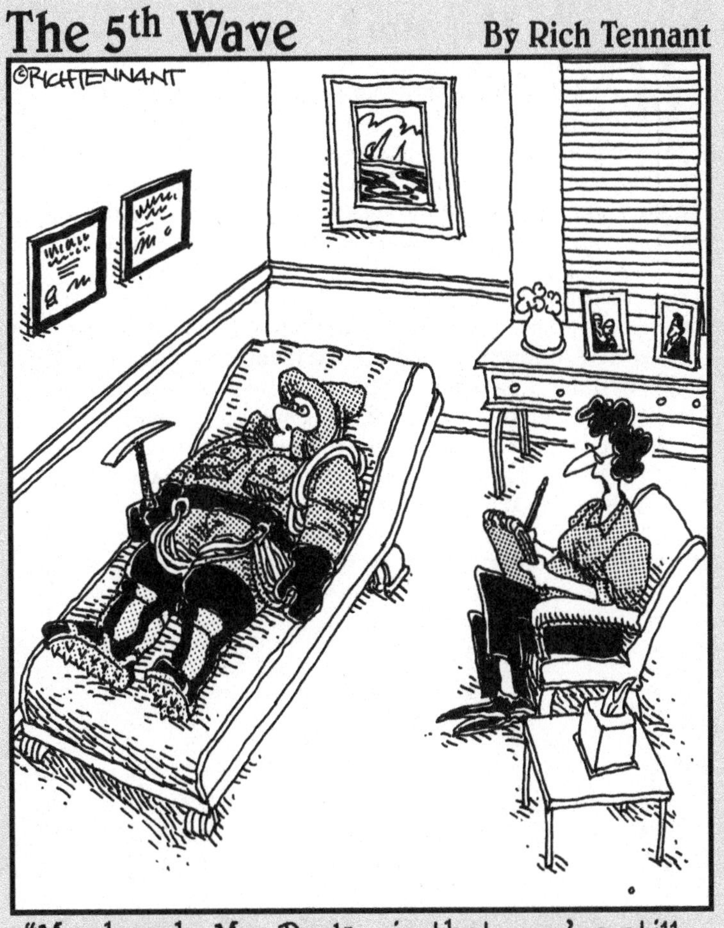

"My hunch, Mr. Pesko, is that you're still making mountains out of molehills."

In this part . . .

We kick things off by giving you an overview of schizophrenia — a no-fault, equal-opportunity disease of the brain that strikes teenagers and young adults in the prime of their lives. Here we dispel some of the myths and misunderstandings associated with the disorder, which have led to unnecessary blame and social stigma. We also show you how to recognize the early warning signs of the disease, outline its risk factors, and cover the range of symptoms and behaviors that characterize schizophrenia. Finally, we tell you how doctors are able to differentiate schizophrenia from other mental disorders with seemingly overlapping symptoms, and discuss the fact that — although treatments have vastly improved the lives of people with schizophrenia and their families — much more remains to be learned.

Chapter 1

Understanding Schizophrenia: The Big Picture

In This Chapter

- Understanding what schizophrenia is, who gets it, and what the symptoms are
- Looking at how schizophrenia is treated
- Getting the support you need

Schizophrenia. If someone you know has been recently diagnosed with schizophrenia, the very word may evoke a cascade of intense feelings: sadness, fear, confusion, shame, and hopelessness. You may ask yourself, how did this happen? Why did it happen to my loved one? It's natural to have these emotions. But take a deep breath. You need to know that the diagnosis isn't as catastrophic as it first appears to be.

Most people know very little about schizophrenia until it hits home, and what they do know is likely to be based on old myths and misperceptions. They need to find out as much accurate information as they can about this complex and misunderstood disease. Knowledge is power — and knowing what schizophrenia is (and isn't) is the first step toward moving beyond your worst fears.

In this chapter, we give you an overview of the brain disorder known as schizophrenia: what it is, who gets it, and what treatments are available. We dispel some common myths about the disorder and tell you how schizophrenia differs from other mental illnesses. Finally, we tell you the good news about the disorder and why you and your loved one have every reason to remain hopeful that recovery is possible.

Schizophrenia is a serious, long-term, life-altering illness, so it's natural to be stunned upon hearing the diagnosis. You may even feel paralyzed, not knowing what to do next. But the first step is clear: You need to gather all the information you can to make sure your loved one is getting the best possible treatment and supports available to him.

Defining Schizophrenia

You're reading this book, which means you probably have a personal interest in schizophrenia — either you or someone close to you has been diagnosed with the disease or you're worried about someone showing signs or symptoms. In this section, we fill you in on what's currently known about schizophrenia and the way the disorder affects the people who have it, as well as their loved ones.

What schizophrenia is

Schizophrenia is a brain disorder characterized by a variety of different symptoms, many of which can dramatically affect an individual's way of thinking and ability to function. Most scientists think that the disorder is due to one or more problems in the development of the brain that results in neurochemical imbalances, although no one fully understands why schizophrenia develops.

People with schizophrenia have trouble distinguishing what's real from what's not. They are not able to fully control their emotions or think logically, and they usually have trouble relating to other people. They often suffer from hallucinations; much of their bizarre behavior is usually due to individuals acting in response to something they *think* is real but is only in their minds.

Unfortunately, because of the way schizophrenia has been inaccurately portrayed in the media over many decades, the illness is one of the most feared and misunderstood of all the physical and mental disorders.

Schizophrenia is a long-term relapsing disorder because it has symptoms that wax and wane, worsen and get better, over time. Similar to many physical illnesses (such as diabetes, asthma, and arthritis), schizophrenia is highly treatable — although it isn't yet considered curable.

But the long-term outcomes of schizophrenia aren't as grim as was once believed. Although the disorder can have a course that results in long-term disability, one in five persons recovers completely. Some people have only one psychotic episode, others have repeated episodes with normal periods of functioning in between, and others have continuing problems from which they never fully recover.

Who gets schizophrenia

No group is risk-free when it comes to schizophrenia, but some people are more likely than others to develop the disorder. The following statistics may surprise you:

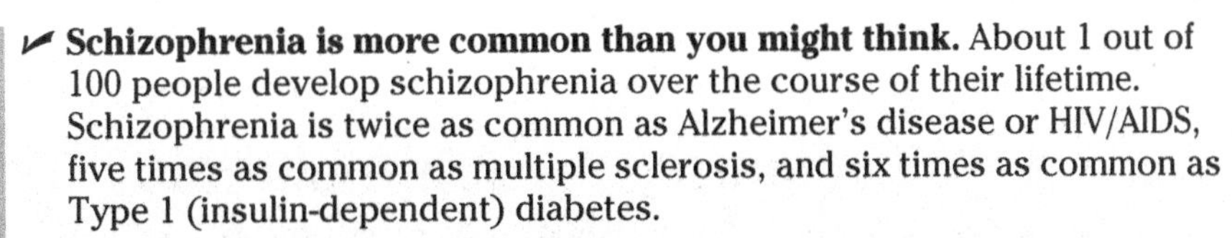

- **Schizophrenia is more common than you might think.** About 1 out of 100 people develop schizophrenia over the course of their lifetime. Schizophrenia is twice as common as Alzheimer's disease or HIV/AIDS, five times as common as multiple sclerosis, and six times as common as Type 1 (insulin-dependent) diabetes.

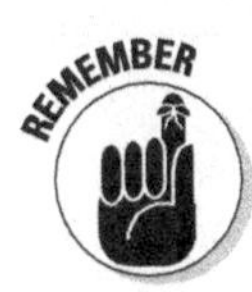

  Although new cases of schizophrenia are somewhat rare, the number of individuals with the disorder remains relatively high because schizophrenia is a chronic disorder that often lasts for an extended period of time.

- **Schizophrenia affects both sexes equally and is found among people of all races, cultures, and socioeconomic groups around the world.**
- **Although schizophrenia is more likely to affect people between the ages of 17 and 35 (the onset tends to be earlier in men than in women), it can begin in children as young as age 5 or have a late onset in a person's 50s, 60s, or 70s.**

  Childhood-onset schizophrenia is extremely rare, affecting about 1 in 40,000 children. Only 1 in 100 adults now diagnosed with the disorder had symptoms before the age of 13. Because the disorder tends to surface more gradually in children, it often goes unnoticed. Chapter 2 lists some of the early red flags to watch for if you suspect that something may be wrong.

  An earlier onset is often indicative of poorer outcomes because the disorder can interfere with education, development, and social functioning. On the other hand, early recognition can help improve outcomes and minimize disability.

Famous people with schizophrenia

Many accomplished and successful people are reported to have had schizophrenia. Here's a short list:

- **Lionel Aldridge** (1941–1998), professional football player on the Green Bay Packers in the 1960s
- **Syd Barrett** (1946–2006), founding member of the band Pink Floyd
- **Jim Gordon** (1945–), drummer and member of Derek and the Dominoes
- **Peter Green** (1946–), guitarist and founder of the band Fleetwood Mac
- **Tom Harrell** (1946–), jazz musician
- **Jack Kerouac** (1922–1969), author of *On the Road*
- **Mary Todd Lincoln** (1818–1882), first lady of the United States, wife of Abraham Lincoln
- **John Nash** (1928–), mathematician, Nobel Prize winner, subject of the film *A Beautiful Mind*
- **Vaslav Nijinsky** (1889–1950), ballet dancer
- **Brian Wilson** (1942–), bass player and singer in the band The Beach Boys

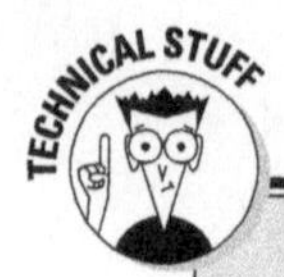

Comparing the schizophrenic brain to the normal one

New imaging techniques — like magnetic resonance imaging (MRI) and positron emission tomography (PET) — have opened virtual windows into the brain. Scientists have been able to visualize the living brain and discern some of the differences in the structure and function of the brains of people with schizophrenia and the brains of their normal peers.

Some of the differences observed in the brains of people with schizophrenia are

- **Enlarged ventricles:** Fluid-filled cavities within the brain
- **A loss of gray matter:** Brain tissue that is comprised of nerve cells
- **Abnormalities in white matter:** Myelin-covered nerve fibers that serve as "wiring" connecting different parts of the brain

In the rare cases where schizophrenia first appears in early childhood, differences have been found in the *cortex* of the developing brain. The cortex forms the surface of the brain.

Functional magnetic imaging studies have enabled scientists to observe the brain while it's performing various tasks. These studies have found that the brains of people with schizophrenia work differently — either harder or less efficiently — than those of people without the disorder.

All these variations are meaningful, but when it comes to diagnosing a particular individual, science is not yet at the point where a diagnosis can be made based on imaging data.

What causes schizophrenia

Schizophrenia is a no-fault, equal-opportunity illness most likely caused by a number of factors, both genetic and environmental. Most scientists now accept a *two-hit theory* for the cause of schizophrenia, which suggests that the genetic susceptibility is compounded by one or more environmental factors:

- **Genetic susceptibility:** Based on family genetic history, some people are more vulnerable to the disorder than other people are.
- **Environmental factors:** In someone genetically predisposed, certain environment factors may come into play, such as:
  - Physical trauma that occurs to the fetus during childbirth
  - Oxygen-deprivation or some psychological or physical problem that occurs to the mother during pregnancy and affects the developing fetus
  - Emotional stress, such as the loss of a parent or loved one during young adulthood

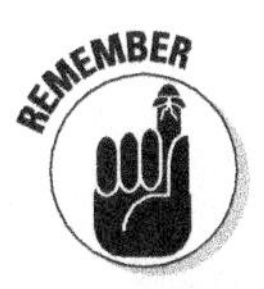

Although schizophrenia is genetically *influenced,* more than genetics is involved in its development. Studies of identical twins show that, if one twin develops schizophrenia, the other twin has only a 40 percent to 50 percent chance of also developing the illness. There's also an increased risk among fraternal twins when one develops schizophrenia, the other has between a 10 percent and 17 percent chance, far less than that of identical twins. Having a parent with schizophrenia also increases a person's risk of developing the disease, to about 10 percent. And if you have a sibling with the disorder — not your twin — you have a 6 percent to 9 percent chance of developing the disorder yourself.

Scientists still don't know the precise causes of schizophrenia for any particular individual, yet family members and patients themselves tend to dwell on (or even obsess about) finding a "reason" or a "cause" for the illness. Although this instinct is a natural one, finding the precise cause or explanation is impossible, not to mention counterproductive — finding a reason doesn't help treatment, and it often creates unnecessary and misplaced guilt, with one family member blaming another.

See Chapter 2 for a full discussion of the possible causes of schizophrenia.

The Symptoms of Schizophrenia

There are almost 300 named psychiatric disorders, and schizophrenia is one of them. Although many mental illnesses have symptoms that overlap, schizophrenia has a distinct pattern of symptoms. No two cases of schizophrenia look exactly the same, but most people with schizophrenia display three types of symptoms:

- **Positive symptoms:** The term *positive symptoms* is confusing, because positive symptoms (as the term might suggest) aren't "good" symptoms at all. They're symptoms that *add* to reality, and not in a good way. People with schizophrenia hear things that don't exist or see things that aren't there (in what are known as *hallucinations*). The voices they hear can accuse them of terrible things and can be very jarring (for example, causing them to think that they've hurt someone or have been responsible for some cataclysmic world event).

  People with schizophrenia can also have *delusions* (false beliefs that defy logic or any culturally specific explanation and that cannot be changed by logic or reason). For example, an individual may believe that there is a conspiracy of people driving red cars that follows his every movement. He will use the fact that there are red cars everywhere he goes as evidence that the conspiracy is real.

- **Negative symptoms:** These symptoms are a *lack* of something that should be present; behaviors that would be considered normal are either absent or diminished. For example, people with schizophrenia often lack motivation and appear lazy. They may be much slower to respond than most other people, have little to say when they do speak, and appear as if they have no emotions, or exhibit emotions that are inappropriate to the situation. They may also be unable to get pleasure from the things that most people enjoy or from activities that once brought pleasure to them. Families often get frustrated when a relative with schizophrenia does nothing but sleep or watch TV — they wrongly attribute this behavior to the patient not being willing to assume responsibility or "pull himself up by his bootstraps."

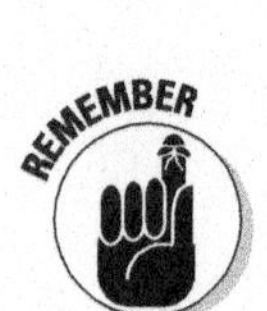

  Negative symptoms are part and parcel of the illness for at least 25 percent of people with schizophrenia.

- **Cognitive symptoms:** Most people with the disorder suffer from impairments in memory, learning, concentration, and their ability to make sound decisions. These so-called *cognitive symptoms* interfere with an individual's ability to learn new things, remember things they once knew, and use skills they once had. Cognitive symptoms can make it hard for a person to continue working at a job, going to school, or participating in activities she may have enjoyed at one time.

In addition to the symptoms mentioned above, people with schizophrenia may also have sleep problems, mood swings, and anxiety. They may experience difficulties forming and maintaining social relationships with other people. They may look different enough that other people notice that something is very odd or strange about them and that they don't quite look "normal." They may have unusual ways of doing things, have peculiar habits, dress inappropriately (such as wearing a heavy coat or multiple layers of clothes in the summer), and/or be poorly groomed, which can discourage other people from getting involved with them.

See Chapter 3 for more about the differences in these types of symptoms.

Dispelling the Myths Associated with Schizophrenia

People wrongly associate the symptoms of schizophrenia with split or multiple personalities (like Dr. Jekyll and Mr. Hyde), antisocial behavior (similar to what we see in serial killers), and developmental disabilities. Others believe that schizophrenia is a character defect and that the individual could behave normally if he really wanted to.

Here are a few of the most common misconceptions about schizophrenia:

- **Schizophrenia is the same as a split or multiple personality.** Schizophrenia is *not* the same as multiple personality, which is an exceedingly rare, totally different disorder that is now more commonly called a *dissociative identity disorder.* (Under stress, people with this disorder often assume different identities, each with different names, voices, characteristics, and personal histories.)
- **People with schizophrenia are violent.** People with schizophrenia are more likely to be victims rather than perpetrators of crimes. Many people believe that most people with schizophrenia have a propensity for violence, but the reality is that most people with schizophrenia don't commit violent crimes, and most violent criminals don't have schizophrenia.

  For example, *serial killers* (people who commit three or more subsequent murders) usually aren't *psychotic* (out of touch with reality); they're likely to be diagnosed with an *antisocial personality disorder* (a disorder in which people disregard commonly accepted social rules and norms, display impulsive behavior, and are indifferent to the rights and feelings of others).

  However, people with untreated schizophrenia, who refuse to take medication and whose thinking is out of touch with reality are at increased risk of aggressive behavior and self-neglect. The risk of violence also increases if someone with schizophrenia is actively abusing alcohol or illicit drugs. For better or worse, the aggressive behavior is usually directed toward family or friends rather than toward strangers.
- **Poor parenting causes schizophrenia.** For many years, clinicians were taught and actually believed that schizophrenia was caused by parents who were either too permissive or too controlling. The term *schizophrenogenic mother* was once used to describe such parents — the blame usually fell heavily on mothers because they tended to spend the most time with their offspring. Another outdated theory is the *double-bind theory,* which suggested that schizophrenia is due to inconsistent parenting, with conflicting messages.

  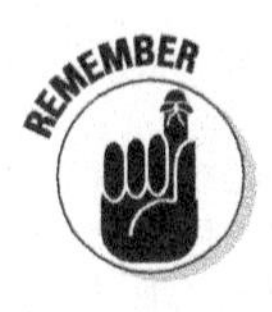

  These ideas were not based on controlled studies, and these theories no longer have credibility today.

  Schizophrenia is a no-fault disorder of the brain.
- **People with schizophrenia are mentally retarded.** Some people think that schizophrenia is synonymous with mental retardation (now called *developmental disabilities*). No. Like the general public, people with schizophrenia have a wide range of intellectual abilities. They may *appear* less intelligent because of the impaired social skills, odd behaviors, and cognitive impairments that are characteristic of schizophrenia. However, they're not lacking in intelligence, and schizophrenia is distinct from *developmental disabilities* (physical and mental deficits that are chronic and severe and that generally begin in childhood).

- **Schizophrenia is a defect of character.** Negative symptoms of schizophrenia give people the mistaken impression that those with the disorder are lazy and could act "normally" if they wanted to. This idea is no more realistic than suggesting that someone could prevent his epileptic seizures if he really wanted to or that someone could "decide" not to have cancer if he ate the right foods. What often appears as character defects are symptoms of schizophrenia.

  When the negative symptoms of schizophrenia are persistent and primarily caused by schizophrenia, they're referred to as *deficit syndrome.*

- **There's no hope for people diagnosed with schizophrenia.** Sixty years ago when people were diagnosed with schizophrenia, they were either kept at home behind closed doors by embarrassed and forlorn families who saw no other alternative, or consigned to long-term stays in distant state hospitals for care that was largely *custodial* (they weren't treated — they were just taken care of). Other than using highly sedating drugs, doctors had few tools available to them to relieve the agitation and torment of their patients or to help restore their functioning.

  In contrast to how things were in the past, schizophrenia is now considered highly treatable. Several generations of new medications and the emergence of new forms of therapies have enabled doctors to treat the symptoms of the large majority of patients with schizophrenia enabling them to live meaningful, productive lives in their communities.

For more myths about schizophrenia, check out Chapter 16.

Finding Out Whether Your Loved One Has Schizophrenia

Schizophrenia doesn't always make its appearance in the same way. Sometimes its symptoms come on suddenly, seemingly out of the blue, and this can be very confusing or even shocking. A very common scenario is that a young person, previously described as an excellent student, standout athlete, or all-around great kid, goes off for college and suddenly calls home after a month or two to report that he's being followed or has been targeted by an alien group. When the individual has had no prior history of a serious mental disorder, the onset of this disorder is called a *first break* or an *acute psychotic break.*

Other times, schizophrenia comes on gradually, or its symptoms are so subtle that the person simply hasn't been diagnosed earlier. Often, it's difficult for the individual and people around her to notice that anything is wrong (because they've come to accept what they view as the person's quirky personality) until things further deteriorate and can no longer be ignored.

Families say that their relative never seemed "quite right"; the person may have had problems at school or work, problems relating to peers, and a history of odd or unusual behaviors. Then she suddenly exhibits delusions, hallucinations, or other signs indicating that she's out of touch with reality. After that, the possibility of schizophrenia can no longer be ignored.

No matter how the scenario unfolds, the key is getting a diagnosis for your loved one and ruling out other possible causes for the symptoms you're noticing. In the section below, we tell you how to do both.

Getting a diagnosis

If you have any suspicion that your loved one may have schizophrenia, it's vitally important that he be seen by a mental-health professional as soon as possible. If the clinician is not a psychiatrist — maybe he's a psychologist or social worker — he'll likely suggest that your loved one be seen by an internist or general practitioner to make sure that the symptoms are not due to any underlying physical disorder (such as a brain tumor, epilepsy, or drug intoxication) and to rule out other medical explanations.

Unlike some physical illnesses, there's no simple blood test or X-ray that can establish the diagnosis of schizophrenia. So the mental-health professional will interview your loved one and take a thorough history to help arrive at an accurate diagnosis. Often they will interview family members to round out their understanding of the patient's history and functioning at home, and to solicit their assistance in filling in details that the patient may have forgotten or be hesitant to talk about.

When mental-health professionals make diagnoses of schizophrenia, they sometimes identify various subtypes of the disorder based on their characteristic symptoms. These subtypes include paranoid schizophrenia, catatonic schizophrenia, and undifferentiated schizophrenia (see Chapter 4 for more information on all these). These subtypes no longer hold the same diagnostic or *prognostic* (ability to predict the future) importance that they once did. Today, more emphasis is placed on designing treatment strategies that address positive, negative, and cognitive symptoms.

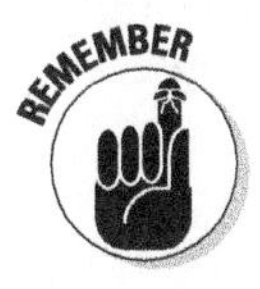

Early diagnosis is important — it leads to better outcomes. Even having a name for the disturbing symptoms people experience enables patients and those around them to better understand and cope with their situation.

Ruling out other explanations

After medical causes are ruled out and schizophrenia is suspected, your next step is for your loved one to see a psychiatrist — specifically, someone who is experienced in diagnosing and treating schizophrenia.

Finding a psychiatrist experienced in diagnosing and treating schizophrenia isn't always easy. Two of the best sources of referrals are academic medical centers and family support groups. (For more on finding a psychiatrist for your loved one, check out Chapter 4.)

One of the reasons that diagnosing schizophrenia can be challenging is that its symptoms sometimes overlap with other mental disorders. Mental-health professionals determine whether a person has schizophrenia or some other psychiatric condition with similar or overlapping symptoms by doing what's called a *differential diagnosis.* For example, to diagnose schizophrenia, some of the conditions psychiatrists rule out include

- **Mood disorders:** People with schizophrenia can have mood swings, become depressed, or exhibit *hypomanic* (persistently elated or irritable) moods or behaviors. People with *bipolar disorder* or *severe depression* can have psychotic thoughts (such as delusions or hallucinations) that resemble those found in schizophrenia. But in schizophrenia, the thought disorder predominates over mood symptoms.
- **Schizoaffective disorder:** Schizoaffective disorder, despite the name, isn't a type of schizophrenia — instead, it's a different diagnosis with a combination of thought and mood symptoms. The diagnosis is sometimes used when the symptoms of the disorder can't be clearly categorized as either schizophrenia or a mood disorder.
- **Substance use and abuse:** The symptoms associated with acute schizophrenia can be caused by drug-induced intoxication, especially from hallucinogenic drugs (like LSD), cocaine, or amphetamines. A significant proportion of people with schizophrenia use alcohol and/or other drugs to mask their symptoms and/or ease their anxiety about their symptoms and have co-occurring mental-health and substance-use disorders.

To determine whether psychotic symptoms are induced by drugs or a symptom of schizophrenia, a clinician may need to see the patient over time and observe the patient when she is not using drugs or alcohol.

- **Borderline personality disorder:** People with borderline personality disorder often have moods that change on a dime, have conflicts with other people, act out inappropriately, or have impaired judgment. They may also behave in ways that hurt themselves (for example, deliberating cutting or burning themselves). However, it's not common for people with borderline personalities to have hallucinations or cognitive impairments.

Sometimes an individual's psychiatric diagnosis changes over time based on whichever symptoms appear to be most prominent at the time the person is seen. It doesn't necessarily mean that the previous diagnosis was wrong.

Normal teenage behaviors and the diagnosis of schizophrenia

Not surprisingly, the teenage years have been called the "roller-coaster years" because of the ups and downs caused by surging hormones, and because adolescents are prone to engage in strange and risky behaviors. Many young people have mood swings, use and/or abuse alcohol, or maintain unusual sleep schedules (reversing day and night, or sleeping too little or too much).

Because the onset of schizophrenia usually coincides with the late teenage years, schizophrenia is often missed and its symptoms are dismissed as behaviors of normal adolescence. It takes an experienced clinician to confirm or rule out a diagnosis of schizophrenia in teens, but some warning signs include the following:

- **A dramatic decline in school performance:** For example, excessive absences or failing subjects at which she once excelled.
- **Having thoughts that often don't make sense:** For example, a teenager with schizophrenia may think his thoughts are being monitored by electronic equipment in the house or that his food is being poisoned.
- **Being suspicious or paranoid:** Lots of teenagers are "paranoid" that their parents are going through their things or spying on them, but that's not what we're talking about here. The suspiciousness or paranoia in a teenager with schizophrenia might lead him to believe that his room is bugged by the FBI.
- **Staying isolated or not having friends:** Not every teen is captain of the football team or homecoming queen — we're not talking about popularity here. We mean having absolutely no friends — not even one — and never socializing with other kids or participating in school activities.
- **Use of drugs and/or alcohol:** Teenagers frequently experiment with drugs or alcohol, so if you find out your teen is doing either of these, that doesn't mean he has schizophrenia. But if you see drug and alcohol use in conjunction with the other symptoms in this list, that can be evidence that he may have schizophrenia. ***Remember:*** Drug and alcohol use in teens is a serious problem whether they have schizophrenia or not, so if you suspect your teen may be drinking or doing drugs, be sure to get him help. Contact the federal government's Center for Substance Abuse Treatment (CSAT) toll-free help line at 800-662-4357 or go to `www.findtreatment.samhsa.gov` for tips on where to start.
- **Family history of mental illness:** Genetics alone doesn't cause schizophrenia, but if you have a family history of mental illness, and you're noticing other symptoms in this list, your teen may have schizophrenia.

Improving the Lives of People with Schizophrenia

Since the 1950s, the mental-health profession has made marked advances in the treatment of schizophrenia. Now most people with schizophrenia are treated in the community as opposed to remaining in hospitals for long-term care. When individuals *do* need to be hospitalized, it's usually for a brief period of time to stabilize their symptoms. In this section, we cover the range of treatments and supports that are essential to recovery.

Medication

Today, medication is considered the mainstay of treatment for most individuals with schizophrenia. However, medication alone isn't enough — it's more successful when combined with psychosocial (see the following section) interventions.

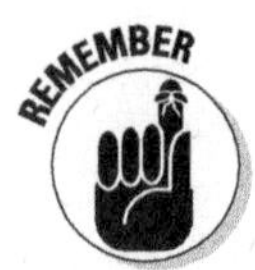

Antipsychotic medications — like medications used to treat many other chronic illnesses (such as diabetes, epilepsy, heart disease, and asthma) — control symptoms. They don't provide a cure.

Good *psychopharmacologists* (psychiatrists who have training and experience in prescribing medications that are used to treat psychiatric illnesses) now are more likely to work along with individuals and families to find a medication regimen that will help keep positive symptoms under control. Also, today doctors are more likely to listen to patients who complain of adverse side effects and to modify doses or the type of medication accordingly, to encourage compliance. Finally, the availability of *practice guidelines* (summaries of best practices based on research evidence or professional consensus), developed by many professional organizations, have improved the overall state of the art of medication management.

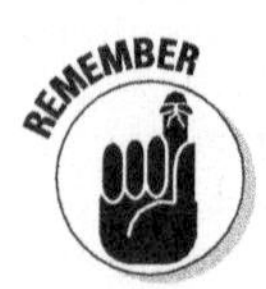

Collaboration between a patient and doctor is less possible when a person with schizophrenia is acutely ill and unable to understand or remember what's being discussed. The approach to medication management is a long-term one.

We cover medication options in Chapter 8.

Psychosocial treatments

Psychosocial treatments include psychological treatments, social approaches, and combined approaches that are especially helpful in restoring confidence and self-esteem, as well as in helping people with schizophrenia develop the skills they never acquired or lost as a result of their illness (which often curtails or interrupts an individual's education or work).

Psychosocial treatments include social skills training, vocational counseling and job training, *cognitive remediation* (compensatory learning strategies that improve neuropsychological functions like memory, concentration, planning and organizing), and assistance with the activities of daily living. Psychological treatments include supportive psychotherapy (talk therapy) and *cognitive behavioral therapy* (CBT), which is focused on changing negative thinking patterns. Self-help approaches and family psychoeducation are important elements of a comprehensive system of care.

Because cognitive problems and the complexity of the service system often make it hard for people with schizophrenia to arrange for their own care, in the past, families were usually thrust into the role of de facto case managers. Increasingly, professional *case managers* (mental-health workers who help people with chronic illnesses navigate the complex system of healthcare and social services) have become part of the landscape of mental-health treatment. Case managers coordinate services, help in the event of crises, and provide ongoing support to enable people live successfully with some degree of autonomy and independence. Assertive community treatment (ACT) programs, comprised of multidisciplinary treatment teams, reach out to the patient and can be particularly helpful to those with a more severe form of the illness.

We cover the variety of psychosocial approaches in detail in Chapter 9.

Family psychoeducation

Although families were once seen as part of the problem, they're now viewed as part of the solution and frequently essential to recovery. With the growth of groups like the National Alliance on Mental Illness (NAMI), family psychoeducation has flourished at national, state, and local levels.

Family psychoeducation groups provide a place for families to exchange information about the illness, learn what works and what doesn't (both in terms of treatment and coping strategies), identify ways to minimize the risk of relapse, and find out how to identify and access community resources. For example, the NAMI Family-to-Family educational program has given countless families the opportunity to learn the things they need to know to be effective caregivers and advocates for their loved ones.

More important, perhaps, family psychoeducation groups help family members recognize that they're not alone and that others are working hard to improve care — not only for their own loved ones, but for all individuals and families affected by serious mental disorders. At the same time, they help people to live their lives without letting them be defined solely by the illness. Families have been instrumental, in turn, in improving public understanding and awareness of the needs of people with schizophrenia.

You can find information on advocacy organizations for dealing with schizophrenia in Chapters 11 and 15.

Peer support and mutual self-help

Another crucial element to recovery is providing people with schizophrenia the opportunity to talk to and exchange information with their peers. Having the chance to know other people facing the same challenges can help people with schizophrenia recover more quickly from acute episodes of the illness and can help them avoid relapse and hospitalization. Clubhouses, drop-in centers, and mutual support groups can play an important role in fostering recovery. For example, NAMI Peer-to-Peer programs offer a recovery curriculum for consumers.

For more on these support groups, turn to Chapter 9.

Basic support: Housing, financial aid, and healthcare

Like everyone else, people with any mental illness need stable and affordable housing, entitlements when they can't support themselves financially, and access to quality healthcare, mental-health treatment, and medications. Often, mental illnesses are associated with poverty and a cascade of personal losses — including friendships, work opportunities, and a place to call home.

Because the resources needed to cope with any chronic disorder are generally beyond the reach of any one individual family, governmental and charitable organizations oversee and fund many of these services and supports, which are cost-saving in human and economic terms.

Chapters 7 and 13 discuss various financing and housing options for people with schizophrenia.

Family and close friends can play a vital role in fostering their loved one's recovery. They're the ones who best know their loved one, including his hopes and dreams. They also are likely to have the greatest stake in seeing him recover and succeed. One advocate we know once said, "No one has the same fire in his belly to make the system work for his loved one."

Recognizing the Challenges That Remain

We'd be less than honest if we said that everything is perfect today for people dealing with schizophrenia — it's not. Here are a few of the problems that remain:

- **Many patients still are unable to find a medication that works for them.** Their persistent positive, negative, and cognitive symptoms are vexing to them, as well as to their families and clinicians. (See Chapter 8 for more about medications and schizophrenia.)
- **Doctors still don't know which drugs work best for which individuals.** The choice of medication still relies on a good deal of trial and error, which takes time and requires patience.
- **Families still have to learn that, despite their best efforts, they can't talk someone out of schizophrenia or wish it away with an abundance of love and caring.** (See Chapter 11 for ways to help everyone in the family live with schizophrenia.)
- **Most communities don't have the full breadth of services and supports to necessary to support recovery.** (See Chapters 12 and 13 for more information on community resources.)
- **The scarcity of appropriate low-cost housing, adequate health-insurance coverage, and competitive jobs undermine progress for many people with schizophrenia.**
- **Mental-health services still tend to be fragmented and insufficient in number, and finding psychiatrists who are experienced and willing to work with individuals with long-term mental illnesses is still difficult (particularly in rural areas).** (See Chapter 5 for information on choosing the right doctors.)

Holding On to Hope: The Good News about Schizophrenia

It's easy to dwell on the negatives when dealing with schizophrenia, but the truth is, there are many reasons for hope:

- **We know, without question, that schizophrenia is a no-fault disorder of the brain and that with appropriate treatment and supports, the illness doesn't necessarily have to have a chronic, deteriorating course.** People do and can recover!
- **Early diagnosis and the availability of community-based treatment and social supports can restore an individual's dignity, improve her quality of life, and enable her to make meaningful contributions to her family and community.** Your loved one may find a different path than you or she anticipated, but it can still be a good one.
- **The ultimate goal of recovery is about more than relief of symptoms.** Recovery entails helping people get back to work or school, live with others, and make their own life decisions. Patients and families should accept no less.

- **The role of families and friends is critical to recovery.** They need to:
  - Support and anchor their loved ones during the acute phases of the illness
  - Help their loved ones find the tools they need to recover and avoid relapse
- Continue to educate themselves to better cope with the challenges they encounter, working individually and collectively to fight stigma and discrimination based on misunderstanding
- **Just as scientists now know that there are many different types of cancer, researchers may one day learn that schizophrenia is a family of similar disorders that are currently lumped under one term.** This discovery could pave the way for more targeted and personalized treatments. Because the precise causes of schizophrenia are still unknown for any particular individual, scientists are exploring a number of possibilities including genetic, viral, infectious, chemical, developmental, and environmental explanations. There has never been more research being conducted on the causes and cures for schizophrenia than there is today. (See Chapter 10 for the latest on research into schizophrenia.)

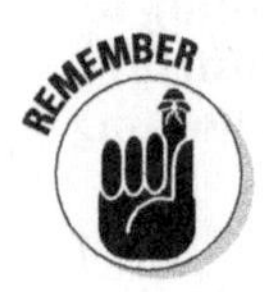

Never give up hope. Just around the corner are answers to questions that can't be answered today and solutions to problems that seem insurmountable.

Chapter 2

Causes and Risk Factors

In This Chapter

- Debunking the myths of schizophrenia
- Understanding the roles of nature versus nurture
- Looking at genetics and environmental triggers
- Understanding the importance of early recognition and treatment
- Examining schizophrenia over the life span

One of the first questions young children ask is, "Why?" But whatever your age, it's human nature to try to find a reason why things happen. When a disease like schizophrenia affects someone you love, your first questions will likely be, "Why did this happen? Was it something I did? Could it have been prevented?" And right after the whys come the ifs: "If only I hadn't eaten that, done that, moved there, neglected this, ignored that . . . then maybe this wouldn't have happened."

In this chapter, we look at the whys and ifs of schizophrenia: what research says about the causes and risk factors associated with schizophrenia. We also examine past theories of why schizophrenia occurred — theories that have now been discredited by research and an expanding knowledge base. You may ask, "Why do I need to know this stuff?" Because the more you understand about schizophrenia, the better prepared you'll be to deal with it.

Searching for a Reason

Disorders like schizophrenia are a result of something going wrong, but just what that something is, isn't very easy to pinpoint. Naturally, patients and families, as well as clinicians, want to know the cause of schizophrenia and what can be done to prevent it. After all, there are vaccines against some diseases like polio and smallpox, and preventive measures that ward off others (such as scurvy, which can be prevented by getting enough vitamin C in the diet).

However, with many chronic physical illnesses (such as diabetes, arthritis, or high blood pressure), even when doctors know the body systems involved, they don't know the specifics of why it occurs. In a person with diabetes, for example, the body doesn't metabolize sugar the way it should, and the body either doesn't produce enough insulin or the insulin that the body does produce doesn't work the way it should to control blood sugar. But no one really knows why. So, although doctors know *where* something is wrong but can't explain what *caused* it to go wrong.

Similarly, when it comes to schizophrenia, scientists still don't know why one person gets the disorder and another doesn't, why someone gets it at one age and not at another, or why one person develops it after some environmental stressor and another person doesn't. Doctors *do* know that the genetic makeup of some people makes them more prone to develop schizophrenia than others, and researchers have identified some of the brain mechanisms that are faulty.

In the following sections we cover what the medical community knows about the brain and schizophrenia. We also debunk some common myths about the disease.

Looking at the human brain

The human brain is composed of billions of cells that are able to connect or communicate with one another by *electrochemical* (electrical and chemical) means. When a cell is stimulated, it releases a very small amount of a chemical known as a *neurotransmitter.* For a brief moment, the presence of that neurotransmitter causes the next cell to be stimulated. Different kinds of cells have different chemical neurotransmitters, and one of the most important neurotransmitters is called *dopamine.* Cells that release dopamine and that have dopamine receptors are found in different areas of the brain.

When certain drugs are given that increase dopamine levels, they cause an individual's dopamine system to become active. If a person with schizophrenia receives such a drug, he temporarily becomes more symptomatic (for example, experiencing more hallucinations or becoming more suspicious). On the other hand, medications that block the dopamine receptors and reduce the activity of the dopamine system are effective in treating some of the symptoms of schizophrenia.

Studies have shown that medications that are strongest in blocking dopamine receptors are also the most potent in treating the positive symptoms of schizophrenia, like delusions, hallucinations, and agitation (see Chapter 3 for more on positive symptoms). This doesn't mean that dopamine is the cause of schizophrenia — it just means that the dopamine system is involved in regulating the symptoms of the disorder, just like insulin is involved in regulating the level of blood sugar. One theory of how schizophrenia symptoms are produced is that there is an excess of dopamine in certain parts of the brain.

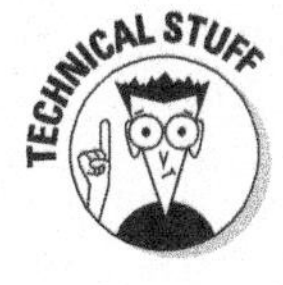

One reason that it's so difficult to pinpoint the cause of schizophrenia may be because the diagnosis may actually describe a *group* of disorders that produce similar symptoms rather than a single disorder. For example, in looking at memory loss, scientists now recognize that similar symptoms are produced by various disorders (including Alzheimer's disease, vascular dementia, and frontotemporal dementia), by traumatic brain injury, or even by certain kinds of poisons.

Separating the myths from reality

Schizophrenia isn't a new disease. Even before the disease had a name, there were numerous theories about its symptoms that later came to define the disorder. In the days of Hippocrates (about 460 b.c. to 370 b.c.), it was believed that people with mental illnesses were possessed by the devil because they heard voices and saw visions. Priests used religious rites and exorcisms in hopes of a cure. In the 17th century, during the Inquisition, people with the same symptoms were thought to be witches and were burned at the stake.

In the late 1800s, a German psychiatrist named Emil Kraepelin called the same symptoms *dementia praecox* — attributing them to "the sub-acute development of a peculiar simple condition of mental weakness occurring at a youthful age."

Swiss psychiatrist Eugen Bleuler coined the term *the schizophrenias,* borrowing the term from the Greek root *schizein phren* or "split mind" and using the plural form. Bleuler didn't think the disorder was a form of dementia, nor did he believe that it was solely a disease of the young.

As recently as the mid-1900s, many mental health professionals were sure that schizophrenia was caused by poor parenting, especially bad mothering. Unfortunately, old myths die hard, and many people who were taught and believed these obsolete theories long ago still practice psychiatry and psychology today.

Here are two of the most common bad-parenting myths:

- **The schizophrenogenic mother theory:** Freudian psychoanalysts theorized that pathological mothers created pathological offspring with schizophrenia. The term *schizophrenogenic mother* was used to describe mothers who were accused of being too aloof, too cold and withholding, or too permissive and doting. Understandably, this made many mothers feel guilty and responsible for something they did or didn't do, led to marital problems (with one spouse accusing the other of causing the illness), and alienated patients with schizophrenia from their mothers. Even well-meaning clinicians erected barriers between mothers and their offspring, creating a climate of mistrust that, to some degree, still exists today.
- **The double-bind theory:** Although mixed messages can be confusing, they don't cause schizophrenia. However, the idea that mixed messages cause schizophrenia was the essence of a theory developed in the 1950s by British anthropologist Gregory Bateson. He believed that the root cause of schizophrenia was the conflicting communications that children receive from their parents. For example, a mother may express warm sentiments in her words but come across sounding cold and detached in her tone. Or a mother and father may respond differently to the same event, one parent condemning and the other condoning the behavior of the child.

  Bateson believed that children, who are unable to make sense of these contradictory messages, act out with delusional symptoms, the outward manifestation of conflict and anxiety created by the *double bind.* After all these years, this theory has never been proven or shown to have a useful application in the treatment of schizophrenia.

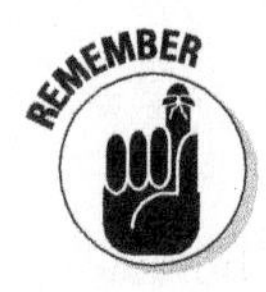

Although these ideas about schizophrenia were once in fashion, they are now considered myths. If any clinician treating your loved one still believes or follows them, your loved one may not get appropriate treatment and care. Finding out if this is the case is easy. If you suspect that a therapist has such an orientation, you might simply ask, "Could I be the cause of my son or daughter's illness?" If he says yes, find another doctor.

Beware of any clinician who blames you for your relative's illness. Schizophrenia is a no-fault illness that isn't caused by parents. Even more important, *insight-oriented psychotherapy* (therapy focused on unconscious psychological conflicts) or *psychoanalysis* (therapy focused on Freud's theories, which include free association, dream interpretation, and transference) can be harmful to patients with schizophrenia. If a clinician proposes psychoanalysis for the primary or sole treatment of your loved one, head for the door.

Over the past 50 years, with advances in mental health research, these myths have been disproved, but new ones emerge all the time (see Chapter 16). For example, many people think that schizophrenia means a split or multiple personality, a myth that's been perpetuated by TV shows and movies like *The Three Faces of Eve.*

Today, assertions about schizophrenia and its treatment are more likely to be subject to empirical study before they're adopted. In fact, one of the most encouraging aspects of schizophrenia treatment is the enormous amount of research currently going on and the many new research tools (such as molecular biology, MRI and PET scans, and cognitive tests) available to study the disorder.

Looking at the Respective Roles of Nature and Nurture

Much like the question "Which came first — the chicken or the egg?", the question "Which has more influence on your development — your genes or your environment?" can be endlessly debated. Is schizophrenia caused by *nature* (biology), by *nurture* (the way a person is raised or the person's life experiences), or by some combination of the two?

One reason that this remains an issue is because, in the search for causes, scientists usually look in the area where they've done most of their work: Biologists look to biology for the answer, psychologists look to psychology, and so on. So who's right? Maybe both.

Searching for the genes that cause schizophrenia

The study of genetics, molecular biology, and the human genome is accelerating at a rapid pace. Many studies have been conducted that attempt to link a single gene to schizophrenia, but none of the studies with positive findings have been *replicated* (repeated with the same results). Because of this, the current thinking is that genetic risk is real, but rather than it being caused by a single "big" gene, it's probably a result of multiple "small" gene problems. This is known as the *multigene theory of causation.*

Even if the genes individually have a small effect, they likely interact with each other and also interact with environmental factors (see "Nurture: Looking at environmental factors," in this chapter). The activity of some of these genes is known to be related to neurotransmitters like dopamine (see "Looking at the human brain," earlier in this chapter), which, in turn, is linked to the positive symptoms of schizophrenia.

Remember: The genetic link in schizophrenia isn't a simple one — it isn't passed on directly like brown eyes or blond hair. It's far more complex, involving multiple genes and other factors.

For example, in studies of the genetics of schizophrenia, studies have clearly shown that, with identical twins, if one twin has schizophrenia, there's about a 40 percent chance that the second twin will have schizophrenia as well. For fraternal twins, the rate is less than half of that. To the biologist, this shows that nature, or genetics, is the cause. For the non-biologically-oriented, these facts offer proof that, even with identical chromosomes, biology doesn't provide a conclusive answer.

There is clear evidence that genetics plays a major role in schizophrenia and, increasingly, that environmental factors also play a role. This evidence has given rise to what is known as the *two-hit theory of schizophrenia,* the idea that genetic susceptibility is compounded by environmental (psychological, social, or physical) factors. This theory has led to a search for risk factors that contribute to the onset of the disorder.

Nature: Focusing on your family tree

Genetic studies of families, twins, and adoptions have clearly shown that having a biological history of schizophrenia in family increases the risk that a person will develop the disorder:

- In studies of identical twins, if one twin has schizophrenia, it increases the risk that the other one will have it too by about 40 percent.
- If one fraternal twin has schizophrenia, there is a 10 percent to 17 percent chance the other one will have it too.
- If one parent has schizophrenia, the risk of the offspring having schizophrenia is about 10 percent.
- If both parents have schizophrenia, the risk of the offspring having schizophrenia increases to between 30 percent to 46 percent.

The risk of developing schizophrenia is greater in people with a history of the disorder in their immediate families than it is in the general population.

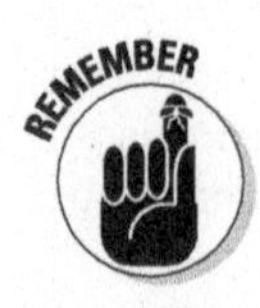

Although family history is an important risk factor, 80 percent to 90 percent of people with schizophrenia have *no* family history of the disease. Additionally, the fact that in the case of identical twins, one may become schizophrenic while one may not, indicates that susceptibility for schizophrenia is determined by more than genetics alone.

Nurture: Looking at environmental factors

No one environmental factor by itself has been shown to cause schizophrenia. But a number of environmental factors may increase the risk or chance of schizophrenia occurring. Many people experience the same environmental factors, but few of them develop schizophrenia. It may well take a combination of genetic vulnerability and environmental triggers occurring together for schizophrenia to develop.

For example, if a person has a parent with schizophrenia, that person's chance of developing schizophrenia is about 10 percent. But if one or more environmental triggers happen on top of this family history, schizophrenia may occur. It's sort of like those proverbial straws being piled on the back of a camel; the camel may be able to stand strong with a few of those straws, but eventually, one of those straws will break the camel's back. The number of straws varies from one person to the next, and medical professionals have no way of knowing how many a particular person will be able to withstand.

In the following sections, we cover some of the environmental factors that may contribute to the development of schizophrenia.

Prenatal factors

What happens to you before you're born — or during the process of birth — can affect you all your life. The likelihood of schizophrenia developing has been linked to several *prenatal* (before birth) factors:

- **The age of the birth father:** One prenatal risk factor that's been linked to schizophrenia is the age of the birth father. Children with fathers who are over the age of 50 are three times more likely to develop schizophrenia than children whose fathers are under 30 years old at the time of their birth. Some researchers have suggested that this may be the result of sperm mutations that occur with advancing age.
- **Influenza:** Studies have shown that children born to mothers who contracted the flu while pregnant (especially during the second trimester) also have a greater chance of developing schizophrenia.
- **Starvation:** Maternal starvation is linked to increased risk of schizophrenia in offspring. Starvation can occur either because of poverty or because of eating disorders such as anorexia.
- **Stress:** Recently, a large epidemiological study looked at stressors such as the death of a close relative or a diagnosis of cancer, heart attack, or stroke in a close relative as risk factors for having children who would develop schizophrenia later in life. Only one of these factors increased risk: The risk of developing schizophrenia or a related disorder was 67 percent greater among the children of mothers who experienced the death of a close family member during the first trimester than those who did not have that stress.

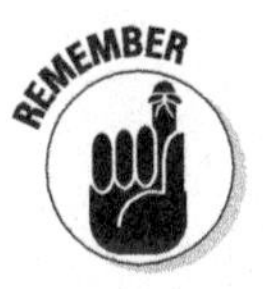

The vast majority of fetuses exposed to these prenatal environmental stressors did *not* develop schizophrenia, leaving the perplexing question of why some did and others didn't still unanswered.

Viral speculations

For many years, researchers have speculated that viral infections can damage parts of the brain, leading to some of the sensory disturbances associated with schizophrenia. One known characteristic of viral infections is that they can attack some parts of the brain, leaving other parts unscathed.

Although these theories are still being investigated, research findings remain inconclusive. No specific virus has been identified that can be considered a cause of the disorder and scientists still do not understand when or under what circumstances viral infections affect the brains of people diagnosed with schizophrenia.

Obstetrical and birth complications

The ways in which birth complications double the risk for schizophrenia are not known. But several studies show that various obstetrical and birth complications do increase risk.

A statistical review of multiple studies looking at the link between obstetric complications and schizophrenia found three groups of complications associated with the disorder:

- **Complications of pregnancy,** including bleeding, diabetes, Rh incompatibility, and pregnancy-induced high blood pressure
- **Abnormal fetal growth and development,** including low birth weight, cardiovascular congenital anomalies, and small head circumference
- **Complications of delivery,** including lack of uterine muscle tone, inadequate oxygen intake by the baby, and emergency cesarean section (C-section)

Other life experiences

Although parents have been let off the hook as far as finger-pointing blame for schizophrenia goes, the current consensus is that other environmental stressors and stress in general may contribute to the onset of schizophrenia. For example, urban life, geographic migration, and poverty are all associated with increased rates of schizophrenia.

Other studies have shown that individuals with schizophrenia smoke marijuana more often than the general population. Some prospective studies now show that smoking marijuana (before the onset of psychotic symptoms) increases the likelihood of schizophrenia by two to four times. On the other hand, the overwhelming majority of people who smoke marijuana don't develop schizophrenia.

Nutritional theories

With so much medical and cultural emphasis on the link between diet and health, it isn't surprising that people wonder whether schizophrenia may be due to eating too much of the wrong thing or too little of something that's good for you. Although some associations have been found that link schizophrenia with increased consumption of refined sugars, it's a far stretch to suggest that refined sugars *cause* the disorder.

In fact, there is no systematic research that suggests that any vitamin, nutrient, specific food, or food allergy can cause schizophrenia.

So is use of marijuana a risk factor for schizophrenia or do people with schizophrenia use marijuana to self-medicate? And is smoking marijuana by itself a risk factor? Some studies suggest that it may only be a risk factor if certain genetic factors are also present. For example, people who have a variant of a specific enzyme (called COMT) that is important in dopamine metabolism (which is implicated in schizophrenia — see "Looking at the brain," earlier in this chapter), develop psychosis more often than those who don't have this specific variant gene configuration. This situation is a very good example, perhaps even a model, of how an environmental influence (the use of marijuana) and a genetic factor may interact together to increase the risk of schizophrenia.

Finding Out More about Risk Factors by Looking at Individual Differences

Schizophrenia can occur at any age — but why? Why do some people develop schizophrenia any time from childhood (which is extremely rare — only 1 in approximately 40,000 children is diagnosed with schizophrenia) to old age (1 percent to 2 percent of cases are diagnosed in people over age 80). Are there genetic differences? Environmental differences? Hormonal differences? Or does a combination of these factors result in some people developing schizophrenia as children and others not until they're senior citizens? Or are there different types of schizophrenia that vary with age?

Childhood schizophrenia can be difficult to diagnose, for several reasons:

- Childhood schizophrenia symptoms tend to surface more gradually than the psychotic break common in adults.

- Often, childhood schizophrenia is misdiagnosed as autism (which generally appears before the age of 3), one of several other pervasive developmental disorders, bipolar disorder, depression, *dissociative disorder* (disruption of memory, awareness, or consciousness), or substance abuse.
- Hallucinations are commonly associated with childhood bipolar or dissociative disorders as opposed to schizophrenia, but the hallucinations of childhood schizophrenia are more pervasive, long-lasting, and continuous (as opposed to being brief and intermittent).

No one is sure about the relative contributions of genetics versus prenatal or environmental stress when it comes to the development of schizophrenia in children or adults. But there is ongoing research looking at schizophrenia across the life span. Some imaging studies have found that children with schizophrenia are more likely to develop abnormalities in brain structure as compared to those with a later onset of the disorder. Recent research supported by the National Institute of Mental Health (NIMH) links a particular gene (called NGR1), which is implicated in schizophrenia in adults, to adverse effects on brain development in children. This suggests a continuum between the child and adult-onset disorders.

Although scientists once believed that the brain finished developing in early childhood, they now realize that connections in the brain are refined well into a child's teens. The parts of the brain involved in planning, decision-making, and reasoning are still taking shape during these years. Based on imaging, scientists know that as the brain develops, certain structures are more involved in mental illness than others. For example, in the brains of adolescents with schizophrenia, there is a significant change in gray matter.

Gender also plays a role in when schizophrenia is diagnosed. Women are more likely to be diagnosed with a later onset of the disorder than men. Some researchers have hypothesized that it occurs later in women because estrogen plays a protective role in warding off symptoms of schizophrenia.

What Science Still Doesn't Know

Clearly, the cause or causes of schizophrenia are still unknown. Scientists aren't even certain whether schizophrenia is one disorder that manifests itself in different ways (referred to as a *spectrum disorder*), or whether schizophrenia is more than one disorder with overlapping symptoms. Similar dilemmas have existed and do exist with other medical problems. For example, is cancer due to one underlying cause, or are there many cancers with many causes?

Even if science finds a single cause for schizophrenia (for example, a specific gene), it won't necessarily lead to a way to prevent or effectively treat the disorder. (In 1993, the Huntington's Disease Collaborative Research Group isolated the precise genetic defect that causes Huntington's disease. But even with that discovery, a strategy for both prevention and definitive treatment still eludes scientists.) Although it may not have the same luster or star power as the discovery of one specific cause, the identification of risk factors and an understanding of the ways that risk factors impact the structure and function of the brain may actually turn out to be a more productive approach.

Some risk factors may be controllable (like cholesterol levels are for coronary artery disease). Other risk factors may lead medical professionals to earlier methods of detection. And by learning the ways that risk factors bring about brain changes, we may actually be able to disrupt the biological or psychological pathways that give rise to the suffering and disability associated with schizophrenia.

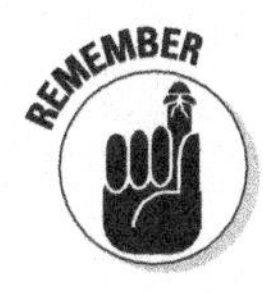

It's vital for scientists to work tenaciously to uncover the causes of schizophrenia. Such investigations are likely to yield important clues about how the disorder can be prevented and lead to improved treatments and care. But wracking your brain about why your loved one developed schizophrenia and searching for specific causes in your particular case is an exercise in futility for several reasons:

- Given the state of current knowledge, neither you nor any doctor will be able to figure out precisely why it happened in a particular situation.
- As much as you might like to, there is no way you can go back and change the past.
- More important, searching for a cause (or looking to place blame) can serve as a distraction from coping with your situation, and moving toward acceptance, treatment, and recovery.

Chapter 3

Suspecting Schizophrenia

In This Chapter

- Recognizing the symptoms and signs of schizophrenia
- Understanding why diagnosis is tricky
- Looking for warning signs
- Taking action when it's needed

If you're like most people, you probably know little about schizophrenia aside from what you've seen on TV or in the movies — much of which was probably sensationalistic and inaccurate. You're more likely to be familiar with stereotypes than facts. Yet, there's no denying it: The symptoms associated with schizophrenia can be truly frightening, especially if the disorder isn't accurately diagnosed and treated.

As is the case in general medicine, appropriate treatment requires an accurate diagnosis. Chapter 4 outlines the criteria that professionals use to diagnose schizophrenia — including the specific signs and symptoms that need to be present for a defined period of time, and that lead to functional impairments. That chapter also describes *exclusion criteria* — criteria that diminish the likelihood of a diagnosis of schizophrenia and suggest something else.

In this chapter, we describe the wide range of symptoms and signs that are seen in people with schizophrenia, as well as some of the telltale warning signs.

Recognizing the Symptoms and Signs of Schizophrenia

Like other medical disorders, schizophrenia is an illness that is characterized by symptoms and signs. *Symptoms* are descriptions of what a person is experiencing (often verbalized in the form of complaints). Typically, when patients visit their doctors, they freely volunteer descriptions of their symptoms (although this isn't always the case with people with schizophrenia who often lack insight; see Chapter 6):

- I feel confused and can't think straight.
- I feel so depressed and have no energy.
- I haven't been able to sleep or get out of bed.

Other times (when people aren't aware of what they're feeling), a friend, family member, or doctor may ask one or more questions designed to elicit symptoms — for example:

- You look very pale. Are you feeling okay?
- How is your mood? You seem so sad.
- You look like you're distracted. Are you hearing voices?
- I'm worried about you. Are you thinking of hurting yourself?

Signs are observations that are made about a person based upon what others see, without the individual necessarily verbalizing his problems. For example:

- You see someone crying.
- You see someone sweaty and shaky.
- You see someone refusing to eat or drink.
- You see someone staring into space.

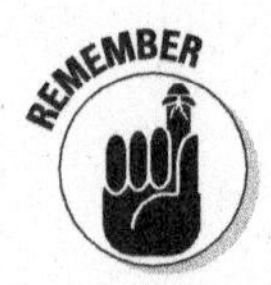

Not every person with a particular disorder will have the same symptoms and signs. And no person will have all of them. For each individual, symptoms and signs may change in severity, reappear, or disappear over time.

The primary symptoms associated with schizophrenia fall into three broad categories: positive symptoms, negative symptoms, and cognitive symptoms. And some other symptoms don't fall neatly into any of these categories. We cover these in the following sections.

Positive symptoms: What's there

Positive symptoms are the easiest to see, the most dramatic, and, in general, the ones that demand attention. One reason they're referred to as positive symptoms is that they *add to,* or alter reality. Twenty years ago, positive symptoms were the only symptoms that were noticed because they're the ones that are most closely tied to psychosis.

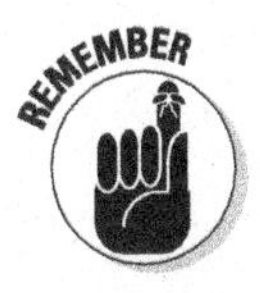

The term *psychosis* doesn't refer to a specific disorder (such as schizophrenia, depression, or bipolar disorder) but rather to the condition of being out of touch with reality. Psychosis is usually a temporary state — one in which a person is having positive symptoms like delusions, hallucinations, or other grossly abnormal distortions of thinking and perception, which we cover in more detail later in this chapter.

Before the availability of antipsychotic medications, persons with schizophrenia, and those who cared for them, spent most of their energies trying to control the tormenting positive symptoms that made patients agitated and unapproachable.

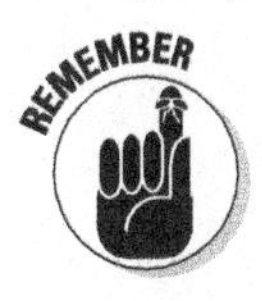

Symptoms may appear slowly over time, or may come on suddenly and intensely like an acute fever. In either case, it's important to recognize when something seems wrong and to seek immediate professional medical and/or mental-health help.

Hallucinations

Hallucinations are false sensory perceptions. They're probably the most dramatic or frightening symptoms of schizophrenia, both to the person with the disorder and to those around her. These false perceptions can affect all the senses:

- Hearing, in the form of *auditory hallucinations:* The person hears voices or sounds that aren't there. Auditory hallucinations are the most common type.
- Sight, in the form of *visual hallucinations:* The person sees something that isn't really there. Visual hallucinations may be visions or signs to which the individual with schizophrenia attaches great meaning or significance.
- Smell, in the form of *olfactory hallucinations:* The person smells odors, usually bad ones, like rotting organic matter, that no one else smells.
- Touch, in the form of *tactile hallucinations:* The person feels the presence or touch of someone or something when no one is actually present. People with both mental illness and substance-use disorders commonly feel bugs crawling over their bodies (sometimes as a result of using cocaine).

Hallucinations are perceptions that are experienced only by the individual with schizophrenia and are not shared by others. Most hallucinations are frightening, especially initially, but then the individual may find some way to incorporate the hallucination into his altered reality in an effort to make it more understandable.

Auditory hallucinations are, by far, the most common type of hallucination. They are experienced differently by different patients, but often, they begin with whispers or mumbling and then become clearer. The person experiencing the voices is unable to recognize that they're coming from within her own head; instead, she attributes them to coming from outside her, like other voices or sounds people hear.

The voices are often threatening or accusatory, blaming the individual for having done something bad. When the voices persistently order a person to do something that he wouldn't ordinarily do, or wouldn't even think of doing, these are called *command hallucinations.* Sometimes a person will initially reject the voices or complain about them, but may later become convinced that the voices are "real" and even try to talk back to them.

Someone who's experiencing auditory hallucinations may seem to be in a world of her own, not listening to others or staring into space. Other times, a person experiencing auditory hallucinations may try to listen to the real person she's with, but "the voices" make it seem as if she's listening to two or more people speaking at the same time, which makes it hard to respond correctly or quickly.

The voices may be very persistent (even interfering with sleep), or they may come and go, with the individual unable to predict when they'll recur — a frightening experience. Stressful situations can make auditory hallucinations worsen, but they can intensify for no reason at all. If a person with schizophrenia is confronted with the reality that no one else hears the same voices, the individual may simply stop talking about them or not tell others that she's hearing them. Treatment with antipsychotic medication usually decreases or removes the voices entirely, or reduces the individual's concern about or fear of them.

Delusions

Delusions are false beliefs that the person with schizophrenia accepts as true; no amount of evidence or explanation can change the person's belief. Most frequently, delusions take the form of a belief that some individual or group is after the person with schizophrenia or wants to harm or control him. Delusions are often accompanied by feelings of suspiciousness, which are then referred to as *paranoid delusions.*

Sometimes the delusions are not clearly formed, and the person feels suspicious or threatened but doesn't attribute it to a particular individual or group. Other times, the individual may believe she has been given great or unusual powers and is able to do things that normal humans cannot do. These delusions are referred to as *delusions of grandeur,* which are often, but not always, associated with religious beliefs. For example, someone may believe that he is Jesus Christ, the devil, or some important person in history.

Voices may tell the person that he has great powers. There may be accompanying visions and signs, which "prove" to the individual that what the voices are saying is true. Generally, no rational discussion can dissuade someone from his false belief. In fact, confronting the individual with the truth often angers the person with schizophrenia and convinces him that anyone who doesn't share his beliefs is against him.

Directly confronting delusional thoughts or beliefs often worsens the situation. Just not agreeing to or not directly confirming the false belief may be a wiser approach.

Because psychotic thinking is the result of a brain disorder, trying to make sense of the content of the hallucination or delusion is as useless as trying to understand the meaning of a kidney stone! Instead of wasting time and energy trying to understand what it means, recognize it as a sign of disturbed thinking and focus on getting your loved one the help he needs.

Antipsychotic medications often lessen or eliminate delusional thinking to the point where a skilled therapist can then discuss the problem of the false belief with the person.

The 2002 Academy Award–winning film *A Beautiful Mind* vividly portrays the delusions and visual hallucinations experienced by mathematician John Nash, who was diagnosed with schizophrenia. It has played a pivotal role in raising awareness about the symptoms of schizophrenia for a generation of moviegoers.

Disorganized thinking

Less dramatic, but just as damaging to a person's ability to function in reality is another positive symptom known as *disorganized thinking,* which can affect speech and/or writing. Instead of being able to hold an organized and logical conversation (thinking about one topic or one issue in a proper sequence), the person with schizophrenia may:

- **Jump from one topic to another.**
- **Make up words that don't exist.** These words are known as *neologisms.*
- **Repeat words or thoughts.**
- **Jump from one word to another that sounds alike but really has no relationship to the first word.**

The individual may sound very earnest, and feel like he's making sense, but other people are unable to follow his train of thought or logic. This situation may be just as frustrating to the speaker as it is to the listener.

When you think about hallucinations, delusions, and disorganized thinking, you realize how severe these positive symptoms can be and how they undermine an individual's ability to think coherently and rationally. (See Chapter 12 for techniques for coping with these symptoms.)

Negative symptoms: What's missing

Negative symptoms are what's missing or lacking in an individual's mind and behavior as a result of schizophrenia. Negative symptoms often aren't as well defined or clear cut as positive ones, so they're often confused with depression or laziness — but they're part of schizophrenia and can be just as debilitating.

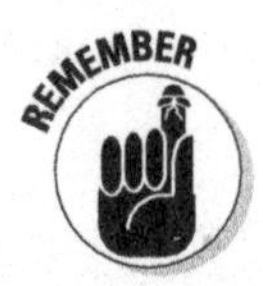

No matter how they look from the outside, negative symptoms are part of a brain disorder. They aren't due to a lack of moral fiber on the part of the person with the illness.

An individual with negative symptoms of schizophrenia may have a blank stare that looks "spacey." She may seem unresponsive to other people and things in the environment. Also, the individual's speech may be monotone or flat, without any inflection offering you a hint of her true feelings. The person with negative symptoms of schizophrenia may also display the following symptoms:

- **An inability to experience simple pleasure from people or things around him:** This is known as *anhedonia.*
- **Lack of initiative, motivation, or willfulness:** This is known as *avolition.*
- **Lack of or limited speech:** The person may be slow in responding, have only a limited range of response, or not even respond at all. This is known as *alogia.*
- **A lack of emotions or feelings:** The person may look expressionless — not showing any signs of happiness, excitement, or anger. This is known as *flat* or *blunted affect.* Some research suggests that this may be more a matter of appearance rather than a reflection of the individual's inability to feel emotions.

After treatment, many families complain that while their relative is no longer psychotic, the person is "wasting her life" watching television in a room with few outside interests. They feel very frustrated because nothing they do or say motivates the person to become more engaged in the world around her. Families need to understand that this isn't something the person has control over or is doing to annoy them — it's part of the illness.

People used to think that these symptoms were the result of the side effects of medication or of institutional treatment (which, in the past, often included long hospital stays). But today, most experts agree that negative symptoms are probably due to brain dysfunction. Some researchers have studied people with schizophrenia early in the course of their illness and found that they had motivational deficits even then. Many believe, in fact, that negative symptoms may emerge before positive ones do.

Although medication is highly effective in treating positive symptoms, it has been less successful in treating negative symptoms, which can remain unchanged or only marginally improved even when positive symptoms go away. It is generally believed that newer antipsychotic medications (see Chapter 8) are just as effective as older ones in controlling positive symptoms, but may be slightly more successful in minimizing negative symptoms.

Approximately one in four patients with schizophrenia may have *deficit syndrome,* persistent negative symptoms that are not secondary or due to other causes (such as depression or medication side effects). The importance of finding ways to treat negative symptoms can't be underestimated. Failure to do so can compromise an individual's quality of life and impair her ability to work and maintain meaningful social ties.

Cognitive symptoms: Changes in mental functioning

Unfortunately, even when positive symptoms are controlled, people with schizophrenia may have severe problems with *cognitive* (thinking) tasks. A person with schizophrenia may be unable to remember things he's been told, and he may have problems following directions or keeping track of time or appointments. For example, a person with schizophrenia may not be able to remember or follow simple instructions like "If you feel agitated, don't drink coffee." Following directions about which prescribed medications to take in the morning and which to take in the evening can be just as difficult.

If the person returns to school or work, tasks that were in the past very doable, can now seem insurmountable. For example, the person may be unable to focus or concentrate. Neuropsychologists have devised and administered very specific tests to identify the particular thinking problems and where they occur in the brain.

Working memory (the ability to hold a fact in mind to be used later — for example, to remember that the 4 p.m. train will be on track no. 5 has been found to be impaired in many people with schizophrenia, as have verbal abilities. Cognitive symptoms make it extremely difficult for some people with schizophrenia to carry out what seem like simple tasks or to be able to hold down a job. For example, people with this type of cognitive problem should choose jobs that maximize their skills and minimize the need for working memory. (It might be difficult for them to be waiters who have to remember complex orders in a busy restaurant.)

In fact, it has been found that cognitive symptoms and negative symptoms (see the "Negative symptoms: What's missing" section, earlier) are more difficult for people to overcome than positive ones, and that they prevent recovery and a return to normal life in a more profound way than the more dramatic positive symptoms.

Because of the importance of cognitive symptoms in preventing recovery, the National Institute of Mental Health (NIMH) is supporting the development of a standard battery of neuropsychological tests to assess the severity of these problems in individuals. The NIMH is also supporting research to discover medications to treat cognitive impairments like the antipsychotic drugs used to treat hallucinations and delusions.

Negative symptoms and cognitive symptoms may sometimes get better or worse together — but they are really separate features of schizophrenia related to different areas and circuitry in the brain. Thus, positive, negative, and cognitive symptoms have to be treated separately, but concurrently, for a truly comprehensive approach to the treatment of schizophrenia. Many people now believe that negative and cognitive symptoms are really the core symptoms of schizophrenia and that, until there are effective treatments, schizophrenia will remain a major public-health problem.

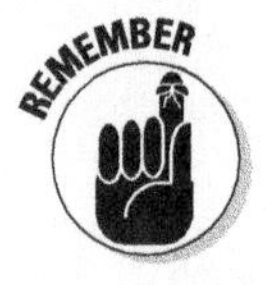

Although there are currently no known effective medications to treat cognitive symptoms, various psychosocial interventions may be of help.

Other disturbing symptoms and behaviors

In addition to the three major categories of symptoms — positive, negative, and cognitive — other symptoms are frequently seen in people with schizophrenia. These symptoms are not specific to schizophrenia — in fact, if these symptoms are seen alone (without the positive, negative, and cognitive symptoms we describe earlier), they probably indicate that the illness being seen is *not* schizophrenia. Typically these other symptoms are more likely to fluctuate in severity than positive, negative, and cognitive symptoms do.

As treatment progresses, these other symptoms tend to emerge, as the more obvious positive symptoms of schizophrenia tend to recede.

Again and again: Obsessive-compulsive behaviors

It is not uncommon for people with schizophrenia to engage in repetitive behaviors like rocking, rubbing their hands together, or getting up and down over and over. Likewise, individuals may complain that the same thought or idea keeps going through their minds even though they don't want it to.

Some of these repetitive unwanted behaviors are made worse when a particular antipsychotic medication, clozapine, is used to treat schizophrenia. Reducing the dosage of clozapine (brand name: Clozaril) will sometimes help. Adding an antidepressant medication like fluoxetine hydrochloride (brand name: Prozac), a selective serotonin uptake inhibitor (SSRI), may also help reduce the behavior.

Sometimes the need to move around and pace is not a compulsive behavior, but a side effect called *akathisia,* which is usually associated with high-potency, first-generation antipsychotic medications like haloperidol (brand name: Haldol). (See Chapter 8 for a more in-depth discussion of psychotropic medications and their side-effects.)

Ups and downs: Mood swings

Shifts in mood, more often in the direction of sadness or depression rather than mania, are fairly common in schizophrenia. Depressive symptoms can be so severe and persistent that the diagnosis may change from schizophrenia to *schizoaffective disorder* (which includes elements of both a thought disorder and a mood disorder). The diagnosis of schizoaffective disorder is even more likely if mood varies between depression and elation (known as *hypomania*). When this is the case, a mood stabilizer such as lithium or valproate (brand name: Depakote) will generally be added to the antipsychotic medication.

Depression sometimes becomes apparent when the person with schizophrenia is showing fewer positive symptoms, and he realizes how sick he's been and how his life has been disrupted by the illness. Depression can become so severe that suicidal thoughts and behavior can occur. If suicidal thoughts become prominent, clozapine (brand name: Clozaril) has been found to be the most effective antipsychotic medication.

If sadness, loss of appetite, and sleeping difficulties become the prominent symptoms, treatment with an antidepressant drug is often indicated. Your loved one's psychiatrist must be careful when starting someone on an antidepressant — they need to make sure that positive symptoms are not made worse or that your loved one isn't moved toward manic behavior. Careful and accurate reporting — by the person with schizophrenia, as well as family and friends — will help the psychiatrist adjust the medication dosage.

Wired: High anxiety

A person with schizophrenia may sometimes feel excessively anxious or nervous, sometimes for no apparent reason. Anxiety may be so severe that it interferes with the person's ability to fall asleep. Then the sleeplessness may exacerbate positive symptoms (especially paranoia). On a very short-term basis, for severe anxiety, an anti-anxiety medication like Valium may be used, but an anti-anxiety med should not be used regularly or long term.

Be sure to report back to the psychiatrist whether your loved one's anxiety (nervousness, worry, sweating) is getting better, getting worse, or staying the same.

Sometimes if an individual is becoming increasingly anxious and positive symptoms are getting worse, the person may begin to display *catatonic behavior,* which is characterized by holding fixed positions for a long period of time. When the catatonic person's arms are moved, there is a feeling of resistance, called *waxy flexibility.* The treatment for catatonic behavior usually entails increasing the dosage of antipsychotic medication.

Sleepless: Going on empty

Sleep problems are very common in people with psychiatric disorders. No one should be allowed to become truly sleep-deprived, because sleep deprivation can worsen the symptoms of schizophrenia. Instead of just prescribing a sleeping pill, the psychiatrist should try to understand why your loved one is not sleeping (for example, she may be afraid of symptoms, hearing noises, or sleeping too much during the day) and recommend an appropriate remedy.

Knowing Why Diagnosing Schizophrenia Is Tricky

If you ask families to describe the onset of schizophrenia, no two stories will be exactly the same. One reason that you're likely to get widely divergent descriptions is because sometimes schizophrenia creeps in slowly until its appearance becomes blatant, and other times it appears to come on suddenly, like a bolt of lightning out of the blue.

The earliest signs of schizophrenia can be subtle and nonspecific, tending to wax and wane over the course of weeks, months, or even years. A person can be fine one morning, overtly psychotic the same evening, and fine again the next morning. When you're living with an individual or seeing him every day, the changes taking place can be so subtle that you may not even realize that something is wrong. Another factor that comes into play: You're always hoping for the best — that the symptoms will disappear on their own. Even looking back, you may be unable to mark the precise time when you could no longer deny that your loved one was ill and desperately needed help.

The term *first break* is used to define the onset of schizophrenia. It's usually marked by both positive and negative symptoms that are serious enough that they obviously necessitate some form of treatment, which may or may not include hospitalization. (For an example of a first break that came on suddenly, check out the "It happened all of a sudden" sidebar, in this chapter. We've changed the names and details to protect people's privacy.)

It happened all of a sudden

Marge Faber, a homemaker and part-time real-estate agent, breathed a sigh of relief when the last of her three boys was ready to go off to college. She and her husband, Frank, would have more time to travel and to visit their first grandchild, whose parents had escaped the brutal winters of Buffalo, New York, and relocated to Tampa, Florida.

Marge's youngest, 19-year-old Brett, was an easy-going kid who was always popular with his peers. Except for the usually sibling rivalry and competitiveness common among boys, the brothers got along exceptionally well. Brett admired his brothers, who were two and four years older than he was.

Brett was always a solid student, so he had his choice of schools to attend. When he was offered a soccer scholarship at a large university in the Southwest, he enrolled in a program in the university's College of Education. The summer before his freshman year, Brett worked at a local day camp as a swim instructor.

A week after Brett arrived on campus, he locked himself in his dorm and refused to eat. His roommates, who had only met him on Facebook (`www.facebook.com`), were concerned and told the resident assistant in the dorm. That same evening, Marge and Frank got a call from the school's student health services alerting them to what had happened. They called Brett and couldn't get a coherent story — he was whispering so low that they could barely hear him.

After a sleepless night, Marge and Frank flew out to check on Brett. When they arrived at the school, he was pacing and looked very nervous. He told them that he hadn't been able to sleep or leave the dorm for meals because people in the next room were plotting a Columbine-style attack on campus. They asked questions, but Brett's answers made no sense. They knew something was wrong.

This was the first time that Brett had been away from his close and very supportive family. Maybe he was having difficulty adjusting, Marge thought. So they stayed at a hotel close to campus for another week and visited Brett every day. But the situation didn't improve. Brett still refused to eat or leave the room. He insisted on doing 250 push-ups to build up his strength, in case he needed to protect himself and his roommates. After doing just 20 push-ups, he fell to the floor in exhaustion. His parents called 911 and accompanied Brett to the emergency room of the local hospital. A psychiatrist on call met with Brett when they arrived. Brett confided to the doctor that voices had been telling him to build his strength to ward off the attackers.

He was diagnosed with paranoid schizophrenia, and the doctor prescribed olanzapine (brand name: Zyprexa), which Brett agreed to take. Marge and Frank took him back to their hotel room for a week to watch over him. He told them that the voices weren't as loud, but they were still there. The Fabers decided to take their son back to Buffalo for care until the next semester.

They were stunned. "He was the perfect child until he became ill," Marge said, as she recounted the story 15 years later. At the age of 34, Brett was never able to complete his education and still lives at home in the same bedroom where he grew up, spending most of his time listening to music or watching TV. Over the years, he has been on a variety of medications, each with different side effects, but none has been able to completely quell the voices.

We always knew something was wrong

"She always seemed different," said Liz Turner as she began to tell us about her daughter Erin, now 41 years old. "Something wasn't right," she said. Erin was Liz's first child, so she really had no yardstick to gauge things by until her daughter Meg was born, ten years later. "There were signs I didn't see or didn't want to see," Liz said.

Erin was oxygen-deprived at birth but "sort of" met all the milestones her mom faithfully chronicled in her baby book. Her speech was a bit delayed, and she wasn't that responsive to other people. Everything annoyed her — from the labels on her clothes to the noise of the vacuum cleaner. By second grade, Erin was afraid to go to school and clung to her mother's apron strings. By fifth grade, she tested high in certain subjects but was lower in others, especially mathematics. Erin was always considered a "cry-baby" by the other kids at school. In fact, she seemed to prefer to be alone and was never invited on play dates or to parties.

By the time Erin was a teen, she looked a bit eccentric — she'd dyed her hair pink and sported a tattoo on her ankle. She suddenly became very outgoing and began hanging out with a group of kids who were always getting into trouble. Liz found some marijuana in Erin's room and knew she had been smoking but figured that kids would be kids — Erin wasn't the only one of her peers smoking pot. Her moods changed on a dime, and her parents were baffled — unsure whether it was the drug use or something else.

One night, Erin stole several $20 bills and a gold necklace from a neighbor's home. She let herself in the open back door and helped herself without thinking about the consequences. When the neighbor returned home and found her exiting the house, she was caught red-handed. The neighbor, who was always irritated by the loud music coming from the Turners' house, pressed charges.

A kind-hearted police officer said he would get the neighbors to drop the charges if the Turners took Erin for a psychiatric evaluation. They were humiliated by the thought of mental illness in their family, but they had no choice. The doctor met with Erin several times, and Erin admitted that she had been hearing voices — they had been such an integral part of her existence since she was a child that she thought everyone else heard them, too. She said that smoking pot made them go away, even for an hour or so.

The doctor spoke to the family and explained that Erin had a diagnosis of schizoaffective disorder. Liz's husband, Tim, said that an aunt on his side of the family had some problems, but people didn't talk about them much at the time. As stunned as they were, the family was happy that they finally could attach a name to what was wrong and get the proper medication to help treat the illness.

Diagnosing schizophrenia is complicated by the fact that the typical age of onset of the disorder overlaps with the tumultuous roller-coaster years of adolescence. In teens, the first symptoms of schizophrenia tend to emerge so slowly or so vaguely that they mimic or overlap "normal" adolescent behaviors. With surging hormones and pressures to fit in with their peers, most teens tend to be moody and restless. Also, the typical teen is often prone to engage in risky behaviors, including experimentation with drugs and/or alcohol.

The average parent — and even the average teacher or pediatrician — usually can't differentiate between the typical turmoil of adolescence and the first warning signs of schizophrenia, especially when the symptoms or signs are masked by illicit substance use. For this reason, most parents of people with schizophrenia say they never understood the disease or recognized its symptoms until long after it hit. (For an example of this, check out the sidebar, "We always knew something was wrong," in this chapter. We've changed the names and details to protect people's privacy.)

When to Worry: The Warning Signs

Before any overt signs of psychosis appear (in a period known as the *prodromal phase*), people with schizophrenia may experience some non-psychotic symptoms that are the very first signs of the disorder. Here are some of the warning signs of schizophrenia:

- Social withdrawal and an increased tendency to remain alone
- A decline in performance at school or work
- Loss of motivation and an inability to concentrate
- Increased irritability, depression, and/or anxiety
- Suspiciousness
- Neglect of physical appearance
- Changes in sleep patterns

Talking about or actually trying to hurt or kill oneself isn't a warning sign. It is a red flag that should be taken seriously. If your loved one is talking about suicide, you should take immediate action — have him evaluated by a mental-health clinician.

One study in Australia followed a group of approximately 100 young people with symptoms that didn't quite meet the criteria for diagnosis, but who had a family history of schizophrenia, to see if they could predict those who would go on to develop the disorder. One-third of the group developed psychotic symptoms within a year, which was predicted with a high level of accuracy based on the research participants' initial symptoms.

There is increasing recognition that the public, in general, needs to become mental-health literate and be able to recognize the earliest signs and symptoms of a mental-health problem. A 12-hour training program called Mental Health First Aid was developed in Australia to help the public identify, understand, and respond to a mental-health problem or crisis. The program is being brought to communities across the United States under the sponsorship of the National Council for Community Behavioral Healthcare. To find out more about the program, contact the National Council at 301-984-6200 or go to www.thenationalcouncil.org.

Taking Action: Getting Treatment for Your Loved One Right Away

The *duration of untreated psychosis* (DUP) is the period of time between the onset of the first psychotic symptoms and the time a person receives treatment. According to a recent study commissioned by the National Alliance on Mental Illness (NAMI), the average duration of untreated psychosis is more than eight years. This lag is due to a number of factors, including:

- Stigma related to mental illnesses
- Lack of health insurance coupled with the high cost of care
- The limitations of *mental-health literacy* (the general public's knowledge and beliefs concerning mental disorders)

Unlike many other physical or mental disorders, schizophrenia is a disorder that is rarely over-diagnosed or diagnosed too quickly. Even when family members are aware of symptoms and signs of the illness, they may fail to do anything, hoping the symptoms will resolve on their own. Plus, family doctors and pediatricians are often uncomfortable suggesting that a patient may have schizophrenia — it isn't something they're used to diagnosing or treating. And even psychiatrists may be reluctant to deliver the message.

If you suspect that someone you know may have schizophrenia, have the individual seen by a psychiatrist who specializes in the disorder. If you're a parent or close relative, have confidence in your gut instinct that something is wrong and get it checked out; you've probably known the person longer and better than anyone else.

Getting a diagnosis is the first step in getting help. In most cases, your fears and suspicions will be allayed by someone who is expert and knowledgeable about diagnosis and treatment of the disorder. (Turn to Chapter 4 for more information on getting a diagnosis.)

Part II
Finding Out What's Wrong and Getting Help

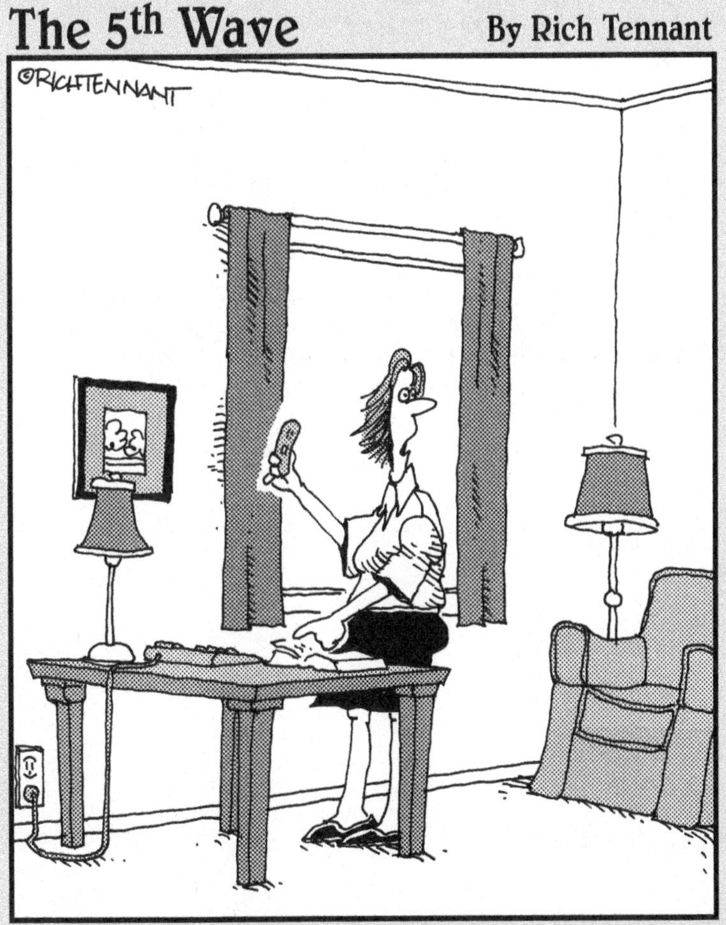

"I made an appointment with a Dr. Douglas Sooner. I know it's silly, but I always heard, the sooner the diagnosis, the better."

In this part . . .

In this part, we explain that arriving at a diagnosis of schizophrenia — and differentiating it from other disorders — can be tricky and demands the training and expertise of a skilled clinician. You find out how to go about finding a psychiatrist and assembling a multidisciplinary healthcare team to provide the full range of coordinated treatments, services, and supports that people with schizophrenia and their families need. Because denial (both by people with schizophrenia and their families) is often a major barrier to treatment and recovery, we explain why denial occurs and how it can be overcome. And we provide you with some of the concrete tips you need to navigate the complex system of care and prepare for the future.

Chapter 4

Getting a Diagnosis

In This Chapter

- Understanding how schizophrenia is diagnosed
- Recognizing different subtypes of schizophrenia
- Differentiating between schizophrenia and other possible diagnoses
- Searching for a second opinion
- Coming to terms with the diagnosis of schizophrenia

Whether you've long suspected that something was wrong or you were blindsided by symptoms that appeared all of a sudden, now the symptoms that worried you finally have a name. This situation is probably somewhat reassuring but it will also raise many questions.

After a loved one is diagnosed with schizophrenia, you want to know more about how the diagnosis was made, how the symptoms of schizophrenia differ from other mental illnesses, and why the disorder is often confused with other health conditions. We wrote this chapter to answer those questions and to give you a glimpse of your loved one's prospects for the future. We also provide some advice on how to adjust to a diagnosis that no one is prepared to hear, and let you know how and when to get a second opinion.

Understanding How Diagnoses Are Made

When you're dealing with any type of disease, one of the first things you want from your doctor — besides getting a prescription to fix the problem — is a diagnosis. Being able to put a name to a set of symptoms helps people understand, accept, and deal with their disorder. At the same time, you may wonder how the doctor arrived at this diagnosis: How does he know it's schizophrenia and not another type of mental disorder?

The next sections describe how doctors obtain information to make a diagnosis, what differentiates schizophrenia from other illnesses, and why people diagnosed with schizophrenia can have such varying symptoms.

Diagnosis: Giving a name to a set of symptoms

Just the word *diagnosis* can sound frightening and clinical. However, diagnoses are nothing more than the names given to various physical and mental disorders or diseases. A diagnosis is a generalization that describes what the average person with that disorder or disease experiences, and what can be expected in the future based on criteria that are periodically revised by the medical community.

The value of a diagnosis is that it provides a shorthand way of communicating important information about a medical condition, such as:

- The characteristic symptoms of the disorder
- The expected *course* (how it may vary over time)
- The prognosis of the disorder (the outlook for the future)
- Most important, options for treatment

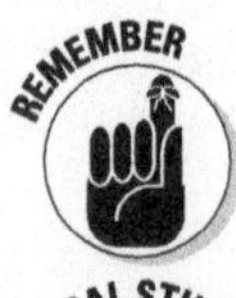

With any illness — whether mental or physical — any one individual is unlikely to show *all* the symptoms and behaviors associated with a diagnosis. Your loved one with schizophrenia won't fit the precise description of the disorder you find in textbooks, because everyone experiences the disorder in a somewhat unique way.

More recently, the term *schizophrenia spectrum disorders* has come into use to describe the variations in illness that fit under the name of schizophrenia.

Inside the Diagnostic and Statistical Manual: The psychiatric bible

The classification of various mental disorders and the criteria used to make diagnoses are found in a book called the *Diagnostic and Statistical Manual of Mental Disorders,* published by the American Psychiatric Association and often referred to simply as the DSM. The DSM is a consensus document, meaning that agreement has been reached by many professionals about what to name a particular disorder that has certain *criteria,* or characteristics, associated with it. It is used by psychiatrists and other mental-health professionals to make diagnoses.

The current DSM is the fourth edition of this official guide to diagnosis, so this edition is logically called DSM-IV. Editions or revisions come into being about every ten years, and the next edition is not expected before 2010. The manual is massive (just under 1,000 pages) and includes 16 categories of mental disorders with multiple diagnoses in each category. Schizophrenia is part of the "schizophrenia and other psychotic disorders" category.

Many of the same symptoms can be found in more than one category or disorder, but every diagnosis is based on a pattern of symptoms as well as the history of the illness.

If you're curious about the other categories of mental illness or want to look up something in the *DSM-IV,* you can find a copy at your local library, or preview portions of the book (search within the book) at `http://books.google.com/books?id=3SQrtpnHb9MC`, or buy a copy at major online booksellers. The list price is $84.

Looking for Schizophrenia

Getting the right diagnosis is as important with mental illness as it is with physical illness, because, in all disease, treatment is determined by diagnosis. A psychiatrist or other mental-health professional makes a diagnosis by determining how closely a patient's "story" fits the pattern of symptoms that have been identified for the particular disorder.

Differentiating among mental illnesses isn't always easy, and a diagnosis may change over the course of years or even months. There are several reasons for this:

- **Different mental illnesses often have overlapping symptoms.**
- **The predominant symptoms may ebb and flow in the same person over time.** For example, when hallucinations and delusions are predominant, the person may be diagnosed with schizophrenia; when mood symptoms, like excitability or depression, dominate, the person may be diagnosed as having a mood disorder.

Diagnoses are made using information gleaned through verbal interviews with the patient, observations of his behavior, and, often, interviews with other people in the patient's life. An accurate diagnosis also requires collecting information about the recent history that led to the current problem, along with the lifetime history of behavioral or emotional problems in the individual and his family. When the individual who's sick is unable or unwilling to accurately articulate his story, family members or close friends can play a pivotal role by augmenting missing information and providing relevant medical records.

A complete examination includes a physical exam as well as general medical laboratory tests. When available, this information may be obtained from the patient's general practitioner or internist. Although there is no specific laboratory test to detect schizophrenia, lab tests are used to rule out the possibility of physical disorders whose symptoms mimic those of mental disorders.

When the clinician — most often a *psychiatrist* (an MD who has special training in mental disorders) or another licensed mental-health professional (see Chapter 5 for more on different types of mental-health professionals) has all this information, the next task is to consider which of the numerous descriptions of mental disorders (diagnoses) best fits the patient's symptoms, behavior, and history.

The elements of a psychiatric interview

When an individual comes to a clinician's office for a psychiatric *assessment* (interview) — either on her own, brought by a family member or friend, or even escorted by law-enforcement authorities — an interview is used for making a diagnosis. We cover the main elements of a psychiatric interview in the following sections.

Determining the reason for the visit

The clinician will ask, "Why are you here?" to determine the person's problems or symptoms and then will follow up with other similar questions to determine the nature of the person's problems. Here a few examples of the kinds of questions the clinician may ask:

- What symptoms are you experiencing?
- When did they start?
- How often do they occur?
- Do your symptoms interfere with your school, work, or ability to take care of yourself?
- Do you hear voices? If so, what do they say?
- How often do you drink alcohol? How much? When?
- Have you ever used marijuana? Cocaine? Other drugs?
- Do you ever feel depressed?
- Do you ever have thoughts of hurting yourself?

Conducting a mental status examination

The clinician will generally conduct a *mental status examination,* which involves both observation by the clinician and direct questioning to determine the individual's thought processes, mood, perception, orientation, memory, and so on.

In addition to listening to the person, the clinician will observe the individual's behavior:

- Is he sitting still, or fidgeting and moving around excessively?
- Does he appear to be distracted by sounds or voices that aren't there?
- Does he cry easily? Laugh inappropriately? Change moods on a dime?
- Is he too talkative or too quiet?
- Does he seem impaired by alcohol and/or other drugs?

The clinician is looking for unusual behaviors or signs that are characteristic of a particular disorder.

Getting a good history

Because patients may be forgetful, anxious, or may not be thinking clearly, the clinician (or an assistant) may request the same information about symptoms, history of the problem, and family history from other reliable informants (such as family members or close friends). This information may be requested either during the initial diagnostic interview or at another time.

If you keep a notebook of detailed observations, that can really help your clinician make an accurate and timely diagnosis. (See Chapter 14 for more on keeping track of your loved one's symptoms and treatments.)

Looking at the criteria for schizophrenia

A pattern of symptoms and behavior over a certain period of time has to be met before the clinician makes a DSM-IV diagnosis of schizophrenia.

The criteria for diagnosing schizophrenia are very specific:

- There must be a mixture of certain *signs* (observable behavior) and *symptoms* (verbally reported experiences) that are present for a significant portion of time (over a one-month period), with some signs and symptoms present (but not necessarily continuously) for a minimum period of six months.
- If the signs and symptoms are present for one month, but less than six months, a formal diagnosis of schizophreniform disorder is made. So between two visits, the diagnosis can change from schizophreniform to schizophrenia, just by virtue of the passage of time, without any change in symptoms.

To make a diagnosis of schizophrenia, certain *inclusion criteria* (required criteria) and *exclusion criteria* (disqualifying criteria) need to be met. Two or more of the following must be present for a significant portion of time during a one-month period in order for someone to be diagnosed with schizophrenia:

- **Delusions:** False, fixed beliefs that cannot be dispelled with logic.
- **Hallucinations:** False sensory perceptions, usually auditory, with no basis in reality.
- **Disorganized speech:** Speech that reflects illogical thinking and cognitive impairment.
- **Grossly disorganized or catatonic behavior:** Observable dysfunctional movements or holding fixed immobile positions for long periods of time.
- **Negative symptoms:** For example, too little emotion for a given situation or no desire to carry out meaningful activities (see Chapter 2).
- **Social and/or occupational dysfunction:** The criterion of social and/or occupational dysfunction must be met, which means the person is unable to function in one or more areas of everyday life (such as self care, work, school, or interpersonal relationships). The person is functioning markedly below the level at which she functioned before becoming ill.

If other symptoms or conditions are present, a diagnosis of schizophrenia cannot be made.

The most common exclusion is substance abuse. A variety of drugs that are often used illicitly — for example, stimulants (such as amphetamines), marijuana, *PCP* (also known as angel dust), cocaine, and hallucinogenic drugs (such as LSD and psilocybin or mescaline) — cause symptoms that mimic schizophrenia.

Other exclusion criteria are

- A history of severe mood swings (elation and/or depression) that would lead to alternative diagnoses of an affective (mood) disorder or schizoaffective disorder
- Evidence of a physical disorder — such as hormonal (thyroid or adrenal gland) problems or a tumor that may have spread to the brain and is giving rise to mental symptoms

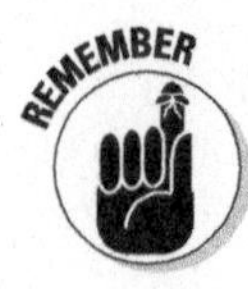

Co-occurring mental-health and substance-abuse disorders are so common that the possibility of both occurring simultaneously should never be overlooked. Because individuals who are diagnosed with schizophrenia often abuse alcohol, drugs, and/or other substances, accurate diagnosis may be complicated if an individual shows up in an emergency room without the clinician being able to obtain a reliable history. If the symptoms are solely the result of drug intoxication, they will usually disappear in a matter of hours or days. However, drug use sometimes triggers or leads to the onset of what will become a schizophreniform disorder or schizophrenia.

Describing different types of schizophrenia

The DSM-IV recognizes four types of schizophrenia: catatonic, paranoid, disorganized, and undifferentiated. Because these terms are still used in the mental-health profession (and you may hear them from clinicians who are treating your loved one), we define them in the following sections, listing their predominant symptoms.

Frankly, we don't think these terms are very useful in describing the severity of the illness or in directing treatment. It's likely that in the next revision of the "bible," old labels will give way to new ones. Instead of these labels, many clinicians prefer to use the terms *positive, negative,* and *cognitive* to describe their patients' symptoms and approaches to treatment, remediation, rehabilitation, and recovery. (See Chapter 3 for more about positive, negative, and cognitive symptoms associated with schizophrenia.)

Catatonic

The term *catatonic* refers to abnormal motor activity. The individual may remain frozen in one position for long periods of time. He may display *waxy flexibility* (allowing himself to be moved) or become rigid and resist being moved, holding the position in which his arms or legs are placed.

Paranoid

The predominant symptoms of paranoia are *delusions* (fixed, false beliefs) and *hallucinations* (hearing voices) — although the individual may seem quite ordinary in other areas of functioning. The paranoid-type patient often believes that some group (such as the FBI, communists, or the Nazis) is after her, and she frequently hears voices that threaten, command, or berate her. No amount of reassurance or "proof" will convince her that she isn't at risk, or that the voices aren't real and are internal, coming from her brain rather than from the outside environment.

Disorganized

The main feature of disorganized schizophrenia is speech that is very disorganized, illogical, and hard to follow, often accompanied by feelings that are inappropriate or too shallow for what's being said or discussed. Coherent delusional ideas are not present (in other words, if the person is delusional, you might not even be able to understand the delusion because of the person's disorganized thinking and speech), and if there are hallucinations, they're fragmentary and disorganized. The person may be so disorganized that he cannot adequately carry on activities of daily living (such as washing, dressing, and eating).

Undifferentiated

If an individual doesn't have the characteristics or features of the other three types, she's classified as undifferentiated. If new symptoms don't emerge over a long a period of time, this type is sometimes also called the *residual type.*

The Great Imposters: Ruling Out Other Mental Conditions

To the casual observer, different mental disorders have similar symptoms. The diagnosis of schizophrenia is made primarily comparing an individual's symptoms to the pattern of symptoms and behaviors characteristically associated with the disorder. However, even mental-health professionals admit that diagnosis is more an art than a physical science, because there are no laboratory tests or diagnostic X-rays that can definitively confirm the diagnosis.

For some physical disorders, health professionals have tools like blood tests and imaging procedures to help make an accurate diagnosis. In mental disorders, reliable diagnoses are achieved by conducting a thorough clinical interview, taking a very good history, and watching the evolution of the illness and sometimes its response to medication. A similar situation occurs in medicine when a patient has abdominal pain, vomiting, diarrhea, and fever and a doctor needs to determine whether it's due to appendicitis, salmonella food poisoning, or a stomach virus. When the pattern of symptoms isn't clear cut, it takes a skilled practitioner, a thorough work-up, and time to recognize the difference. Sometimes internists say that an illness needs time "to declare itself."

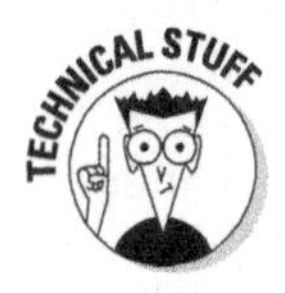

Magnetic resonance imaging (MRI) and *positron emission tomography* (PET) are two brain imaging techniques that allow scientists to visualize the structure or function of the brain in great detail. Although many studies have demonstrated structural differences in the brain between groups of people with or without schizophrenia, the differences are not large enough that they can be used clinically at this point in time to make or confirm diagnoses in any one individual.

In the following sections, we cover some of the disorders that make it challenging to distinguish between two or more disorders or conditions with similar symptoms.

Schizoaffective disorder

Despite the similar sounding names, schizoaffective disorder isn't a type of schizophrenia. Rather, it's another diagnosis that falls under the same *DSM-IV* category, "schizophrenia and other psychotic disorders."

Many of the symptoms that characterize schizoaffective disorder overlap with those of schizophrenia, and differentiating between the two is often difficult. The big difference is that, in schizoaffective disorder, there has been an uninterrupted period of illness that meets the criteria for a *mood disorder* (characterized by major depression, mania, or a mixture of the two). This is in addition to, and concurrent with, the symptoms of schizophrenia (such as delusions and hallucinations).

There is an increased risk for suicide in people with schizoaffective disorder (which is often associated with profound depression). Also, appropriate treatment for schizoaffective disorder often requires the use of mood stabilizers (such as lithium) or even antidepressant drugs, as well as antipsychotic medications.

One of the reasons for using medication in any illness is to relieve or reduce symptoms. Regardless of the specific diagnosis, the same medications or combinations of them may be used to treat similar symptoms.

Bipolar disorder

The onset of bipolar disorder (also called *manic-depressive disorder*), another severe mental disorder, is sometimes quite abrupt, beginning with manic or *hypomanic* (mildly manic) behavior. Although mental-health professionals used to believe that bipolar disorder occurred only in older people (unlike schizophrenia, which usually begins in a person's teens or early 20s), it's now recognized that even children and adolescents can have bipolar disorder.

Mania is characterized by an excess of energy (for example, staying up all night for days at a time without tiring), having grandiose ideas that border on delusions, and, perhaps, even having hallucinations. These symptoms overlap with those seen in sudden-onset schizophrenia, so the diagnoses can easily be confused.

The onset of bipolar disorder can also begin with depressive symptoms, such as a profoundly sad mood, sleeping too much or too little, a lack of interest in anything, the inability to experience pleasure (called *anhedonia*), and suicidal thoughts. Someone with bipolar disorder can also have delusions, especially of a self-deprecatory type, where the individual believes he's responsible for many of the ills of the world, or that his body is rotting inside or is riddled with cancer.

A diagnosis of bipolar disorder is made on the basis of at least one episode of both manic and depressive symptoms, not necessarily alternating or in equal numbers. The overlap of symptoms with schizophrenia can initially lead to misdiagnosis, but usually the prominence of the mood symptoms (depression or mania) leads to the correct diagnosis and appropriate treatment. For example, it's not uncommon over a long period of illness for individuals to be diagnosed sequentially with schizophrenia, schizoaffective disorder, and bipolar disorder if their symptoms change. To learn more about bipolar disorder, see *Bipolar Disorder For Dummies,* by Candida Fink, MD, and Joe Kraynak (Wiley).

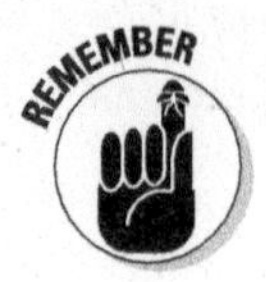

Because symptoms fluctuate, don't be surprised if an individual's diagnosis changes over time. This doesn't necessarily mean that there has been a diagnostic error. It just means that the pattern of symptoms is different now, so a different diagnosis and treatment are indicated.

Severe depression

Some individuals may become severely depressed (see the preceding section) but never go on to exhibit manic behavior. They may experience repeated episodes of depression with delusions (sometimes called *delusional depression*) and/or hallucinations.

The person with severe depression shows no interest in things around her and may barely speak. Even if the severity of the episode decreases, the individual may remain aloof, slow-moving, and appear preoccupied. These symptoms can sometimes be confused with the symptoms of schizophrenia.

In severe depression, depressive mood symptoms are more prominent than deficits in thinking. It's important to differentiate between the two disorders because antidepressant medication is a necessity in treating severe depression, but the use of antipsychotic medication is needed to treat schizophrenia. Less commonly, individuals with either depression or schizophrenia may require both types of medication (see Chapter 8).

Substance use and abuse

The widespread use of so-called *street drugs* (illegal drugs) can give rise to symptoms and signs that are similar to those seen in schizophrenia. Because drug experimentation frequently begins in someone's late teens or early 20s, also the peak time when the symptoms of schizophrenia appear, one can be mistaken for the other — at least initially.

Use of stimulant drugs, such as amphetamine or methamphetamine (also known as *crystal meth*), over a period of time frequently causes extreme paranoid feelings and behaviors. As a result, individuals on these drugs often are brought to a hospital emergency room by law enforcement authorities. Usually, keeping them safe, providing supportive care, and sometimes administering sedative medications relieves the acute paranoid symptoms in hours, and what looked like schizophrenia is diagnosed instead as drug intoxication and acute amphetamine psychosis. Testing for drugs in the person's blood or urine helps confirm the diagnosis.

A class of drugs known as *hallucinogens* — that prominently includes marijuana, LSD, and PCP (also known as *angel dust*) — gives rise to visual distortions and illusions, a sense of loss of control, and, sometimes, disorientation. This can lead to extreme fear, or what is commonly referred to as a "bad trip." Although this may initially be mistaken for schizophrenia, the symptoms are usually short-lived and soon recognized as a drug-induced phenomenon. However, in some individuals, what starts as a drug-induced bad trip gives way to continued hallucinations, delusions, and inappropriate mood and winds up continuing and being diagnosed as schizophrenia. Scientists still aren't sure about how or why this occurs.

Use of street drugs or alcohol in individuals known to have schizophrenia frequently leads to an exacerbation or worsening of the symptoms. Chapter 6 provides more information about co-occurring mental-health and substance-use disorders.

Personality disorders closely linked to schizophrenia

There is another totally separate category of disorders in *DSM-IV* known as *personality disorders.* Ten specific personality disorder diagnoses are outlined in the manual, but only three of them are closely related to the symptoms of schizophrenia:

- **Paranoid personality disorder:** The personality of someone with this disorder is characterized by a persistent pattern of distrust and suspiciousness with thoughts that other people's motivations are directed against him.
- **Schizoid personality disorder:** A person with this disorder is distant or detached from ordinary social relationships, and shows very little emotional expression or responsiveness compared to what you would expect in a given situation.
- **Schizotypal personality disorder:** A person with this disorder is uncomfortable with close relationships and has thinking and perceptual difficulties, along with what is seen as eccentric behavior.

One other *DSM-IV* personality disorder that may be considered during a workup for schizophrenia is borderline personality disorder (BPD), which is characterized by intense instability of relationships, mood, self-image, and self-esteem and is marked by impulsivity. The impulsivity is often characterized by extreme risk-taking behavior, self-mutilating behavior, recurrent suicidal behaviors, and wide swings in loving or hating individuals with whom the individual is involved. The hatred can be so intense at times that it can be considered paranoid.

Such intense and impulsive feelings and actions can cause clinicians to consider a diagnosis of schizophrenia, but the absence of persistent organized delusions and hallucinations and the absence of consistent depressed or manic mood differentiates this personality disorder from schizophrenia and bipolar disorder (see "Bipolar disorder," earlier in this chapter).

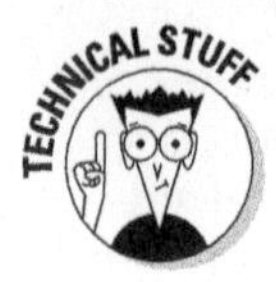

Some clinicians feel BPD fits more closely with the "schizophrenia and other psychotic disorders" and "mood disorders" categories rather than with "personality disorders."

Personality disorders often begin in early adulthood and remain stable and persistent over the years; they don't wax and wane. People with personality disorders behave in ways that don't fit society's norms, which can lead to their being very distressed and/or somewhat impaired; they don't, however, suffer the profound disability and loss of function seen in people with schizophrenia.

People recognize that the individual is somewhat eccentric, but they don't characterize the individual as out of control or out of contact with reality (having hallucinations and delusions).

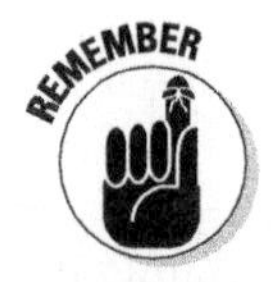

In general, the presence of clear-cut psychotic symptoms (delusions and hallucinations) is what distinguishes schizophrenia from these personality disorders.

Receiving the Diagnosis of Schizophrenia

Few diagnoses are as initially frightening as schizophrenia. Your fears are understandable; you may remember hearing about people years ago with schizophrenia who were placed in custodial care and never seen or talked about again, or you may recall sensational news stories of people with homicidal tendencies or multiple personalities. Many people today don't realize that these news reports are generally overblown and that schizophrenia is a treatable illness. Moreover, the disorder often goes into remission, and its symptoms can often be controlled by medication.

If your child is diagnosed with schizophrenia, you may blame yourself and wonder what you did wrong. Was it your genetics, your parenting, or both? Along with guilt, you may feel angry, ashamed, or terrified about the future. You wonder whether your son or daughter will ever be able to work, marry, or have children.

Some families compare being diagnosed with schizophrenia to being diagnosed with a potentially fatal illness, like cancer or heart failure — and in many if not most cases, the diagnosis is more difficult to deal with, because society is less accepting and sympathetic toward mental disorders than physical conditions. Many times, families have told us they were in shock in the doctor's office and came home and cried.

Doctors don't always deliver the diagnosis of schizophrenia well or easily. They may be slow to put a name to it, waiting to be more certain before delivering what they consider "bad news" — many disorders (such as bipolar disorder, personality disorders, substance abuse, depressions, or schizoaffective disorder) look alike when they're assessed within the confines of an appointment that often only lasts 50 minutes. Other times, patients don't fully reveal their symptoms to their doctor and appear to be far more organized and lucid than they normally are outside his office.

Families can be guilty of contributing to confusion of diagnosis. They may ignore, overlook, or minimize symptoms that are right before their eyes. This can result in long delays before diagnosis. Many patients and families are afraid of hospitalization, having to take medication for the rest of their lives, or being labeled with a stigmatizing illness, so they actively avoid seeking professional help.

Ignoring or minimizing these symptoms will not help them go away. All you're doing is prolonging the time before your loved one gets the help she needs.

Trust your instincts. Even if pediatricians, teachers, or internists tell you that your adolescent or young adult will grow out of the problem, if you feel something is very wrong, be sure to see a specialist to get a diagnosis. The earlier you identify and intervene in schizophrenia, the better the chances of reducing impairment and disability.

People react to an initial diagnosis of schizophrenia in a range of different ways. The following sections describe the difficulties people typically encounter in moving past denial to a state of acceptance.

Accepting the diagnosis

Because of the myths and misunderstandings associated with mental illnesses, in general, and schizophrenia in particular (see Chapter 1) — as well as the uncertain course that schizophrenia may take — an initial diagnosis is often met with fear, denial, disappointment, and guilt. This occurs almost universally even though the individual or his family may have been aware that "something was very wrong" for some time. Acceptance is a process that doesn't take place overnight.

Attaching a name to an illness is one of the first steps that enables people to move forward, to learn more about the disorder, to seek help, and to find support from other patients and families (see Chapter 17). A diagnosis gives them a shorthand way to talk about the disorder and communicate with mental health professionals who are in a position to help.

In the best of circumstances, acceptance allows a patient and his family to learn everything they possibly can about schizophrenia; find the very best experts to help them; and surround themselves with people who care, understand, and accept them.

Because of their extensive experience in dealing with large numbers of people, the clergy, particularly those members trained in pastoral counseling, can play an important role as natural supports to help families come to grips with the diagnosis. Clergy can also help you find understanding professionals in the community and provide support for the person with schizophrenia.

Denying the diagnosis

Although acceptance is the best way to move forward in any difficult situation, denial can be a formidable roadblock. Initial denial is a typical reaction to any life-changing event. When denial becomes a permanent coping mechanism for dealing with a chronic illness such as schizophrenia, however, crucial time can be lost before treatment begins.

Some patients and families are in such denial that they go doctor shopping to get a more palatable diagnosis. One family we know went to four different doctors and wound up with four different diagnoses; this gave them the ammunition they needed to rationalize that doctors don't know anything anyway. (In reality, each of the doctors observed similar symptoms and signs in the patient, but in different proportions, at different points in time — and each of them suggested similar classes of medications.)

We've also met families who were so upset by a diagnosis of schizophrenia that they begged the doctor to change it. In this situation, many doctors comply and change the diagnosis to one that is more socially acceptable (such as depression or bipolar disorder). This strategy can backfire, undermining treatment and the patient's own acceptance of and/or understanding of her illness.

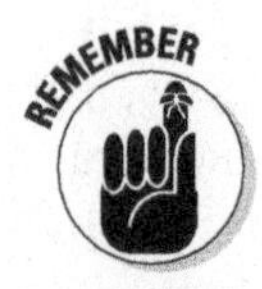

A diagnosis doesn't change who your loved one is. Just as a person who is diagnosed with cancer is not solely defined as a cancer patient, a person diagnosed with schizophrenia is more than her diagnosis. It's sometimes easy to forget this when you're in the throes of a crisis.

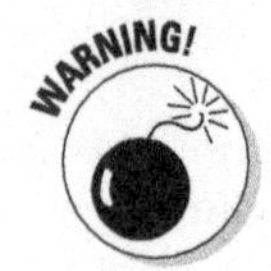

From time to time, schizophrenia is misdiagnosed. This is more likely when a doctor has limited understanding of and experience with serious mental disorders — for example, someone who tends to see the *worried well* (people who are high functioning but with relatively minor problems) or when a patient is seen during a *first break* (the first time a person is psychotic and out-of-contact with reality) and there's little history to rely upon.

Others times, lack of acceptance is manifest by patients' and families' refusal to accept *evidence-based treatments* (treatments that have a scientific basis). Instead, they search for unproven treatments, thinking that changes in diet or the addition of vitamin supplements can restore mental equilibrium, while symptoms persist. This can delay treatment and, in some cases, it may even increase losses and worsen the course of the disease.

Lack of insight on the part of the patient can also be a formidable barrier to treatment. For more information on denial, turn to Chapter 6.

Predicting the Course of the Illness

When an individual is first diagnosed with schizophrenia (sometimes referred to as the *first break*), it's natural to wonder if it will go away or last forever, and whether the symptoms will become more severe or dissipate over time. Unfortunately, for any particular individual, there are no definitive answers.

The most common course and outcome for people with schizophrenia is that it's variable, with *exacerbations* (worsening of symptoms) and *remissions* (periods of relative wellness with minimal symptoms). Some individuals only have a single psychotic break (sometimes called a *nervous breakdown*) and then never have another clear episode. Other people continue to have symptoms, which may either remain stable or deteriorate over time.

Although doctors can't accurately predict the extent to which your loved one will improve, stay the same, or get worse, they can make generalizations about the progression of the disorder.

Keep in mind, though, that these are generalizations, and may not apply in your situation. In addition, even individuals with the most severe variants of the illness can live productive lives with the help of medication and other supports.

Factors that predict a better course

Certain people are more likely to have only a single episode, or to remain stable for long periods of time. Some factors that tend to predict a better course and outcome include the following:

- Female gender
- Presence of a precipitating event (for example, a stressor, such as the death of a parent, which precipitated the break)
- Predominance of mood symptoms (for example, depression) over psychotic symptoms
- Insight into and understanding of the illness
- Good adherence to medication
- No prior family history of schizophrenia

Predictors of poorer outcomes

Although everyone hopes for improvement or at least stabilization, the symptoms of some individuals don't improve or may even worsen over time. The following factors can point toward a more severe course and outcome:

- Individuals with an earlier age of onset
- Poorer adjustment prior to diagnosis
- Lower educational achievement
- More negative and cognitive impairments

Seeking a Second Opinion

If you have any nagging concerns about diagnosis or treatment, don't hesitate to get a second opinion. Many people feel embarrassed about seeking another opinion because they're worried that they'll offend their current doctor. If you're of that mindset, change your way of thinking — because doctors are changing theirs. Most doctors aren't insulted when a patient with a complex problem wants to seek a second opinion. In fact, many doctors welcome another professional's perspective — two heads are better than one! — and choosing healthcare providers who encourage you to seek out additional information, including information from other doctors, is wise.

When to get a second opinion

Not every situation calls for a second opinion — when diagnoses and treatment choices are relatively straightforward, a second opinion usually isn't necessary. Second opinions add expense to your medical bills and can be time-consuming. However, they're clearly in order under certain circumstances:

- If the diagnosis or course of treatment is unclear or ambiguous
- If the patient wants to take advantage of experimental or additional treatment options that are only available elsewhere
- If a patient or her family has doubts or concerns about a doctor, or questions about the illness or its treatment that the doctor hasn't answered satisfactorily
- If a patient shows no signs of improvement
- If a patient or his family simply thinks it may be useful for someone else to take a look at the case with fresh eyes

Even if the second opinion doesn't shed new light on an old problem, it may help buy peace of mind.

How to find a second opinion

There are a number of options for finding a psychiatrist for a consultation:

- Ask your own psychiatrist or internist for a reference.
- Check with your local hospital or an academic medical center to find someone with the expertise you require.
- Check lists of "best doctors" in regional magazines.
- Seek the names of good physicians from family and friends, or from people who have had a similar illness.
- Check with your local NAMI affiliate to see if it maintains a list of practitioners (To find your local affiliate, go to `www.nami.org/Template.cfm?section=your_local_NAMI` — or go to `www.nami.org` and, under the "Find Support" section click on "State & Local NAMIs.") or contact one of the other organizations listed in the appendix.

Going for a second opinion

When you decide to go for a second opinion, be sure to tell your current doctor that you're doing so. Your current doctor probably will need to provide the second doctor with information. Here's how to do this:

- Respectfully explain your rationale for getting a second opinion, without directly challenging your current doctor.
- Explain that you'll be asking the other doctor to speak with him, to solicit his opinion, and see if they can come up with any alternative diagnoses or treatments, as the case may be.
- Leave the door open to returning because, in all likelihood, that's probably what you'll want to do.

Depending on the type of insurance you have, some insurers reimburse the cost of a second opinion, but it's always a good idea to check in advance with your insurance provider.

If you're uncertain about your relationship with your doctor, her reaction to your seeking a second opinion may actually help you decide whether to stay or leave. Client-centered, confident doctors don't resent second opinions, and may even suggest it to you.

Chapter 5

Assembling a Healthcare Team

In This Chapter

- Recognizing the importance of finding the right mental health professionals
- Choosing a psychiatrist
- Meeting the rest of the team
- Fixing a team that's not working effectively

If you've ever had to find a doctor in an emergency, you may have experienced the unsettling feeling of having to pick a name out of that proverbial hat, with no other options. Although this situation may be unavoidable under certain circumstances, for a chronic medical condition like schizophrenia, you need to — and will have the time to — carefully assemble a well-versed, experienced team of professionals who know you and your loved one well (and vice versa). Odds are, you're going to be spending a lot of time with these people over the years, so you need to be comfortable with each other.

In this chapter, we help you find the professional help your loved one needs. We tell you what kind of mental-health professionals are involved with treating schizophrenia, how to check out credentials, and how to ensure that your team will work well together. We also help you through the trying times when the team isn't working out — how to approach the problem and how to improve a stressful situation.

Putting Together a Healthcare Team

Just as a baseball team needs a skilled pitcher, catcher, batters, and various other team members in the right positions — as well as a skilled manager to pull them all together — you and your loved one need a variety of professionals to help you handle different aspects of your journey.

Finding the right group of mental-health professionals to help you and your loved one can be a lot of work, and can be a draining experience involving phone calls, research, and sometimes money spent to interview different people. So why should you make the effort to assemble a team of professionals? Being able to choose people you and your loved one like and understand — and who like and understand the two of you — is important because any type of mental-health treatment requires close collaboration between a patient, a therapist, and, to some extent, the family. Things go much more smoothly when you're working with a group of people you trust and respect.

Many people feel that even seeing a mental-health professional is an admission of weakness. The terms *shrink* (derived from head-shrinker) and *head doctor* are widely used disparaging terms applied to psychiatrists, psychologists, and social workers by the media and the public. Some people fear that these professionals can read and control their minds — which is far from the truth! (Honestly, most healthcare professionals would be delighted if Mind Reading 101 could actually be added to their medical-school classes.)

Mental-health professionals are ordinary people who are trained to understand the mind and behavior — and to use that knowledge to improve mental health or diagnose and treat mental disorders. Any healthcare professional who comes across as knowing all the answers — or as someone who's condescending — is a person to delete from your healthcare team roster permanently.

In the next sections, we describe the different types of mental-health professionals, starting with the person who'll be your team manager — your psychiatrist.

Your First Priority: Finding and Interviewing a Good Psychiatrist

Finding the right psychiatrist is essential to the management of schizophrenia. Not only is your psychiatrist the coordinator of all your team members; he's also the person who makes most of the medical decisions relating to treatments and medications. You want someone you feel comfortable with, whose judgment you trust, and whose reputation in the medical community is stellar. Where do you find such a paragon? Not to worry — many wonderful psychiatrists are practicing today. This section is all about finding the right one for your loved one and you.

Who's on first?

You probably already know the answer to this question — your psychiatrist is. She's your first line of defense against schizophrenia, and part of the reason is because she knows and prescribes the drugs used to control the most troubling symptoms of the disorder. Research shows that medication is the single most essential element of treatment for schizophrenia and that identifying the right medications for your loved one is vital to recovery. For this reason, your first priority should be finding the right psychiatrist.

Be sure to invest as much time as necessary to identify an expert who's knowledgeable about *psychopharmacology* (the medications used to treat mental disorders) and about your loved one's disorder (schizophrenia).

Psychiatrists are physicians whose training enables them to diagnose and treat mental disorders. After medical school, they complete an additional four years of residency in psychiatry and some take written and oral examinations to become board-certified. Some go on for additional specialty training in fields such as *geriatric psychiatry* (specializing in the care of older persons) or *child and adolescent psychiatry* (specializing in the care of younger ones).

The large majority of them have an MD (Doctor of Medicine) degree after their name, although some psychiatrists are trained as osteopathic physicians and have a DO after their name (for Doctor of Osteopathy). Psychiatrists who are Doctors of Osteopathy have also completed psychiatric residencies.

There are many excellent mental-health practitioners, but psychiatrists have the medical training to understand the complex relationships between the mind and body — and are best trained to rule out or make sure that there is no underlying medical basis for the psychological symptoms a person is experiencing. The amount of training a psychiatrist has in conducting various types of psychological therapies (for example, psychotherapy or cognitive behavioral therapy; see Chapter 9) varies based on where and how he was trained.

In most states, only a physician can involuntarily hospitalize an individual, although he need not be trained as a psychiatrist (see Chapter 6).

Looking for a specialist in serious mental illness

A psychiatrist is a psychiatrist is a psychiatrist? Not at all. Because only about 1 out of 20 individuals diagnosed with a mental disorder is likely to have what is considered a "serious mental illness" like schizophrenia, it makes sense that the majority of psychiatrists maintain practices that are geared toward patients with less severe mental-health problems. For example, many psychiatrists focus on treating people with less severe symptoms of depression and anxiety, or on counseling couples with marital problems.

You want to make sure that the doctor you select is experienced and comfortable working with individuals with schizophrenia. You also want to find out about the doctor's educational background and training, whether he's certified by the American Board of Psychiatry and Neurology (meaning, he has passed a national examination), and whether he sees a large number of people with serious mental disorders in his practice.

You wouldn't want to choose a surgeon for an operation that rarely does the procedure you need to undergo, and the same logic applies to choosing clinicians for treatment of a complex disorder like schizophrenia.

Starting your search

Whether you're looking for an auto mechanic or a baby sitter, the best way to find a reputable referral is usually through word of mouth. The same thing can be said about finding a psychiatrist or any other mental-health professional. Although there are places where you can find names and directories of individuals, vetting a clinician by checking him out with other families, trusted friends, or relatives who've used him and were satisfied is always prudent.

Compiling a short list

The vast majority of psychiatrists practice in larger cities; if you live in a small city or town, you may have to travel to a larger city or an academic medical center. Either way, you want to first compile a list of possibilities. Here are some suggestions for doing that:

- **If you're being referred for help by a physician or another mental-health professional (for example, a psychiatrist you met in an emergency room), ask the doctor to provide you with the names of several psychiatrists she would recommend.**
- **Speak to your primary-care doctor, internist, family doctor, pediatrician, or gynecologist, and see if one of them can recommend one or more psychiatrists for you to consider.**

- **Check with your local or state medical or psychiatric societies (which are usually listed in a phone book or on the Internet) and ask them for names of doctors who are convenient to your home.** For a complete list of district branches of the American Psychiatric Association (a professional specialty organization of psychiatrists), go to `http://online-apa.psych.org/listing/`.
- **If you have health insurance that covers mental-health and substance-abuse (sometimes called *behavioral health*) treatment, find out the names of doctors who participate with your private insurance plan or accept Medicaid or Medicare.**
- **Contact public mental health clinics or other outpatient programs in your community.** Many of them may function under the umbrella of the state mental-health authority or county/city mental-health department (also listed in the phone book or on the Internet).
- **Contact your state mental-health authority or state department of education to find out the names of licensed practitioners in your area.**

A number of sites on the Internet provide different types of information on doctors. For example, the American Medical Association (AMA) has a DoctorFinder service (`http://webapps.ama-assn.org/doctorfinder/home.html`), which allows you to search for a doctor by name and location or by specialty and zip code. Unfortunately, this site, like most others, has its limitations: It only includes doctors who are members of the AMA, and the information provided is too limited to use in selecting a psychiatrist. (For example, it may say that the doctor has an office-based practice, without providing information about the types of patients she sees or her knowledge of psychiatric medications).

An increasing number of Web sites — including HealthGrades (`www.healthgrades.com`) and Revolution Health (`www.revolutionhealth.com`), among others — also offer directories of psychiatrists and other physicians, some free and some at cost. But these sites only enable you to build a list of possibilities — they don't provide specific advice on how to narrow your list to make an informed choice. See the appendix for other suggestions on finding mental-health providers on the Web.

Google Maps (`http://maps.google.com`) can be useful for pinpointing the location of various mental-health professionals after you have their names (and may even help you with directions for getting to your first appointment).

Making a selection

After you've compiled a short list, your best bet is always to go with a psychiatrist who comes recommended as knowledgeable and trustworthy by someone you trust and who has your interests in mind. Check with trusted friends or relatives to see if they can suggest names and are willing to tell you about their own experiences.

Call the office of a local affiliate of the National Alliance on Mental Illness (NAMI), and ask to speak with consumers or family members who have experience with psychiatrists in your community and who can share their opinions with you. They can help you figure out who's good, better, and best where you live on the basis of their own experiences. (To find your local NAMI affiliate, go to `www.nami.org/Template.cfm?section=your_local_NAMI` — or go to `www.nami.org` and, under the "Find Support" section click on "State & Local NAMIs.")

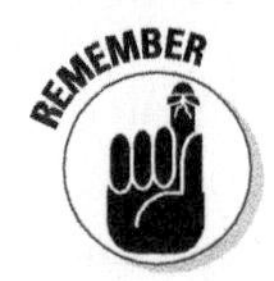

Having preferences concerning age, gender, religion, race, or language is perfectly acceptable, if that makes you or your loved one feel more comfortable. However, because experienced psychiatrists are in short supply, you may have to set priorities about what characteristics are most important to you and your loved one.

A picture is worth a thousand words: If you can't find an online bio for the person, sometimes you can be your own investigator and use Google Images (`http://images.google.com`) to find the person's picture. Just looking at the doctor's photo may give you a sense of gender, age, or other considerations that are important to you but that you might be reluctant to ask about.

If you or your loved one has special needs, you'll want to find someone with the appropriate specialty. For example, if you're seeking care for an elderly parent, you may want to look for a geriatric psychiatrist. If your teenage son is abusing drugs and has signs of a mental disorder, you may want to look for a psychiatrist who has a specialty in addiction psychiatry or experience treating people who have both mental health disorders and substance abuse problems.

Preparing for the first meeting: Questions to ask

We always tell families that, whenever possible, they should either speak to a psychiatrist before their loved one does or meet with the psychiatrist in person to make sure that he's the type of person your loved one is likely to feel comfortable with. This advice is particularly relevant with children and adolescents — you don't want to expose your child to someone you don't respect and trust.

After you talk to or meet with the psychiatrist, your loved one may want to have a no-obligation, first-time meeting with the psychiatrist to make sure that she feels comfortable with the individual's style and approach.

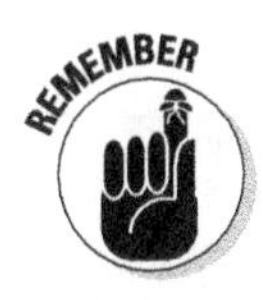

We can't overstate the importance of doing everything you can to enhance the odds of making the first visit work. Many families tell us about loved ones who had bad initial experiences that turned them off from getting help for a long time afterward. Finding someone who is respectful to your loved one as well as to family and friends is essential.

If a person's first experience with a psychiatrist is negative, it can turn him off from treatment, a situation that can be very hard to undo. You want to avoid this scenario, if at all possible.

The following is a list of questions that your loved one (depending on her condition) or you can ask to find out more about the doctor:

- **What are your hours for seeing patients?** If you're working, it may be difficult for you to take your loved one to see a psychiatrist who only sees patients during the day. Try to find someone whose hours work with your schedule.
- **What are your fees and what kind of insurance do you accept?** If she doesn't accept insurance, ask whether she has a sliding fee based on income.
- **Where is your office located?** Some doctors practice in multiple locations and one may be more convenient than another. (The importance of having a place to park if you drive or being close to a bus route if you don't shouldn't be overlooked.)
- **What's your philosophy and approach toward treatment?** Is he a biological, psychosocial, psychoanalytic (see Chapter 2), or *biopsychosocial* (someone who combines biological, psychosocial, and social concerns) psychiatrist?

  Ideally, it would be nice to find someone who can both prescribe medication and provide supportive therapy. Often, a doctor will only do medication management, and you will need to see another individual for therapy. This is perfectly acceptable if the care is coordinated.

  Psychoanalysis is generally not the treatment of choice for people with serious mental disorders like schizophrenia or bipolar disorder. If someone recommends psychoanalysis for the treatment of schizophrenia, leave the office as quickly (but politely) as you can.
- **What types of patients are you most comfortable working with?** Some psychiatrists specialize in certain disorders (for example, schizophrenia, mood disorders, anxiety, marital problems, and so on) or in working

with special groups (such as older people, children, or adolescents). Ideally, you want your loved one to have a psychiatrist who specializes in people like him! The fit doesn't need to be perfect, but if someone rarely sees people with schizophrenia, the psychiatrist probably has less experience in using antipyschotic medications.

- **How long will it be before I can schedule an appointment with you?** Many good psychiatrists balance clinical responsibilities with teaching or other commitments so they have tight schedules. But most doctors have the flexibility in their schedules to see people within a day or two if it's an emergency. (This may be more difficult in the case of a new patient.) If the wait is too long for you, you might ask the doctor to recommend another psychiatrist who can see you sooner.
- **What arrangements do you have in place to handle overnight or weekend emergencies?** There should always be someone on call in the event of an after-hours emergency (either a covering doctor or an answering service that can reach the doctor).

Unless you're in an emergency situation, invest your time upfront to avoid disappointments. Of course, if your loved one needs to see someone right away, you'll need to streamline the process for the time being.

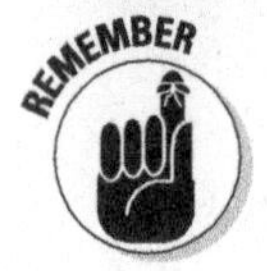

You can always change doctors when you have more time to do so. Your need may be so urgent that an emergency-room doctor is your only recourse in the short run, but after the crisis is over, you can evaluate whether you want to make that relationship permanent or look elsewhere.

Meeting a psychiatrist: What to expect

At this first meeting, the psychiatrist is likely to speak to your loved one alone at first and then probably will ask to speak to both of you together (either at this meeting or a subsequent one). The doctor will be trying to learn about her (see Chapter 2) and may ask you to provide additional information. It may take one, two, or perhaps a few meetings for the doctor to have enough information to decide on a working diagnosis and on an approach to treatment. With your loved one's permission, the psychiatrist may want to gather records from other physicians or mental-health professionals.

When this evaluation is completed, the doctor will share his ideas about diagnosis and treatment. The doctor will play an ongoing role in monitoring your loved one's medication and in determining if she ever needs hospitalization or an alternative to hospitalization. If your loved one is very psychotic (out-of-contact with reality), you may need to be more involved in treatment decisions.

Some of the questions your loved one needs to ask if they still remain unanswered include:

- How often do you expect to be seeing me?
- How long will each session last?
- Will you be prescribing medication for me and supervising it? Will you be providing supportive therapy as well?
- What are the potential benefits, risks, and side effects of any therapies you're prescribing for me?
- What other mental-health professionals do you think need to be on my team? How will you communicate with each other?
- Will my confidentiality be protected? (See Chapter 6 for more information.)
- Do you need me to sign releases for any other additional information that would assist you in my treatment?
- What role do you expect my family to play in my treatment? How can they communicate with you?
- How would you handle my care if I had a psychotic break? Are you affiliated with a particular hospital?

If things seem to be going well up to this point, your loved one should be able to make a commitment to treatment.

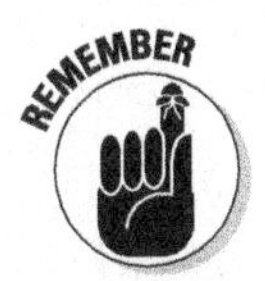

It takes time to get to know someone, and many people are uncomfortable during the first few months of treatment. But if your loved one continues to feel extremely uncomfortable with the psychiatrist, it may be appropriate to try someone else on your list to see what another clinician would be like. If you live in a small town, your options may be limited unless you're willing to travel, which may not be practical.

If no one seems to please you or your loved one, you both need to seriously consider the possibility that you're actively avoiding getting help.

Identifying Other Members of the Team

You can use the same method to find other professionals you'll need on your team as you used to find a psychiatrist (see the preceding sections). The bad news: The process is just as tedious, except that your psychiatrist may be another person who can now help you with referrals.

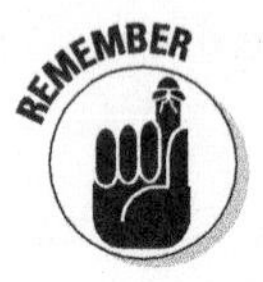

If you or your relative participates in a program like an outpatient psychosocial rehabilitation program or a clubhouse (see Chapter 9 for more about these programs), the composition of your team (both in terms of individuals and their specialties) may be dictated by the staffing of the program.

An array of other mental-health professionals can play different roles in your care. We introduce you to them in the following sections.

Psychologists

Although psychiatrists and psychologists (with doctoral degrees) are both called "doctors," psychologists have graduate training in psychology that leads either to a PhD (Doctor of Philosophy) or PsyD (Doctor of Psychology). Some psychologists only have master's-level training.

After graduate school, depending on the state where you live, most psychologists complete a one- or two-year internship before they can get a license from the state. An essential distinction between psychiatrists and psychologists is that, in most states (except Louisiana and New Mexico), only psychiatrists are able to prescribe medications. Often psychologists practice collaboratively with psychiatrists, who supervise medications, while the psychologist provides psychotherapy.

The title *psychologist* can only be used by an individual who has completed this education, training, and state licensure. Informal titles such as *counselor* or *therapist* or *psychotherapist* are often used as well, but other mental-health professionals with far less training also use these same titles.

Psychologists often provide psychotherapy to individuals or groups. Many have particular specialties (for example, working with special populations like children, adolescents, or victims of abuse) or using particular methods (such as psychodynamic, cognitive behavioral, or supportive therapy; see Chapter 9).

Most states have no special educational or training requirements to call yourself a *therapist* or *psychotherapist.* Anyone with a PhD (doctoral degree) in English literature or political science can call himself a "doctor." Some people hang out a shingle or advertise in the local newspaper without any specialized training. It's essential to ask and check into a professional's background if you aren't sure of her training or licensure.

Social workers

Social workers, also called *clinical social workers,* either have MSW (Master of Social Work) or DSW (Doctor of Social Work) degrees. After their training, many sit for a licensing test and become accredited by their respective states as LCSWs or ACSWs.

Like other mental-health professionals, social workers can work in private practice or as part of a mental-health facility, such as a hospital, clinic, or rehabilitation program. They can't prescribe medications, but if they have experience working with people with mental illness, they often help oversee the use of medications, working closely with a psychiatrist.

Many clinical social workers are trained to serve as advocates for patients and their families. They can assist with referrals, help you obtain benefits and entitlements, and help you navigate the mental-health system. They also can provide support and help educate families and consumers. In fact, many *case managers* (see "Coordinating Treatment and Care," later in this chapter) are trained as or are supervised by social workers.

The National Association of Social Workers (NASW) has an online directory of social workers at `www.helpstartshere.org`.

Psychiatric nurses

Generally, a psychiatric nurse is an RN with a bachelor's, master's, or doctoral degree who has specialized experience and training in working with people with mental-health problems. Psychiatric nurses also may work with individuals or groups in private practice, clinic, or hospital settings.

Because of their nursing background, psychiatric nurses are often attentive to many of the health problems experienced by people with serious mental disorders (see Chapter 15) and are alert to the side effects of psychiatric medications. Some *nurse practitioners* (RNs who are licensed to practice medicine in collaboration with a physician), depending on the state where they practice, are allowed to prescribe medications.

Some additional members of the team

A number of other professionals, including occupational therapists, vocational therapists, recreation therapists, rehabilitation specialists, and peer counselors are called upon to work with people with schizophrenia who have broad needs that transcend treatment alone — which is usually the case. Some of these professionals may be part of your loved one's treatment for only a short time; others may work with them longer.

Licensed professional counselors

Counselors can either have a master's degree in counseling, pastoral counseling, or psychology — or a PhD in counseling psychology. They can provide diagnosis and counseling to individuals or groups and work under a professional license obtained from their respective state. They may also be certified by the National Academy of Certified Clinical Mental Health Counselors. You need to ask.

Although most counselors tend to focus on people with less serious problems, many are experienced in working with people with serious mental disorders like schizophrenia.

Marriage and family therapists

Marriage and family therapists (MFTs) bring a family-oriented perspective to care. They're graduates of master's or doctoral programs or study MFT after earning another mental-health-related graduate degree. Currently 46 states license or certify MFTs.

MFTs work with couples and families and can be helpful in providing consultation, education, and support to families.

Occupational therapists

Depending on the age of onset of their illness, some people with schizophrenia never learned to manage the activities of daily living or, after a long period of illness, lost the skills they once had. The goal of occupational therapy, performed by individuals with OT degrees, is to help restore the skills a person needs to socialize and function appropriately at home, at school, or in work settings.

Vocational therapists

So many people define themselves by what they do. Nothing feels worse than seeing yourself — or being seen — only as a patient; no one wants his primary identification to be that of a person with mental illness or with schizophrenia. Vocational rehabilitation (VR) is a set of services offered by vocational therapists to people with disabilities — mental or physical — to help them secure and maintain meaningful employment.

VR is a state program that is often free to people who meet the established criteria of need. Generally, clients have a long-term disability that is a barrier to employment and that can be overcome with the help of a vocational therapy or rehabilitation. (See Chapter 7 for more on VR.)

Vocational therapists also work privately, paid for by insurers. If you're able to choose a vocational therapist, you want to look for someone who's oriented toward the needs of the individual, who builds upon natural supports like peers and family, and who's oriented toward real work as opposed to *make-work* (repetitive tasks that are boring and offer little opportunity to enhance self-worth).

One specialized type of vocational therapist is a *job coach,* an individual who works side by side with a disabled person to help that person acclimate to the workplace and the tasks that a particular job entails. *Job developers* work with programs to identify real work opportunities in the community for people with schizophrenia.

Recreation therapists

Recreation therapists are trained, certified, and registered and/or licensed to develop recreation resources and opportunities (also referred to as *therapeutic recreation*) for people with illnesses or disabilities. The goal is to restore, remediate, and rehabilitate the patient's functioning. As part of the team, a recreation therapist designs individualized interventions that will contribute to the health and overall well-being of the person with schizophrenia, and that will help her cope with such common symptoms as boredom, depression, and anxiety.

The recreation therapist prescribes activities to meet people's specific social, emotional, cognitive, and/or physical needs. These activities run the gamut and include fitness programs, photography, woodworking, horticulture, stress-management training, computer training, pottery-making, arts and crafts, games, relaxation training, working with animals, and more.

Rehabilitation therapists

Rehabilitation therapists include a broad range of mental-health professionals who work to assist people with vocational skills, job training, social skills training, and money management.

Some rehabilitation therapists (as well as psychologists) specialize in *cognitive remediation,* a teaching technique that tries to restore an individual's ability to learn and function based on neuropsychological evaluation and intervention. (See Chapter 9 for more on cognitive remediation.)

Peer counselors

People who have experience living with various serious mental illnesses and who are in recovery can help by sharing their experience and serving as role models. Many municipalities and voluntary organizations have developed peer-counseling programs to provide support and inspiration, and many states train and/or certify peer counselors. These counselors generally work as members of a professional team and are respected for the unique perspective they bring to treatment and rehabilitation.

Sometimes mental-health peer counselors work in a group setting with multiple individuals. This is one type of *self-help group* (see Chapter 9).

Coordinating Treatment and Care

Most people with schizophrenia require a range of health, mental-health, and supportive services (including appropriate housing, decent medical care, access to entitlement benefits, and so on). These services need to be in place for an individual to live in the community with independence and dignity. Unfortunately, the service system is so complex and fragmented — and the symptoms of schizophrenia create so many barriers — that people with schizophrenia may not always have the ability or insight to recognize, access, and use the services they need.

Having one person to coordinate all needed care and services is an ideal solution to a disease that can seem to sprout new complications and dragon heads at every turn. *Case management* assigns responsibility to either an individual or team to coordinate all these services on behalf of one individual so that services are accessible and accountable.

The terms *case management* and *clinical case management* are generic ones, referring to a variety of different models. Some case managers work individually; others work as part of interdisciplinary teams. Some case managers link clients to services; others provide services directly (usually as a team). A case manager may or may not serve as the patient's primary clinician.

One of the most popular and well-known models of case management is the Assertive Community Treatment (ACT) program. The first ACT program, called PACT (Program for Assertive Community Treatment) started in Madison, Wisconsin, in the late 1960s. At the time, it was referred to as a "hospital without walls."

The defining characteristics of ACT programs include:

- Use of multidisciplinary teams (which draw upon several areas of medicine and practice) rather than individual case managers
- 24/7 availability, 365 days a year, with a high frequency of contact

- Low client-to-staff ratios (10:1 rather than 30:1 or more)
- Assertive outreach to meet clients wherever they are in the community rather than in a clinic setting
- Providing direct services (including emotional support and crisis intervention, as necessary) rather than brokering services only
- Using peer counselors and family members as outreach workers
- Promoting self-management skills, so the client can assume responsibility for her illness
- A practical orientation that includes providing assistance with activities of daily living (ADLs) and linking to social-service benefits and entitlements

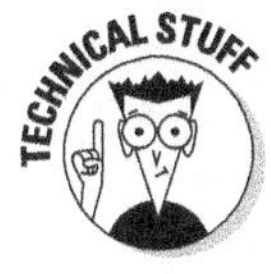

Some consumers find the use of the term *case management* derogatory. Rightly so, they preferred to be viewed as individuals rather than "cases."

The results of empirical studies over more than three decades have shown that ACT programs reduce hospitalization, homelessness, and inappropriate housing; increase housing stability; control psychiatric symptoms; and improve quality of life. Most of the studies took place in urban areas and focused on the most severely ill subset of people with schizophrenia.

In fact, the ACT program model has been proven to work so well that it's been implemented in most states, but not in the numbers necessary to serve all the people who could benefit from these intensive services. State and local programs often establish narrow eligibility criteria to meet the needs of those who are most disabled rather than all those who may benefit from such services.

Those who qualify for ACT programs generally include people who:

- Have a history of multiple hospitalizations
- Have been dually diagnosed with co-occurring mental health and substance use/abuse problems
- Have mental illness and are involved with the criminal justice system
- Have severe mental illness and are homeless

Because of high demand and limited availability, most case management programs do not advertise or look for new clients. You need to contact your public mental-health authority at the state or local level to find out how you or your loved one can obtain these services. Be persistent — and if that doesn't pan out, contact patient, family, or citizen advocacy organizations in your community to learn about these programs (see the appendix).

When families are case managers

One of the unfortunate legacies of deinstitutionalization (see Chapter 15) is that, by not providing funding for high-quality, coordinated resources for community care at federal, state, or local levels, families of people with serious mental illness have become de facto case managers of last resort, trying to patch together different resources for their family members.

Families assume the de facto roles of housing and case management providers, performing a host of critical functions in support of their loved ones, including:

- Monitoring therapeutic and adverse effects of medications
- Providing companionship to fill empty hours
- Offering housing, money, or other crisis assistance to avoid disruption and dislocation
- Securing psychiatric hospitalization (when necessary)
- Serving as individual advocates for their family members (by helping them access high-quality mental healthcare)
- Serving as systems advocates, trying to improve the overall mental-health system to assure availability, access, adequacy, and coordination of health, mental-health, and social-welfare services

These overwhelming responsibilities leave caregivers little time for work, outside interests, or their own social relationships, and it can exacerbate their feelings of loss. This is an emotionally exhausting and difficult role for any parent, sibling, spouse, or friend to assume. Aside from their having to help the patient with day-to-day tasks, they have to learn about the range of resources available in the community. When family members are placed in this role, it often adds another layer of complications to the already strained dynamics between them and their loved ones.

Bottom line: You and your loved one will be fortunate if you can find a case manager who can assist you.

Although case-management programs are costly, multiple studies have shown that they reduce the utilization of more expensive services such as hospitalization, emergency-room use, and incarceration in jails. Equally important, the programs improve quality of life for both the person with schizophrenia and his family.

Redrafting the Team: When Things Aren't Working

If your team is floundering, you or your loved one are likely to be floundering, too. Schizophrenia is a complex disease that requires *integrated* (coordinated) treatment and that takes the input and cooperation of many people.

About one-third of cases of schizophrenia are more complex and difficult to treat than most. If your loved one has *treatment-resistant schizophrenia* (schizophrenia whose positive symptoms don't respond to currently available medications), it may seem like your team isn't working well, when in reality the seriousness of the disease and the limitations of treatment are the problems, not the team members and certainly not the individual.

On the other hand, things may be going badly because you have the wrong team members, or because they're not working together. You're the one most likely to recognize problems, and you'll probably also be the one who has to figure out how to fix them.

Treatment resistant is a term used to describe symptoms that do not respond to conventional treatments. Sometimes people confuse the term *treatment resistant* and incorrectly use it to describe patients who are not adherent to treatment.

Spotting the signs of team dysfunction

How do you know when the problem is with the team rather than with the person with schizophrenia? Some of the signs that the team may be adrift include the following:

- **Failure to listen:** It's vital that all members of the team (including psychiatrists) be active listeners, so they understand their patients' needs and preferences and respect them as individuals. Cookie-cutter approaches to treatment generally don't work and make patients and family members feel dehumanized.
- **Failure to communicate openly with the patient and/or the family:** The concept of *shared decision-making,* a tool now gaining popularity in general medicine, encourages patients and doctors to become active partners in sharing information, clarifying medical options, and choosing or redirecting a course of care. The need for this approach is particularly important in the care of patients with schizophrenia because of the long-term nature of the disorder, the complexities of treatment, the need to prevent *learned helplessness* (the tendency among patients to become passive), the need to encourage compliance, and the role of family and friends in supporting the individual. Both patients and families have the right to expect periodic meetings with the team to discuss and assess progress.
- **Poor communication between team members:** Members of the team need to be talking to each other periodically (or at least communicating by e-mail). For example, if you realize that the psychologist who meets with your loved one every week has neglected to report troublesome side effects to the psychiatrist (who is overseeing medication) or that your loved one seems to be on a progressively downward spiral and that the psychiatrist has no clue, you know there's a communication problem.

- **A team with too many pitch hitters or staff on the bench:** Some turnover of staff is to be expected, but if a program is constantly losing staff members, it's a sign that something's amiss. This is particularly important for patients with schizophrenia who find it difficult to forge new relationships and adapt to change. If the primary clinician changes every few months, your family member may receive disjointed or fragmented care. If a program seems unstable in terms of its ability to recruit and retain staff, you may want to look for other options.
- **Gaps in treatment or care:** For example, if a program provides no opportunities for the patient to participate in rehabilitative or vocational opportunities, or other vital support services are missing, you need to assess why that's happening and how that gap can be addressed.
- **Missing the mark on the appropriate level of expectation:** The bar for expectations shouldn't be set too high or too low. Ideally, you want the team to set realistic and achievable goals. The team has to have experience and wisdom to discern whether a patient who appears to be lazy is really experiencing negative symptoms associated with the illness (see Chapter 3), has low-self-esteem, is depressed, or is simply giving up and needs to be encouraged to do more.

Working to improve your team

After you've identified a problem, you need to find ways to fix it. If you feel that something's amiss, here are some tips on how to change the team in a positive way:

- **Find the right person to talk to.** If the problem is with a private practitioner, call or e-mail him and explain your concerns. You're paying the doctor or other professional directly, so you have some degree of leverage. If the problem is with a program, start at the bottom before you move up the ladder — for example, if the problem is with a mental health counselor, start with that person before going to her boss.

  Whenever you or your loved one enrolls in a new program, ask who you should speak to in the event of a problem. Many facilities, including hospitals, have patient advocates, patient-rights coordinators, or ombudsmen.
- **Choose the best way to communicate.** It may be in person, over the phone, by letter, or by e-mail, depending on your preferences, the preferences of the other person, and the options available to you. If you're meeting in person, always address the person by name, arrive on time, keep it simple, speak firmly but audibly, and don't shout.

- **Put your best foot forward.** Even if you' re angry or hurt on the inside, remember that the problem may be a simple misunderstanding. Stay calm, never threaten, but remain firm and persistent. Use praise, humor, and diplomacy where appropriate, and don't forget to listen to what the other side is saying. You want to be part of the solution, not part of the problem.

  Many families tell us that simply by saying that they're members of NAMI opens the door so that professionals are willing to listen and meet with them. Instead of name-dropping, drop NAMI into the conversation!

- **Put it in writing.** Keep records of your communications. Include the date, the person you spoke with, and what you both said. If your request was accommodated, follow up with a thank-you note. If it wasn't, after an appropriate wait, follow up with a reminder.

- **Resort to desperate measures.** If you don't feel like you're being heard or if you feel the needs of your loved one are being ignored, file a report with the appropriate oversight agency. You may be able to figure out who and where by calling your city, county, or state mental-health authority. In most states, the state regulates and licenses all mental-health programs.

  Contact the state agency overseeing protection and advocacy programs (see Chapter 7) and communicate with your elected officials to see if they can help you. In extreme cases (for example, if there are conditions threatening the health and safety of vulnerable people), the best approach may be to contact the media.

  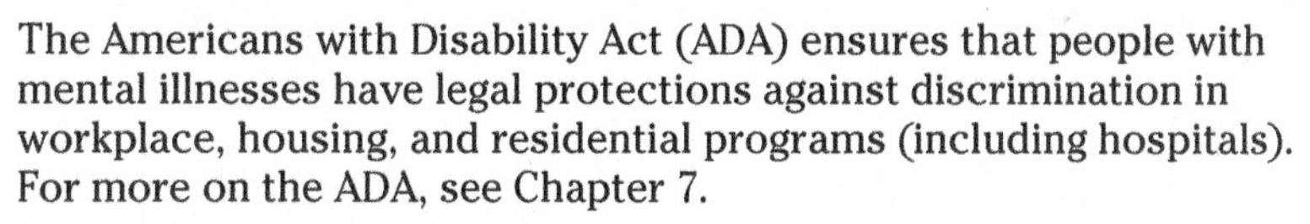

  The Americans with Disability Act (ADA) ensures that people with mental illnesses have legal protections against discrimination in workplace, housing, and residential programs (including hospitals). For more on the ADA, see Chapter 7.

- **Don't sweat the small stuff.** Keep in mind that most people who work in human services are motivated by the desire to help people rather than make money, and that many of them work in difficult settings with only limited resources. Try to always give mental-health workers the benefit of the doubt and keep things in perspective.

- **Remember to reward successful efforts.** It's always motivating and heart-warming when a mental-health professional receives a note from a consumer or family member telling of their successes. Don't forget to tell your team when good things happen; it helps everyone retain their enthusiasm for working through the rough spots.

- **Never give up.** As an important corollary to the preceding bullet, remember that, as with Dorothea Dix who reformed mental hospitals in the mid-1800s, it only takes one committed person to initiate change. If you're having problems with a clinician or program, you probably aren't the only one, and your efforts may help many people in similar circumstances.

Chapter 6
Beginning Treatment

In This Chapter

- Getting your loved one started with treatment
- Encouraging your loved one to become an active participant
- Trying different treatments
- Coping with side-effects
- Knowing what to do if your loved one denies being sick
- Looking at schizophrenia in children, older people, college students, substance abusers, and women

Although getting a diagnosis and being able to attach a name to your loved one's set of perplexing symptoms and behaviors can be a relief, it can also lead to a number of new concerns, challenges, and conflicting feelings as your loved one begins treatment. Sadly, although treatment is the first step toward recovery, as many as two-thirds of those individuals with schizophrenia never receive any treatment at all.

In this chapter, we examine the issues that arise as a person begins treatment for schizophrenia, including the importance of actively participating in care, the frustrations of finding the right psychotropic medications, and the special problems of schizophrenia at different ages and stages.

Starting a Long and Complicated Process

Treating schizophrenia isn't as simple as treating a cut, bruise, or minor infection. But a diagnosis of schizophrenia is definitely *not* a cause for hopelessness, as was once commonly assumed. A range of treatments and supports are available to control, or at least lessen, positive symptoms and to minimize potential losses created by negative or cognitive symptoms (see Chapter 3 for more on symptoms). Starting treatment is difficult in many ways, but it's a time for renewed hope for a more normal life.

Treatment for schizophrenia tends to be long term, with many decision points along the way. If your loved one has been diagnosed with schizophrenia, think of your own self-education as an ongoing process. Decisions will begin to flow more easily over time, when you have more experience and information under your belt.

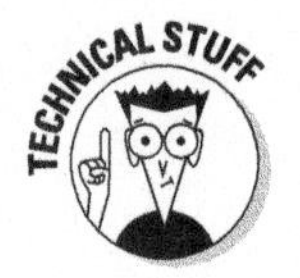

The *beginning of treatment* generally occurs after a person has a first *psychotic episode* (a loss of contact with reality, often signaled by hallucinations or delusions). But it also can refer to the time when a person reinitiates treatment after previously stopping.

Putting the what if's and why's behind you

The relief of having a diagnosis doesn't negate all the questions and concerns you have about schizophrenia. You may still be frustrated because you don't know what caused things to go awry. If so, recognize that there's nothing to be gained by searching for explanations, which are only speculative anyway. Even brain researchers aren't quite sure about the causes of schizophrenia. (See Chapter 2 for more about the causes of schizophrenia.)

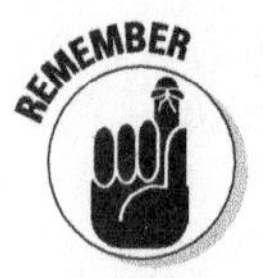

There's no room for placing blame after receiving a diagnosis of schizophrenia. No person is responsible for causing this brain disorder — not patients, family members, or anyone else. Looking for elusive causes is useless as well as distracting, because it places your focus on the past rather than the future.

It's human nature to want answers, but in the case of mental illness, the causes are far more likely to lie in the brain than in the outside influences and events of a person's life. After you have a diagnosis, put the "what if's" and "why's" behind you and help your loved one move into treatment with the positive belief that things can only get better from this point forward.

Developing a positive approach

Accepting the challenges you face and thinking positively about the future is essential — for both you and your loved one. In fact, you really have no alternative! No one likes to think of himself as being sick or being in the role of a patient, especially if the disease is long term — and this feeling is exacerbated in the case of mental illnesses, because of the strong stigma associated with them. But part of acceptance is recognizing that schizophrenia isn't going to go away on its own and that losses can be minimized or even avoided by taking advantage of the resources available to you in your own community.

The symptoms of schizophrenia, like those of many other chronic illnesses, are likely to get better and worsen over time, and they aren't likely to respond to treatment in a week or two. But with appropriate treatment, schizophrenia doesn't necessarily have a deteriorating course. In fact, the large majority of people with schizophrenia can go on to lead meaningful and satisfying lives.

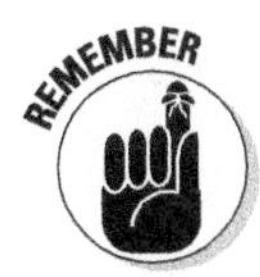

Many myths and misperceptions discourage people from seeking mental-healthcare (see Chapter 16). Many people fear that seeing a mental-health professional is an admission of weakness. Others fear that these professionals can read and control their minds. Both of these myths are untrue.

You or your loved one may be uncertain or concerned about the risks and benefits of using powerful psychiatric medications — this uncertainty is understandable. But one of the most important tasks in the first weeks and months after diagnosis will be understanding the specific risk-to-benefit ratio of using powerful psychiatric treatments in your loved one's particular circumstances so she can take the steps needed to minimize losses and maximize opportunities. This is something your loved one should discuss with her psychiatrist, others on her healthcare team, and you (see Chapter 5 for more on how to assemble a top-notch healthcare team).

Any treatment for any illness isn't without side effects, but weighing the pros and cons, you'll find that treatments for schizophrenia are generally worth the risks and may even be life-sustaining.

Getting comfortable in an uncomfortable setting

Starting anything new — even something positive — always feels uncomfortable at first. When your loved one meets a new psychiatrist or starts a new program, awkwardness, discomfort, and some anxiety are to be expected. You may have experienced the same feelings when you visited a new family doctor or dentist for the first time. After all, you're potentially exposing yourself, whether it's your warts, your cavities, or something else that embarrasses you about yourself. But unless your loved one is candid with a clinician about what he's feeling, he'll be cheating himself and wasting time and money.

Some of the questions that may go through your loved one's mind include the following:

- **Can I trust this person with my feelings?** Two people don't always hit it off or connect from the get-go. Your loved one may find out that this person isn't the type of individual who allows him to feel comfortable and forthcoming about his personal demons. But make sure your loved one gives the person a chance, recognizing that it'll be hard at first and that most people feel uncomfortable when they start treatment. If the feelings don't dissipate over time, your loved one may want to change treatment providers. However, if your loved one doesn't feel comfortable with *anyone,* it may be due to the disorder itself.
- **Will the information I share be kept confidential?** Professionals are often overzealous about protecting someone's confidentiality, but because confidentiality is important, your loved one should ask the clinician about whether she'll be sharing the information with anyone else without explicit permission. Knowing the answer should help allay many concerns. This also applies to various programs your loved one might be attending. Generally, in most programs and ACT teams (see Chapter 5), the team will often share information with each other because they're working collaboratively on your loved one's behalf, but they won't divulge the information to other people or programs without your loved one's permission.

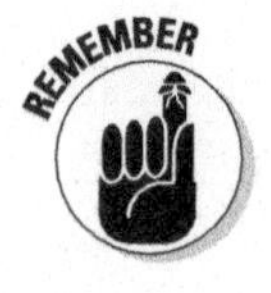

If you or your loved one has concerns about confidentiality or any other questions about your loved one's care, raise those concerns directly with the doctor and discuss it with each other. For example, it's appropriate to question whether information will be shared with educational institutions, employers, or insurers. On the other hand, keeping families completely in the dark about a loved one's diagnosis is generally counterproductive and should be avoided, when possible. (See Chapter 14 for more information on the Health Insurance Portability and Accountability Act and confidentiality.)

- **Will I meet someone in the waiting room whom I know?** Maybe. And if that happens, the person is there for the same reason as your loved one is, so she just needs to do her best to get over that fear.
- **Will I play any role in my own treatment?** Yes, an active one! The days of lying down on a couch and talking to an omnipotent analyst who only nods or says, "Hmm, I understand how you're feeling" are just about over when it comes to state-of-the-art treatment for schizophrenia. Your loved one's doctor or other clinician should involve him in all decisions about his treatment.

For example, the doctor will explain the risks, benefits, and potential side effects of any medication that's prescribed, and your loved one will be able to make choices about the medication that seems most appropriate to him from the ones approved for treatment. In subsequent visits, the doctor should be open and responsive to feedback from your loved one about how the medication is making him feel. The doctor should also be explicit about the consequences of not taking or stopping medication. When medications aren't working, the doctor should suggest and discuss other treatment options with your loved one.

Shared decision-making is a term used today to describe the increasingly popular process of involving patients in making healthcare decisions with their clinicians, based on the best available evidence.

- **Does seeing a psychiatrist when I'm symptomatic automatically mean I'll be hospitalized?** There's a rather high bar for hospitalization these days — in fact, many people think it's too high, with people being refused hospitalization when they need it. Only a very small proportion of people seen by clinicians require involuntary hospitalization, and most hospitalizations, whether voluntary or involuntary, are for relative short periods of time (days or weeks rather than months).

  Even people who hear voices or see things that aren't there are rarely hospitalized, and if they are, it isn't for long. If your loved one's behavior and symptoms don't represent a danger to herself or others, then she's likely to be treated on an outpatient basis. If there's a threat to her own self or danger to others, she probably would want to be treated in a secure setting for her own protection.

- **Will I need to take medications for the rest of my life?** Depending on your loved one's diagnosis and the course of her illness, this is a distinct possibility, but the answer remains to be seen. Taking certain medications or taking medications at all is something that can be re-evaluated periodically, and you and your loved one can have a vital say in that decision.

Drawing On Local Resources

Until schizophrenia hits home, families generally aren't aware of the community resources available to help them. When your loved one has an acute psychotic break out of the blue, you may not even know a psychiatrist, especially a psychiatrist who specializes in treating serious mental disorders like schizophrenia. Even if you do, the person may not be immediately available — the emergency may occur at night or on a weekend, and you'll have no alternative but to use the local hospital emergency room or call the police.

Many families find it helpful to check out the facilities in their neighborhood before a crisis occurs, so they can make an informed choice about where to go in different types of situations.

Scouting out local hospitals

Obviously, the best time to prepare for a crisis is when things are stable. If your relative has been showing signs of a serious mental disorder, you need to you do your legwork to identify the best place to go for acute emergency care, in case your loved one needs it. (Chapter 14 gives you tips on how to cope with psychiatric crisis.)

If your community has a crisis response team, you can call and find out what services are available to you. Be sure to ask if they offer alternatives to hospitalization.

If you ever have trouble getting through and it's a psychiatric emergency, clearly tell the person who answers, "This is a psychiatric emergency." If it isn't an emergency and you're having trouble reaching a human, ask for the director, CEO, or commissioner (in other words, the head honcho), depending on the agency or organization. Although that person isn't likely to answer the phone, you're likely to get a knowledgeable and responsible person who can help you.

Whether you're looking for a hospital, an outpatient treatment program, or a rehabilitative program, navigating the mental healthcare system can be tricky — it's often a complex and fragmented mix of public (federal, state, and local) and private resources. For example, some of the options for inpatient hospitalization include

- Private hospitals that focus on behavioral health issues (usually mental health and addiction)
- Psychiatric wards in local community hospitals
- Psychiatric wards in teaching hospitals affiliated with a medical school
- State-supported psychiatric hospitals
- Veterans' hospitals administered by the Veterans Administration

No matter how ill a person may be, getting into a psychiatric hospital is no easy feat these days. (For more on hospitalization, turn to Chapter 14.)

Connecting with community services

Because of the high costs of inpatient care and restrictions placed by third-party insurers, people who are hospitalized are likely to be discharged "sicker and quicker" than anyone might have thought or wanted. So the minute your loved one is hospitalized, start looking into discharge planning. Here are some items to add to your to-do list:

- **Make sure that the staff knows the specifics of your loved one's insurance coverage and that they're explicit about the goals of hospitalization.**

To double-check your loved one's coverage, your loved one (or you) can independently verify his mental-health benefits, co-pays, and lengths of stay with the insurer.

- **If your loved one has a private therapist or sees a psychiatrist in a public program, make sure that the clinician knows that your loved one has been hospitalized.** Provide the outpatient clinician with the name of the inpatient doctor, and vice versa. This will help assure continuity of care.
- **Inform the staff that you'll need ample time before discharge to coordinate arrangements in the community.** Walking in one day for a visit and finding the staff packing your loved one's things can be disconcerting.
- **Always stay one step ahead.** Look into day programs, partial hospitalization programs, case management programs or ACT teams, or residences in the community.

Some hospitals have social workers, case managers, or discharge planners to help you make plans for after discharge. If one is on staff, ask to talk to this person.

Finding other resources in the community

When your loved one is on her own in the community, identifying local resources can be difficult. But when you start to look for mental-health facilities, you may be surprised to see them everywhere! Here are some options for finding services and supports:

- **If your loved one already has a psychiatrist, psychologist, social worker, or clinician, ask for their help!**
- **Most cities or counties have either free-standing mental-health departments or ones that are under broader health or social services department.** Check the government listings in your telephone directory or online to find out the name of the agency that oversees mental health in your local community.
- **Solicit help from your state of local NAMI affiliate (`www.nami.org`) or from a family you know who has experienced mental illness firsthand.**
- **Contact your local affiliate of Mental Health America (`www.nmha.org`) or any other local mental-health program or citizen-advocacy group.** Ask where you can find a directory of mental-health resources in your community.
- **If you still have trouble finding the information you need, contact your state mental-health authority (see the appendix) and ask where you can access local information.**

- **Use print telephone directories or online ones (such as `www.switchboard.com` or `www.googleguide.com`) to find information.**

See the appendix for other resources to help you locate clinicians and programs.

Trying Different Treatments to Find What Works

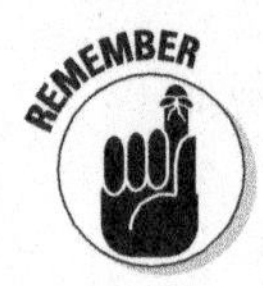

Numerous treatments options are available for schizophrenia. But as is the case with many other chronic illnesses, these treatments control symptoms rather than provide cures. Plus, treatments (both medicines and psychosocial approaches) must be tried and evaluated for each individual. If one treatment doesn't work, it can be replaced by another treatment. This trial-and-error approach is the rule rather than the exception for medical disorders (including high blood pressure, asthma, diabetes, Parkinson's disease, and even cancer).

With progress being made in genetic research, the goal is for medical treatment to be *personalized* (known as *personalized medicine)*. The idea of personalized medicine is that based on an individual's genetic profile, clinicians will be able to select from among known effective treatments and know the one best-suited to the person's genetic makeup, thus reducing the amount of trial and error necessary for a successful treatment outcome. In other words, doctors will be able to get it right the first time!

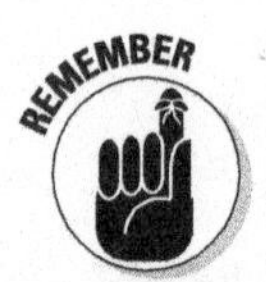

Don't expect this kind of personalization to be available anytime in the next year, or possibly even the next decade. Even with all the advances that have been made, genetic research is still in its infancy.

For now, your loved one and his clinician (and sometimes involved family or friends) will first select a treatment and try it out to see how effective, safe, and tolerable it is. At the beginning of treatment, it's especially important that your loved one stick to the prescribed treatments religiously and provide feedback to the clinician on whether symptoms and function are improving or not. With this information, your loved one and his doctor can gauge whether continuing the treatment regimen is the right thing to do.

People sometimes stop taking medications for what might sound like trivial reasons to others. But some side-effects — such as dry mouth and decreased sex drive — can be very annoying. If side-effects are a problem for your loved one, remind her that there are many choices of medications, each with different side-effect profiles, and sometimes just changing the dose will do the trick.

Your loved one needs to be persistent in sticking with his doctor until they find a treatment that works. It's also important to put things in perspective. Your loved one will be living with schizophrenia and participating in treatment for a long time, and although it's going to be part of his life, he doesn't want it consume his *whole* life. In fact with appropriate treatment, your loved one will be able to forget the first unsuccessful stabs at treatment and recover to the extent that his illness fades more into the background of his life.

Finding a psychiatric medication that works for your loved one

The mainstay of treatment for schizophrenia is antipsychotic medication, and there are many to choose from (see Chapter 8). Here are some of the questions that your loved one and his psychiatrist will want to discuss in considering which medication to try first:

- **If your loved one hasn't taken antipsychotic medications before, has anyone else in the family ever taken them?** If so, which one(s) worked best?
- **If your loved one has taken antipsychotic medications before, which ones worked and which ones didn't?**
- **If your loved one has taken antipsychotic medications before, did he experience any troubling side effects,** such as:
  - Tremors or other abnormal movements
  - Stiffness of arms, legs, or face
  - Feeling like he couldn't remain still and had to move around
  - Dry mouth
  - Blurred vision
  - Significant weight gain
  - Drooling
  - Faintness when quickly standing up
- **If your loved one has insurance that covers medications, are there any medications that *aren't* covered by the company?**
- **If your loved one doesn't have insurance or other coverage, can she afford to pay for newer more expensive medications?**

  Newer and/or more expensive doesn't necessarily translate to "better" or "best."
- **Would your loved one prefer taking an injection once or twice a month rather than having to take medications by mouth one or two times a day?**

If your loved one discusses these points with his physician, they'll be able to work together to select a medication that has the greatest chance of being the right one for your loved one.

Rx: Take as directed

After medication is prescribed, your loved one will need to take it as directed on a regular basis. Remind her that medication is used to control her symptoms so she can lead a more satisfying and hassle-free life. Although she may see and feel some of the effects of the medication right away (less agitation, fewer hallucinations), it's not unusual for the medication to take one or two weeks to begin working, and she shouldn't expect miracles overnight — and neither should you!

More improvement will be seen over the course of the following weeks and months. However, if after several weeks no improvement is seen or felt, your loved one should talk to her doctor and ask whether this is the right medication for her.

We usually recommend that individuals see their clinician, or at least touch base with them on the phone, at least once a week when they first start a new medication.

Your loved one should never stop or abruptly change her medication on her own. She should *always* let the doctor know what's going on, and they should decide together what to do. If your loved one doesn't have an appointment scheduled and wants to go off her medication right away, encourage her to call her doctor first.

Help! I can't stand the side effects!

What should your loved one do if the medication is working to control the symptoms but he's encountering undesirable side-effects? Whenever a person is starting medication, it's common to encounter some side-effects, such as drowsiness, blurred vision, or dry mouth, which go away over a short period of time. Other side-effects are slower to come on (like weight gain or some unexpected mouth and tongue movements). Side-effects are more often annoying or troubling, rather than dangerous.

When your loved one's doctor prescribes a medication, have him ask what side-effects to be on the lookout for and what to do about them. (See Chapter 8 for a list of common side-effects.) If your loved one has already left the office, there's no harm calling the doctor or asking the pharmacist when you go to get the prescription filled.

Your loved one's doctor should alert him to medically dangerous side-effects that need to be dealt with right away (as opposed to ones that are just annoying). A rapid drop in blood pressure, a rapid rise in temperature (not caused by another medical illness), stiffening of the back and neck, or eyes rolling up in the head are possible side-effects that need immediate medical attention. If you think your loved one is having an adverse side-effect that could be life-threatening, call 911 and seek emergency attention.

Symptom control (especially positive symptoms such as delusions, hallucinations, disorganized thoughts, and agitation) is the most immediate beneficial effect that your loved one will experience after taking medication. However, if the positive symptoms of schizophrenia have been controlled and the illness is still disrupting his school, work, or other important social roles, the addition of psychosocial and other support interventions can help facilitate recovery (see Chapter 9).

Considering therapies in addition to medications

A number of psychosocial, psychotherapy, and self-help approaches can be instrumental in your loved one's recovery; these proven techniques can help overcome some of the remaining symptoms (sometimes called *residual symptoms*) and problems with daily living that can't be helped with medicine alone.

Be sure to ask your loved one's clinician, case manager, or rehabilitation specialist about these treatment resources. Depending on who you ask, your loved one will be directed either to another program or to other resources within the same program. Frequently, there will be an initial assessment of your loved one's skills, and then specific exercises, tasks, and role-playing opportunities will be prescribed until your loved one achieves competence in these areas.

For example, if your loved one can't keep up a basic conversation or know to make use of and enjoy leisure time, psychosocial skills programs can be effective in addressing these problems. A first step is usually an initial assessment of the individual's skills and then specific exercises, tasks, and role-playing opportunities are prescribed until your loved one achieves competence in these areas.

If your loved one is having cognitive problems (for example, with memory, decision-making, verbal skills, and so on), cognitive remediation programs (some of which are computer-based) can improve functional impairments.

If your loved one needs help in knowing how to complete job applications, prepare a résumé, participate in a job interview, maintain consistent work and attendance habits, or otherwise function effectively in a work setting, vocational rehabilitation and clubhouse models (see Chapter 9) can provide these kinds of experiences.

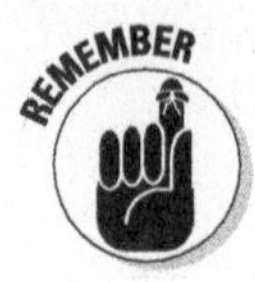

Medical and other psychosocial and self-help interventions go hand in hand. They don't conflict with one another. In fact, when they're used together, they enhance the possibility of positive outcomes. Knee replacements wouldn't be as successful without physical rehabilitation and vice versa — think about the marriage between antipsychotic medications and other treatments in the same way.

Treating schizophrenia and substance abuse

Another important aspect of treatment is the need to simultaneously address the symptoms of schizophrenia and alcohol and/or drug abuse. Unfortunately, because of lack of awareness of some professionals and the scarcity of integrated treatment programs, it's more typical for these individuals to be treated for only one condition or the other. (Those who specialize in mental health may know little about addictions, and those who specialize in addictions may know little about serious mental disorders.)

Yet patients with schizophrenia are five times more likely than the general population to be abusing one or multiple substances. If an underlying substance-abuse problem isn't addressed simultaneously, it leads to poorer outcomes, including relapse, re-hospitalization, and arrest.

What to Do If Your Loved One Won't Accept the Diagnosis

People with serious mental illnesses are often unable to recognize that they're sick — even though it's apparent to others. This situation is more than just *denial* (blocking out of conscious awareness things that are too painful). In the case of schizophrenia, this lack of recognition — which scientists now believe is the result of a brain dysfunction — is a symptom of the illness itself. It's estimated that more than half — some say as many as 80 percent — of all individuals with schizophrenia lack awareness of their illness. Sometimes, lack of insight is worse during acute phases of the illness; other times it is a more consistent problem.

The technical term used to describe this condition of being unaware of one's own illness is *anosognosia.* This condition also occurs with certain types of traumatic brain injuries and strokes, for example.

Because lack of insight is so closely associated with refusing treatment and not adhering to medication plans, it can quickly become a battleground between patients and their frustrated families. There are no simple one-size-fits-all solutions. Lack of insight usually can't be addressed overnight, but there are some practical strategies for coming to terms with the need for treatment that may be worth trying:

- **Exercising empathy:** Flat-out confrontation rarely works and stands a better chance of exacerbating symptoms than reducing them; conversely, empathetic understanding can help. Find ways to communicate that you understand your loved one's point-of-view. Typically, for people with schizophrenia, their delusions and hallucinations feel so real that they can't be convinced otherwise. In this case, you can explain to your loved one that you want her to get help to better cope with these problems.

  For example, you might say, "I know how frightened you are of the soldiers who keep watching you." You're not saying that you buy into the delusion — you're just showing your empathy and concern. Then say, "Maybe you can speak to a psychiatrist who can help you cope with the burden this has placed on you." Again, you're not accepting the delusional thinking, but you're also not rejecting your loved one's point-of-view.

- **Encouraging symptomatic treatment:** Although some people have no insight into their illness, they may have other annoying symptoms associated with schizophrenia that make them amenable to seeing a doctor (for example, insomnia or depression). You could suggest that your loved one see a psychiatrist or internist to address these symptoms without confronting the issue of schizophrenia or strange thinking head-on.

- **Negotiating an agreement:** Your loved one may be refusing to take her medicine, but she may ask you to take her shopping for some new clothes. Perhaps you could strike a bargain with her. If she consistently takes the medication for a week, you'll take her out shopping. In the case of a teenager, you might make receiving her allowance contingent upon taking his medication or you might think up an interim reward, such as a new video game, for taking medication consistently over a certain period of time.

  To bargain effectively with anyone, you must understand his motivations and desires.

- **Simplifying dosing strategies:** Although scientists still don't completely understand the neurobiological mechanisms associated with lack of insight, simplifying dosing strategies helps lessen the problem to some extent. Physicians can help by prescribing once-a-day pills or longer-term injectable medications for patients who have problems complying with more complicated medication schedules.

- **Doing everything you can to stay connected:** This strategy is probably the most important one for encouraging compliance. Whatever your role, the worst thing you can do is cut off your relationship with someone with schizophrenia because he's not taking his medication. Sometimes, taking medication only comes after developing a trusting relationship. A person with schizophrenia may need to make repeated visits to a doctor before he finally agrees to take his medication — even though you and everyone around him want it to happen more quickly.

If one of these strategies doesn't work, try another. Sometimes they need to be used in combination or sequentially.

When someone doesn't realize the need to take medications, encouraging the person to start a consistent medication regimen often requires the support of family members, friends (peers) and professionals.

As a friend or family member, you need to clearly distinguish between your nonsupport of the person's decision to *not* take medication and your support for helping her recover from the illness. Things may seem hopeless now, but you never know when your loved one will change her mind.

If you learn that a case manager has terminated your loved one from program participation because of lack of insight, you need to remind the case manager that this is one of the problems associated with schizophrenia that the program is here to address. Some research suggests that psychosocial programs may benefit patients who lack insight, and that participation in these programs and the accompanying social supports may enhance a person's self-awareness of their illness.

Patients are often more willing to accept a diagnosis when they're among peer role models who are succeeding in managing the symptoms of their illnesses.

If you have the unfortunate experience of encountering a psychiatrist who discharges a patient for being unwilling to take medication, you can gently ask the doctor to build a relationship with the patient and find out the reasons why she's so adverse to medication. Often, patients have had bad experiences with medications or negative experiences with other clinicians in the past, and they need to talk through them.

When people start the routine of taking medication and their symptoms are more controlled, they may be less adamant about not taking it. In fact, they may begin to recognize the benefits. If someone is completely out-of-touch with reality, these strategies are less likely to work. Unfortunately, your loved one may actually have to *be* on medication to realize that she *needs* it.

Some research suggests that the use of the antipsychotic medication clozapine may improve patient insight. Similarly, some cognitive-behavioral approaches have been shown to be effective (see Chapter 9).

As people gain insight into their schizophrenia, the insight is often associated with depression because of their new recognition of the real losses they've experienced due to the illness. If your loved one is gaining insight into his illness and, at the same time, exhibiting signs of depression (particularly if he's talking about or threatening suicide), immediately bring this to the attention of his clinician.

Because lack of insight in schizophrenia is associated with poorer outcomes (such as higher rates of relapse, re-hospitalization, and more impaired functioning), it remains a very important clinical and research issue that requires more attention. In the meantime, don't give up on your loved one. What didn't work yesterday may work tomorrow.

I Am Not Sick: I Don't Need Help, by Xavier Amador, PhD, with Anna-Lisa Johanson (Vida Press), has made a significant contribution to the literature on this topic. Dr. Amador weaves together the story of his own brother's schizophrenia with research on lack of insight and provides helpful practical tips to family members and clinicians who struggle with this problem.

Treatment Considerations for Special Populations

Although schizophrenia usually strikes people in their teens or young-adult years, it can occur at any age or stage during a person's life and the criteria for diagnosis remain the same regardless of age. However, different people may require different treatment — for example, a child may need different treatment than an older adult. Also, an increasing number of people with schizophrenia are being diagnosed with co-occurring substance-abuse problems, which are complex to diagnose and treat in the presence of a serious mental disorder.

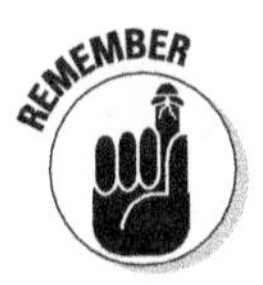

Although scientists are learning about the differences among various special populations, these findings don't apply to every case. In the following sections, we make some generalizations that apply to large groups rather than to individuals. Your loved one may fall into one of these categories but exhibit different symptoms or need different treatments. This is just a starting point for a conversation with your loved one's doctor.

Children

Schizophrenia affects children from families of all socioeconomic classes and cultural backgrounds. It's often more challenging to diagnose schizophrenia in children because of the rapid developmental changes that they experience and their inability to describe the symptoms they're experiencing.

As a result, the disorder typically goes undiagnosed for many years. Often, doctors are also reluctant to stigmatize a young child with a diagnosis of schizophrenia even though that's what it looks like; unwittingly, the child is diagnosed with a disorder that is more acceptable to parents (such as depression) but doesn't receive the proper treatment.

The median age of diagnosis in children is 14 — but the average duration of symptoms before diagnosis is nine years! Schizophrenia is rarely diagnosed in children under the age of 5 and is far less common than most other mental disorders in children, affecting about 1 in 40,000 children under the age of 13. Because children spend a major portion of their day at school, teachers and other school personnel often play an instrumental role in identifying serious mental disorders and in referring families for evaluation, diagnosis, and treatment.

Childhood schizophrenia usually appears gradually but can also have a sudden onset; many of its symptoms often overlap with other childhood disorders such as autism, developmental disorders, conduct disorders, and learning disabilities. Here are the most common warning signs of childhood schizophrenia. ***Remember:*** Different children may experience these symptoms differently.

- **Delusions:** For example, believing that monsters are in his room at bedtime. (For more on delusions, see Chapter 3.)
- **Hallucinations:** Eighty percent of children with schizophrenia have auditory hallucinations such as hearing voices telling them to do things. (For more on hallucinations, see Chapter 3.)

  When children experience hallucinations or delusions, particularly after the age of 7, they should be evaluated by a mental-health professional.
- **Social withdrawal (severe problems in making or keeping friends)**
- **Very detailed, bizarre thoughts and ideas**
- **Confused thinking**
- **Suspiciousness or paranoia (thinking that someone is going to harm them)**
- **Language delays**
- **Poor social and self-care skills**
- **Extreme moodiness, diminished emotions, or lack of emotional expression when speaking**
- **Distorted perceptions of reality (such as an inability to distinguish dreams or TV from reality)**
- **Poor personal hygiene**

- **Suicidal thoughts**
- **Extreme fearfulness or clinginess**

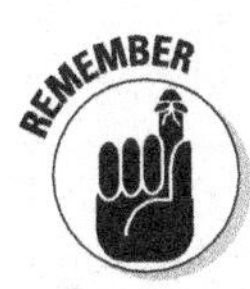

It takes a trained individual to make a diagnosis of childhood schizophrenia. Don't panic if your child has one bad dream or your child seems more clingy than her playmates. However, if your child has a number of these warning signs, you should bring them to the attention of your pediatrician to see if they warrant immediate further evaluation (by a child and adolescent psychiatrist) or whether you should simply monitor for the time being to see how things progress.

Although medication is the primary treatment for childhood schizophrenia, many of the drugs prescribed for children are approved for use only in adults and are used off-label for children. Because children aren't just little adults, they need to receive treatment from an experienced child and adolescent psychiatrist who is specifically trained to diagnose and treat children with schizophrenia.

Witnessing a child with the disturbing symptoms of schizophrenia is horribly frightening for the entire family, especially siblings. Things can quickly spiral out of control, leaving families feeling helpless. For this reason, psychiatrists generally prescribe medication right away — sometimes even before making a definitive diagnosis — to treat the psychotic episode.

Because children are less able to give feedback about how they're feeling and less likely to be able to identify side-effects, their medication needs to be monitored more closely during treatment than it does in adults. If the psychotic behaviors don't respond to medication, the child may have to be hospitalized for a short time.

The same medications used for adults are effective in reducing hallucinations and delusions (which tend to be more transitory in children). Although *second-generation antipsychotic medications* (see Chapter 8), like clozapine (brand name: Clozaril) and olanzapine (brand name: Zyprexa), are less likely to produce movement disorders than first-generation antipsychotics, they often lead to excess weight gain, which can cause other serious health problems. These side effects can be especially troubling to teens who are already overly-concerned about their appearance and what others think about their looks. Work with your child's doctor to consider the pros and cons of different medications and try to find one that not only relieves the symptoms but produces the fewest troubling side effects.

In addition to medication, family psychoeducation can be very helpful in assisting a family learn to learn how to adjust and cope with the illness. Children should be given age-appropriate information about the disorder as well, so they can better understand what's happening to them or their sibling. Children also can benefit from other types of psychotherapies and psychosocial therapies that provide support and skills training.

Schools can play a pivotal role in meeting the educational and social needs of children with schizophrenia. Many children with schizophrenia can benefit from special education and other accommodations in school, including an individualized education plan (IEP). When children are unable to attend school, they may require in-home services and supports. To find out more about IEPs, go to `www.ed.gov/parents/needs/speced/iepguide`.

The disease process of schizophrenia is similar in children and adults, but in children, schizophrenia is

- More likely to have a severe course
- More likely to *recur* (come back again)
- Associated with greater functional impairments (because it often interrupts schooling and normal developmental tasks of childhood and adolescence)

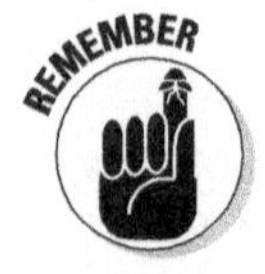

Despite these warnings, *many children fully recover,* showing no apparent signs of the illness as adults. Unfortunately, little is known about how to predict which children will or will not be disabled by their illness.

College students

Because the age of onset of schizophrenia often coincides with the time when kids head off to college, it's not surprising that many families have to grapple with sons and daughters who have their first break on college campuses, which are often far away from home. Also, because of improved treatments, many young people with prior histories of schizophrenia (who may not have otherwise had the opportunity to do so before the advent of newer medications) are heading off to college after having been diagnosed and treated.

The college years can be stressful ones for a variety of reasons such as moving away from friends and family for the first time, more difficult coursework and studying for exams, irregular patterns of eating and sleeping, tendency to experiment with alcohol and/or drugs, and pressure to compete and conform. These stresses can precipitate a first break in someone who is genetically vulnerable or provoke relapse in someone who has already been diagnosed.

Parents of children with a genetic history of schizophrenia, whose teen has shown no signs of schizophrenia, may want to take extra steps to ease this difficult transition:

- **Talk to her about schizophrenia and mental disorders.** A number of Web sites provide just enough information for teenagers (see the appendix). Remember, though, that lack of insight may still interfere with a college student's ability to recognize her early symptoms.

- **Arrange to see your teen every other month or so and to check in more frequently by phone.** You don't want to be a helicopter parent, hovering over his every move, but you want to watch for significant changes in thinking, mood, and behavior. Parent days on campus, holidays at home, and summer vacations can allow you the opportunity to unobtrusively check in on your college student.
- **Introduce your teen to the student health services office or counseling center at the college so he knows that help is available if he needs it.**
- **Tell your teen about Active Minds on Campus, a nonprofit that helps raise mental health awareness among young adults between the ages of 18 and 24 (see the appendix).**

If your son or daughter has already been diagnosed with schizophrenia, discuss his or her choice of colleges in advance. Here are some things to look for:

- **A college that's closer to home:** Try to find one that's within a day's drive, so you can be there to help if necessary.
- **A college that is less stressful:** Some schools have ultra-competitive environments; others are more laid back. You want a school where the emphasis isn't 100 percent on grades and competition, so your son or daughter can learn without any added stress.
- **A college that provides more support:** Find out about the psychological services available on campus. Ask whether any special accommodations or supports are available to people with mental or emotional problems. The way your questions are handled and responded to will give you a feel for the degree of understanding and acceptance of mental-health issues by college mental-health administrators. Increasingly, institutions of higher education are providing mentors or coaches to provide support to people with disabilities. The more support, the better.

  Make sure there is at least one practicing psychiatrist on staff. Introduce yourself and your son or daughter to the psychiatrist before school starts. Ask to be kept informed about any significant problems. Make sure that the college has your son or daughter's written permission to inform you of any problems.

  A survey found that one in four college students report experiencing suicidal thoughts. Don't let patient confidentiality keep you out of the loop when it comes to your child's mental health.

- **A college that has a student health center with a fully stocked pharmacy:** If your son or daughter is currently taking psychotropic medications, make sure the school pharmacy has an adequate supply (or send him or her to school with enough medication to last until the next visit home) or make sure that your student has access to a local or mail-order pharmacy.

The large majority of colleges and institutions of higher education have limited knowledge about schizophrenia. Don't be surprised if you or your loved one needs to teach certain educators and administrators about the disorder.

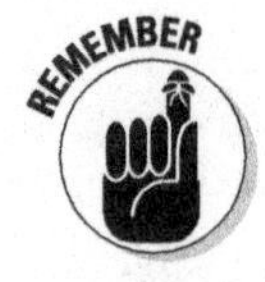

Before your kid leaves for college, talk with him openly about what to do in an emergency. Decide whom he should call first, perhaps you or a therapist. Make sure he has the phone number of a nearby hospital with a psychiatric unit or the contact information for a help line or crisis center. If you're confident that the information will be kept confidential and only shared with your permission, make the emergency plan available to the college health office as well.

A growing number of college campuses are sprouting NAMI clubs, where people with major mental disorders can get peer support and practical assistance from other students. You can find out about them at the NAMI Web site (`www.nami.org`).

People with schizophrenia and co-occurring substance abuse problems

Between one-quarter and one-half of people diagnosed with schizophrenia also have co-occurring alcohol and/or drug problems (sometimes referred to as a *dual diagnosis*). Like schizophrenia, substance-abuse disorders tend to be *chronic* (long-standing) with a pattern of multiple relapses and remissions. These dually diagnosed individuals have a higher risk of self-destructive and violent behaviors, which often results in homelessness, housing instability, incarceration, poor nutrition, inadequate finances, and medical problems.

It can be challenging for either a mental-health professional or an addiction professional to diagnose the other disorder in the absence of multiple contacts with the individual over time. But an integrated assessment, by someone trained in both mental-health and substance abuse, can help better identify co-occurring disorders by systematically looking at the symptoms, history, and course of each disorder in the same individual.

In order to manage and treat co-occurring disorders effectively, a long-term, multidisciplinary team approach — comprised of medical, mental-health, and addiction-treatment specialists — is necessary to provide integrated services based on a single individualized treatment plan addressing both disorders. Unfortunately, many treatment programs are still organized and funded to treat one disorder or the other.

Some of the special approaches used with this population include

- **Psychoeducational classes** that help consumers recognize their symptoms and identify the triggers that precipitate relapse
- **"Double-trouble" groups** and self-help recovery groups that acknowledge both co-occurring disorders and provide useful forums for consumers to discuss and understand them
- **Special 12-step programs** that are sensitive to the needs of individuals with both disorders

Because of the extraordinary barriers these individuals face in accessing and keeping housing and also because of their intensive treatment needs, many individuals with co-occurring disorders benefit from long-term residential treatment facilities and modified therapeutic communities.

Another serious problem plaguing people with schizophrenia (and worrisome to their loved ones) is nicotine addiction. It has been estimated that 75 percent of people with schizophrenia smoke despite the obvious health risks. This is another issue to be tackled by psychiatrists trained in addiction.

Older adults

Although schizophrenia is thought of as a disorder of young people, it can begin in later life or extend into later life when diagnosed earlier. Approximately 0.05 percent of the population (or 1 in 2,000 people) over the age of 65 has schizophrenia, making it about half as common as it is among those between the ages of 18 and 54. With people living longer, the numbers of older people with schizophrenia are likely to increase.

Generally, schizophrenia that occurs after the age of 45 is characterized as having a late onset.

Some people suggest that the late-onset form of schizophrenia is less severe than its early-onset counterpart. Other researchers hypothesize that late-onset schizophrenia is a distinctly different type of disorder. Because psychotic symptoms can also occur in people with Alzheimer's disease, the disease is sometimes initially misdiagnosed.

Some of the distinctive characteristics of the illness when it first appears later in life include the following:

- Late-onset schizophrenia is more common in women than in men.
- The symptoms of late-onset schizophrenia are less severe overall.
- A person with late-onset schizophrenia is more likely to include symptoms of suspiciousness or paranoia.

- Less cognitive impairment is seen in those with late-onset schizophrenia.
- Negative symptoms (see Chapter 3) are less likely to appear with late-onset schizophrenia.
- Lower doses of psychotropic medications are required to manage the symptoms of late-onset schizophrenia.
- Late-onset schizophrenia has a better prognosis.
- Fewer suicide attempts are seen among those with late-onset schizophrenia. That said, the rate of successful suicide attempts is especially high in elderly men.

Older individuals are less likely to self-refer for mental-health treatment for a variety of reasons, so outreach efforts are important to identify the disorder. Seniors may resist treatment, be unable to afford it, or be unable to access it because of mobility problems — and their relatives may think they're too old to get started now. For this reason, it's vitally important that general practitioners who tend to see older patients often, recognize the symptoms of schizophrenia and how they differ from the symptoms of dementia and suggest specialized treatment by a geriatric psychiatrist.

The most significant challenge in treating older adults with schizophrenia has to do with the potential adverse effects of psychotropic medications. Older people can be sensitive to very small doses of medication, so medication needs to be monitored closely, and psychiatrists generally begin treatment with small doses and increase it slowly. Also, because older people tend to have other chronic illnesses, there's always an increased risk of drug interactions that needs to be considered.

Finally, as a group, older people are more sensitive to movement disorders (such as tardive dyskinesia; see Chapter 8).

But it is important to remember that mental illnesses are treatable conditions in older adults.

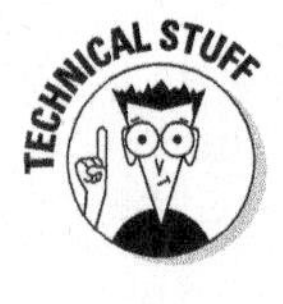

Like children, older adults tend to be excluded from many treatment research studies, so scientists don't know as much about the effectiveness and safety of medications and other treatments in this group. Much of the information that guides the use of medications comes from studies of younger people with schizophrenia or from the practical experience of clinicians who work with older adults.

About half of all older people who receive mental health care receive it from their primary doctors, who may not be best equipped to provide it. If possible, seek out a *geriatric psychiatrist* (a psychiatrist who specializes in the treatment of older people) for your loved one. Geriatric psychiatrists are usually more experienced in making diagnoses in this population. Plus, because of their experience, they're also more familiar with the range of medications that work effectively, appropriate dosing, and potential side effects and interactions with other drugs.

Because of a number of factors including their limited income, curtailed mobility, and social isolation, only half of older adults who acknowledge mental-health problems receive any treatment at all. And although the use of nursing homes and state hospitals for treatment has declined considerably for younger populations, the decline has been far *less* dramatic with older people. Sometimes psychiatric nurses can make home visits, often paid for by Medicare, to help older people with schizophrenia remain with their families or in their homes. (See Chapter 7 for help with financing mental health care.)

If an older person with schizophrenia is suspicious or unwilling to take antipsychotic medications for other reasons, she'll often reconsider if she's told that the medication will improve her sleep (often a problem and concern in older people) or will help alleviate her anxiety.

Women

Although there are tremendous variations among individuals, schizophrenia affects women differently than it does men:

- In general, women experience a later onset of the illness than do men.
- Often, but not always, women have delusions that are less bizarre than those of men. Female delusions often involve sex, pregnancy, and/or romance.
- The course of the disorder tends to be less severe in women, with less functional impairment, than is seen in men.
- Women typically experience more profound mood symptoms than men do.
- Women are less likely to concurrently abuse drugs and/or alcohol than men are.
- Women are slightly more responsive to psychotropic medications, often requiring smaller doses.
- Women experience more favorable outcomes, in general, than men.

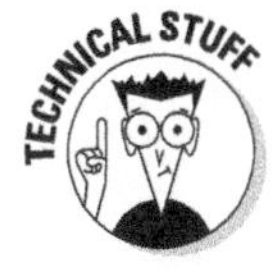

Some research suggests that estrogen has a protective effect for women before the age of menopause and that, after menopause, women develop schizophrenia at about the same rate as men.

Treatment of women with schizophrenia is more complicated because of hormones, pregnancy, and their role as mothers. Women often need less medication, because of their weight and the effects of hormones. Plus, because mood disorders are more likely to be prominent in women, they may be more likely to require antidepressants or mood stabilizers in addition to their antipsychotic medication.

Women benefit from the same psychotherapies, psychosocial strategies, and self-help programs as do men, but if possible, your loved one should take advantage of opportunities to address her special needs as a woman. For example, women with schizophrenia aren't always able to care for their offspring, which can be a cause of severe distress to them. This issue needs to be sensitively addressed by mental-health workers so women learn to understand the limitations their illness might pose in terms of their ability to maintain custody of their children — without making them feel guilty. In many cases, mental-health staff will want to encourage a more realistic, but meaningful, relationship between mother and child. Many women resist treatment for fear that their children will be taken away when someone learns about their illness. Also, women who have been mothers may have had little opportunity to hone their career skills and can benefit from additional help in this arena.

The issue of pregnancy is always a serious one and more so for a woman with schizophrenia. The offspring of a woman with schizophrenia has an increased genetic risk of the disorder (see Chapter 2). Also, the added stress that comes with being responsible for an infant can increase the potential for relapse. If your loved one with schizophrenia wants to have a child, she should discuss the possibility and timing of a pregnancy with a trusted healthcare professional *before* becoming pregnant.

If your loved one decides to get pregnant, decisions about taking or stopping psychiatric medications during pregnancy are often fraught with confusion. Although, in general, anyone should try to use as little medication as possible (especially early in the pregnancy), stopping antipsychotic medication does increase the risk of relapse in people with schizophrenia. Because there's no ironclad data on the effects of antipsychotic medication on the fetus, this is something a woman will want to discuss with her psychiatrist. It appears that first-generation antipsychotics pose *more* risk of miscarriage and genetic defects than second-generation antipsychotics do, although the incidence is quite low for both types.

Care must also be exercised after childbirth when breastfeeding, because medication can make its way into the mother's breast milk, which can result in infants experiencing some of the side effects seen in adults. Also worrisome: Possible effects on the developing infant brain and subsequent behavior are still unknown. To improve the odds, both mother and child should be followed carefully by a knowledgeable psychiatrist before, during, and after the pregnancy.

Like other things in life, there are no guarantees, and your loved one's decisions should be based on the best information she can get from her healthcare team. Prior to becoming pregnant, some women with schizophrenia decide to consult with a *genetic counselor* (a specialized professional who reviews the medical and family history to assess genetic risks and evaluate them with the patient).

Separate from pregnancy considerations, virtually all first-generation antipsychotic medications and some second-generation medications (especially risperidone [brand name: Risperidal]) cause a large rise in the hormone prolactin. There are no known serious health effects resulting from increased levels of this hormone, but it can lead to lactation (milk being produced in the breast), which is a disturbing side effect, especially in men. (Generally this is less a problem in women because they naturally have higher levels of prolactin than men do.)

Cultural Variations

Some people feel more comfortable speaking to someone who shares a similar background and whom they perceive is better able to understand where they're coming from. For some people, this may mean seeking out a therapist of the same age, gender, race, sexual orientation, or country of origin — although having these characteristics in common may be relatively unimportant to others.

This applies to treatment settings, too. We met a mother who told us about her 40-something son with schizophrenia who lived in a supervised residence. One of the most difficult things for him to adapt to was the fact that most of the workers in the home were almost 20 years younger and less educated, and were in a role of telling him what to do.

People who have schizophrenia and are members of minority groups face a number of barriers when it comes to receiving appropriate, high-quality mental health care:

- **Problems with access:** These problems may arise because of poverty, lack of health insurance, problems with transportation, and so on.
- **Reliance on emergency rooms rather than outpatient care often due to lack of insurance to pay for routine psychiatric care and medication.**
- **Pervasive stigma against mental illness and its treatment by family and friends among certain groups:** For example, in some cultures mental illness is sometimes seen as a sign of moral weakness rather than a brain disorder.
- **Lack of mental-health personnel who speak the same language and understand their culture or who are sensitive to an individual's sexual orientation.**
- **Poor mental-health literacy:** They may not understand or recognize the signs and symptoms of mental disorders.

- **Intrinsic differences in help-seeking behavior:** Some groups of people simply don't go for medical help as soon or as often as other people do.
- **Lack of trust in the professional mental-health system:** Certain groups may feel more comfortable turning to their families or their churches for help in coping with their problems.

Finally, because minorities are underrepresented in research, treatment approaches often are not focused around their special strengths and needs.

Schizophrenia around the world

The symptoms that any person with schizophrenia experiences need to be interpreted within the context of his background and culture. Certain thoughts or behaviors, for example, that are considered delusional in the United States may be acceptable somewhere else around the world — in some cultures or religions, it's common for people to experience "visions" or to speak to the dead. If a therapist is a nonbeliever and doesn't understand this, he may misdiagnose the person.

Also, in some cultures, different types of delusions tend to be more prominent. For example, in Ireland, people often have delusions of sainthood; in Japan, delusions of public humiliation are more common. Such differences point to the need for clinicians to be attentive to culture in diagnosing schizophrenia.

To learn more about the differences in schizophrenia in different parts of the world, the World Health Organization has studied people with schizophrenia in both developed and developing countries. They found that the disorder tends to be more severe in developed, industrialized countries — speculating that it might be because undeveloped countries provide more social support and have less stressful and less competitive environments.

The same research team found that people with schizophrenia in developed countries tended to have disorders that came on gradually, while those in developing countries had more acute episodes that were shorter-lasting.

Chapter 7

Paying for Your Loved One's Care

In This Chapter

- Checking out the costs of care
- Tapping into private insurance
- Taking advantage of public programs
- Making the rules work to your benefit
- Exploring other options: VA benefits, college mental health care, and clinical trials
- Planning for the future

Unless you're independently wealthy — and maybe even then — the costs of treating schizophrenia (or any other chronic illness) over time will stagger you. The good news is that, with help from your insurance company and government programs, the whole cost won't fall on you or your loved one. The bad news is that you'll need to be persistent and patient to receive the government benefits that are out there — and will likely have to pitch in to cover the gaps in what's available.

Ideally, you and your loved one will find a social worker, case manager, or other mental-health advocate to help you navigate the murky waters of financing mental health care, but much of the burden of finding and funding care falls on the person with schizophrenia or, more often, his family.

In this chapter, we give you a primer of where to look and who to ask for additional information on financial issues related to the care and treatment of people with schizophrenia, to make navigating these waters a little easier.

Paying for Care

When you consider the cost of treatment for schizophrenia, you may be thinking, "That's what insurance is for," but even private insurance has pitfalls when it comes to funding mental-health treatment, and many people with schizophrenia have no insurance at all.

The complicated world of mental healthcare

Mental healthcare, like general medical care in the United States today, is characterized by a byzantine labyrinth of treatment facilities, private and public programs, charities, and religious and volunteer organizations that include

- Hospitals and outpatient care
- Primary care (family physicians) and specialty care (such as psychiatrists, therapists, and social workers)
- Health, rehabilitative, and support services

The mental healthcare system is fragmented among different programs, each supported by different sources of funding, and different eligibility and application requirements that may require endless paperwork and the patience of Job to complete. (Keep in mind that this is fragmentation is no different than that encountered by people taking care of older parents with chronic health problems. Because of the diverse payers for different types of care, a family caregiver may be coordinating care among five different specialty doctors, a hospital, home health aides, and a hospice program.) The patchwork maze of healthcare in America can be dizzying to anyone and mental healthcare is no different except that the person requiring care may be more mentally incapacitated during an acute crisis.

Programs often have lengthy waiting lists. And these programs usually don't communicate with each other or maintain continuity of care for the consumer. Unfortunately, when it comes to mental health, it's safe to say that there is no such thing as one-stop shopping. If only there was a mental-health dollar store that was open 24/7. And like cancer, diabetes, or heart disease, the cost of specialized care for schizophrenia is exorbitant and can easily devour the savings of most ordinary families. In addition, family caregivers often lose time at work and may even lose their jobs because of their personal stake in being there for their loved one whenever needed — which may occur often, and which is generally unpredictable.

Because resources vary from one community to the next, there's no simple handbook or Web site that enables people to easily learn the "system" that they'll need to rely upon. Moreover, because of changing laws and regulations, the system is often in flux. Navigating the system can be particularly challenging for people who aren't sophisticated in dealing with bureaucracies or for whom the system poses language or cultural barriers. Patients, friends, and families usually find out about affordable, accessible, and high-quality resources in their respective communities simply by talking to each other and to savvy clinicians.

The stigma, discrimination, and lack of understanding associated with mental disorders historically have made mental-health treatment pretty unpopular among taxpayers. Over the last 50 years, states have drastically reduced the number of state-supported psychiatric beds (transferring costs to national and local governments) to the point where there are even waiting lists for the relatively small number of individuals who require long-term supervised residential treatment.

Often, because of gaps in community care, individuals wind up in more costly skilled nursing facilities, jails, and homeless shelters. Based on this situation, many mental-health advocates and legislators have reframed the question from "How can we afford to pay for mental healthcare?" to "How can we afford not to?"

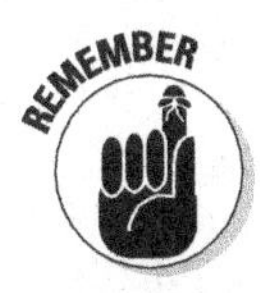

An estimated 47 million Americans have no insurance, and many fall into the lower socioeconomic brackets. Because of this, many people avoid or simply can't afford necessary care, which leads to more costly and complex problems down the road.

Finding adequate treatment is only the first step in living with schizophrenia (and one we discuss in detail in Chapters 5 and 6). The second and often more difficult step is finding the resources to pay for it. A poll conducted by the American Psychological Association and Harris Interactive in 2008 reported that 42 percent of those queried said that cost is the leading factor that discourages people from seeking out mental-health services.

The cost of treatment poses a formidable barrier for anyone with a chronic illness. Many middle-class families experience extraordinary financial strains trying to provide help and pay for care for their relatives over the long term — especially when the individual isn't able to support himself or has no health insurance or disability insurance.

In the following sections, we look at your options for paying for care for your loved one.

Although they're a complement to — rather than a substitute for — professional care and treatment, self-help and support groups (see Chapter 9) can be invaluable in providing information and support — and they're usually free! A self-help group may also help you better understand how to take advantage of the financial resources available to your loved one — members generally are happy to share information on navigating the mental healthcare system.

Private insurance

If your loved one is fortunate enough to have some type of private health insurance, you need to understand its provisions for coverage of *behavioral healthcare* (a term commonly used to include mental illness and substance-abuse treatment). Here are some of the ways in which private health insurance plans vary:

- **Which practitioners your loved one is allowed to see:** If your loved one's insurance plan is a point-of-service (POS) plan, he'll be able to go to any practitioner he wants. If his plan is a health maintenance organization (HMO) or preferred provider organization (PPO), he'll have to choose providers from a preapproved list.
- **Out-of-pocket costs of seeing an out-of-network physician:** If your loved one chooses to see someone who *isn't* on her HMO or PPO preapproved list, she may have to pay a large percentage of the cost herself. These percentages vary from one provider to the next.

- **Whether your loved one must have a referral from a primary-care doctor or case manager before he sees a psychiatric specialist:** In general, HMOs require referrals in order to see specialists, whereas PPOs do not. These individuals are often called "gatekeepers" because they try to minimize costs by preventing unnecessary or more expensive than necessary care. Some insurers have a person see the case manager before he is referred to a specialist; other times, this is handled over the phone.
- **The number and/or frequency of outpatient visits and/or days of hospitalization allowed yearly or in a lifetime:** When a person is facing a chronic illness like schizophrenia, those limits can be reached quickly.
- **The maximum dollar limits on the amount of lifetime coverage:** Again, chronic illnesses are costly, and although it may seem impossible that your loved one would ever reach the limit, it can actually happen quite quickly if your loved one needs inpatient care on a repeated basis.
- **Whether the costs of your loved one's care will be fully paid for:** Some insurance plans cover 100 percent of the cost of care. Most plans require the patient to pay deductibles, co-payments, or other types of out-of-pocket costs.
- **Whether hospitals on the plan are conveniently located and offer high-quality mental healthcare:** Just as your loved one's plan may have a list of preapproved doctors, only certain hospitals may be covered on the plan. You need to find out which hospitals are covered, and whether they offer the kind of care your loved one may need.
- **Whether psychiatric emergency care is covered and how:** If you go to an emergency room and your loved one isn't considered to be an immediate danger to himself or others, you may be sent away and referred to outpatient care.

Your insurer may define a "psychiatric emergency" according to an overly strict standard. If this happens, you may need to provide explicit evidence that your loved one is dangerous to herself of others. It's always helpful to find an ally in a physician who understands the illness and is willing to go to bat for your loved one.

- **Whether medications are paid for under the plan:** Not all plans cover all medications. Some have a list of medications that are preferred, and if your loved one needs to take a medication not on that list, he may have to pay more than he would otherwise. (See Chapter 8 for more information on medication formularies and prescription assistance plans.)

  Talk to your loved one's psychiatrist about which medications are approved by his insurance plan. She may be able to prescribe a medication that's just as effective and is covered by his insurance.

- **The age at which offspring are no longer considered dependents under family policies:** Depending on your insurer and the laws of the state where you reside, the age at which a full-time student is no longer covered under his parents insurance varies.
- **Coverage of preexisting mental conditions:** If your loved one was previously treated for a mental disorder and you change insurers, you may find that your new insurer is unwilling to cover a preexisting condition.

In general, many insurers deny claims because they are filed with insufficient information or documentation, or improper codes provided by the practitioner. This means that your loved one or you may need to take on the task of appealing denials within certain fixed periods of time. Because this entails keeping prior documentation, communicating with the healthcare provider, and responding within a timely manner, it may be a burden that you suggest helping your loved one with.

When you're selecting a plan, you need to weigh the pros and cons of each in relation to the needs and resources of your family. These are also important considerations to look into whenever *anyone* changes jobs or seeks new employment. Choose plans that provide mental-health coverage (just in case you or someone in your family becomes one of the 25 percent of Americans suffer from a diagnosable mental disorder each year). Opt for plans that allow you to choose your own practitioners if you can afford it. On the other hand, HMOs may simplify the burden of filing claims.

There are often unfair disparities in coverage for mental, behavioral, and emotional problems as compared to physical health problems. For example, a plan can set limits for mental healthcare coverage at $50,000 and set limits for physical health at 20 times that amount.

Mental-health parity is a legislative reform being enacted in many states and at the federal level that tries to restore parity (equality) so insurance benefits for mental and physical illnesses are covered equally. The federal law enacted in 1998 is imperfect — it has too many exceptions. State parity laws have attempted to close the gaps, but these laws vary from state to state. Some of the goals of mental health parity include the following:

- A single deductible for both physical and mental illness
- Equal out-of-pocket costs and/or co-payments
- No yearly or lifetime limits to the number of visits or dollars paid

Remember that even if you aren't concerned about health parity now, you never know when you or someone in your family will need mental healthcare. When you advocate for mental-health parity (and we hope you will), use this factoid: A study of health parity for federal workers found that it increased employer costs by less than 0.5 percent.

To find out about your specific mental-health benefits and coverage, check with either the human resources office of your employer, a union official if you belong to a union, or directly with your insurer. If your health plan is only subject to federal law (for example, if you're a federal employee), you can get more information from the Department of Labor by calling 866-275-7922.

If you feel that you or your loved one has been unfairly denied coverage under the terms of the insurer's contract, contact the customer service department of your insurer (preferably, in writing so you have a paper trail to document your efforts). If the insurer is still unresponsive, you can file an appeal with your state insurance commissioner. If you still get no help, contact your state and federal legislators, your state attorney general, or a private attorney or legal advocate.

Don't be completely discouraged by the costs of private mental healthcare. Whether your loved one has comprehensive insurance or not, there are usually ways to obtain the care she needs. You may be able to negotiate payments with a doctor or program so you can afford it. Even if they aren't advertised or mentioned, always inquire about sliding-fee scales or reduced fees. Don't be shy — it never hurts to ask!

Although a small proportion of people pay for their own insurance, health insurance is often unaffordable except through employer-paid coverage. Premiums for employer-sponsored health insurance have increased four times faster than employee earnings since 2000. At a time when health-insurance costs are rapidly escalating and the number of uninsured is growing, this means that many individuals and families are being priced out of necessary mental-health treatment.

Employee assistance programs (EAPs) can be a valuable resource for people who are employed. These workplace benefit programs, which are often free, provide confidential evaluation, treatment, and referral for individuals who may have personal, mental-health, financial, legal, or substance-abuse problems that might otherwise adversely affect their employment. EAPs are often limited in terms of the number of sessions made available to the employee, however. Check with your employer to find out whether you have an EAP and how to take advantage of it.

Public services for the uninsured or underinsured

Many publicly funded treatment and support programs operate on a sliding scale based on an individual's ability to pay. These programs are often operated directly by local government or funded by contracts or grants awarded to private organizations that are designed to serve individuals either with limited income or no income at all. They can be supported by local tax levies, state funds, *federal block grants* (grants that allocate money to states on the basis of some formula set by the federal government), or some combination thereof.

To find out about programs and their respective eligibility requirements, contact your city or county mental-health department. The available programs may include:

- State-supported outpatient treatment programs
- Community mental-health centers
- Nonprofit mental-health associations
- ACT or other case management programs (see Chapter 9)
- Self-help or peer-support programs
- Psychosocial rehabilitation programs
- Family psychoeducation programs
- Substance abuse treatment and recovery programs
- Clubhouses
- Consumer-operated service programs

Often, local affiliates of the National Alliance for Mental Illness (NAMI) provide consumer or family peer support services and are a valuable resource for information and referral. To find out more, go to www.nami.org or call 800-950-6264.

When someone receives treatment at a clinic, they may be assigned to see whomever is there on the day of their appointment. Try to encourage your loved one to request appointments with one clinician who will see him regularly and get to know him, helping providing continuity in care. If the person is going on vacation, have him ask the clinician to brief whomever will be covering on whatever issues are likely to arise.

Veterans' benefits

If your loved one served on active military duty, he may qualify for health-care benefits provided by the Veterans Health Administration (VHA). The VHA provides inpatient psychiatric services at 132 medical centers and outpatient mental-health services at 689 medical centers and community-based outpatient clinics. In addition, readjustment counseling services are available for veterans and their families at 209 vet centers across the nation. To find out about benefits, go to www.va.gov/health or contact the VA healthcare benefits office by phone toll-free at 877-222-8387.

The VA also maintains a staffed hot line with suicide prevention and mental-health professionals. If a veteran is in crisis, he can call the suicide hot line at 800-273-8255.

Entitlement programs

Because of the high cost of care and difficulties keeping a steady job with health benefits, most people with schizophrenia depend on benefits from Social Security, Medicaid, and Medicare. We cover all three in the following sections.

Social Security

Like people with physical disabilities, people with mental illnesses may also only be able to work intermittently, be unable to work for a lengthy period of time, or be unable to work at all. It's estimated that about 1 out of 20 people receiving Social Security benefits are people with mental disabilities.

There are two types of benefits available through the Social Security Administration (SSA):

- **Supplemental Security Income (SSI)** pays benefits to disabled adults and children based on financial need. People over the age of 65 who meet financial limits do not have to prove a disability.
- **Social Security Disability Income (SSDI)** pays benefits to people who have previously worked and paid into the Social Security system. An adult may qualify for benefits based on her parents' earnings if her disability started before age 22. Payments average about $900 per month.

Some people are entitled to both SSI and SSDI if their SSDI income is below a certain threshold.

Unfortunately, none of these benefits comes automatically (or easily), and there are criteria for determining disability based on four standards:

- Earnings
- Severity of illness
- Type of work
- Meeting the criteria on an established checklist

In general, to obtain benefits, an individual has to have a disability that interferes with his ability to work (which is expected to last at least one year) or who has a very low income. The individual also cannot have assets that exceed the limits set by the federal government.

To find out more about Social Security benefits, contact the SSA at 800-772-1213, go to the SSA Web site (www.ssa.gov), or visit your local SSA office. (You can find your local SSA office in the blue pages of your local phone book or by going to www.ssa.gov and clicking on Find a Social Security Office.)

SSA offers a Social Security Online Disability Planner at www.ssa.gov/dibplan/index.htm, which explains the benefits available, how to qualify, and how to apply. The application process entails an in-depth interview, either in person or on the phone.

Some patients and families find it hard to admit that they need help. It's a natural tendency to try to present yourself in a positive light, but when it comes to accessing benefits, you and your loved one need to present an honest — even if it's negative — portrayal if you want to qualify. On the application, make sure you list every disability that applies to your loved one. Carefully read the requirements before applying and make sure your written application shows that your loved one meets them.

For example, many individuals with schizophrenia have a co-occurring substance-abuse problem. If substance abuse is determined to be your loved one's primary problem, she'll be turned down for SSI or SSDI because the laws were changed in the 1990s so that people cannot receive disability payments on the basis of addiction alone. On the other hand, if mental illness is considered the primary disorder, your loved one *will* be eligible for these benefits. By denying the primacy of their son or daughter's mental disorder, parents may be inadvertently sabotaging that individual's chance to receive benefits that could support treatment and recovery.

The application process for benefits can be complicated, especially if the person applying is unable to respond to questions appropriately or accurately because of the symptoms of her illness. If your loved one is in this situation, she may need someone to assist her — a friend, relative, or lawyer, for example.

Expect to be turned down on your first application; it happens frequently. The government apparently looks at the application process as a type of weeding-out process, where only the truly needy or deserving who persist long enough wind up getting benefits. Initially, two out of three applicants are turned down — but upon appeal to an administrative law judge, more than two-thirds of those denials are overturned. People are often discouraged because it can take many months to process an application for disability, but don't let it dissuade you.

Local governments can provide temporary public assistance (called Temporary Assistance for Needy Families) during this waiting period in the form of healthcare, food stamps, transportation, and rental assistance. If at first you don't succeed, appeal! You may need to find a legal advocate or attorney to help you.

If you need assistance filing your claim or making an appeal, there are two national groups who maintain lists of people who can assist you:

- **The National Association of Disability Representatives (NADR):** 800-747-6131 or www.nadr.org
- **The National Organization of Social Security Claimants' Representatives (NOSSCR):** 800-431-2804 or www.nosscr.org

Applying for public benefits can be a tedious and cumbersome process. Whenever possible, ask for help from a case manager or social worker. Make friends in every office you set foot in; fair or unfair, people will go out of their way for people they like. Also, many benefit forms require similar information — keep copies of every form you file in one place so you can easily retrieve the information the next time you need it.

After your loved one qualifies for SSI, it paves the way for his eligibility for other benefits such as Medicaid and food stamps.

Work incentives

People with schizophrenia want more than a paycheck; they look toward employment as a path to self-sufficiency. Many people fear, however, that if they work, they'll lose the very benefits that provide a safety net for them if they become too sick to work again. Under certain conditions, it's possible for people with mental illnesses to work and still receive monthly payments (either SSI or SSDI) as well as Medicaid or Medicare. This is called the *work incentive program.* Further information about work incentives can be found at www.ssa.gov/disabilityresearch/wi/generalinfo.htm. You can also order publications by calling 800-772-1213.

Another resource on the Web: The Ticket to Work Program (www.yourtickettowork.com) is intended to provide people with disabilities with the services they need to land competitive jobs.

Medicaid

Medicaid is a form of health insurance for individuals and families with low incomes who are considered "medically needy" and meet other eligibility requirements. Although the program is governed by the federal government and has some uniform requirements, Medicaid is administered by states so the eligibility requirements, services covered, and rates of payment differ from one state to the next.

Help your loved one get on Medicaid as soon as humanly possible. Get over the stigma or shame you may feel about having to rely on public benefits; you'll only be doing your loved one a disservice by procrastinating. Medicaid opens the door to an array of services that may not be available from any other payer, including private insurers. These include case management, community treatment, and residential treatment services. And remember that Medicaid eligibility is based on your loved one's income, not yours. The sooner he's on Medicaid, the sooner he'll be able to take advantage of these resources.

Unlike SSI or SSDI, which are paid to individuals, Medicaid is paid to the practitioner or program providing the services; in some instances, a patient co-pay is required.

You can find information about Medicaid at `www.cms.hhs.gov/home/medicaid.asp`. For contact information for state Medicaid offices, go to `www.cms.hhs.gov/home/medicaid.asp`. You can also obtain state-specific information in person by going to local welfare or medical assistance offices in your community.

The types of mental-health and rehabilitative services eligible for Medicaid reimbursement vary depending on the state Medicaid plan. To find out more about services funded by specific states, go to `http://mentalhealth.samhsa.gov/publications/allpubs/sma07%2D4301`. The report includes a table of the specific services funded by each state.

Medicare

Medicare is the health-insurance portion of Social Security. To qualify for Medicare, your loved one must be over the age of 65, disabled, or blind. Medicare has hospital insurance (Part A), medical insurance (Part B), and prescription-drug coverage (Part D). Similar to SSDI, eligibility is based on your loved one's history of paying Social Security taxes when he worked or those paid by her parents or spouse.

To find information about Medicare, go to `www.medicare.gov`. Also, the Center for Medicare Advocacy provides a detailed summary of Medicare coverage for mental health services at `www.medicareadvocacy.org/FAQ_MentalHealth.htm`.

Some Medicare health plans (like HMOs and PPOs) cover prescription drugs as part of the plan. The Centers for Medicare & Medicaid Services (CMS) have made available a Prescription Drug Plan Finder (`www.medicare.gov/MPDPF/home.asp`) to find and compare drug plans that meet your personal needs, but because Part D is extremely tough to figure out, you may want to ask a case manager or other mental-health advocate for advice and assistance.

One bit of good news: The newly enacted Medicare Improvements for Patients and Providers Act of 2008 lowers co-payments for people with mental illnesses. Until now, Medicare beneficiaries had been paying a 50 percent co-pay for mental-health treatment, including therapy. Over the next several years, the co-pay will gradually be lowered to 20 percent, the same as beneficiaries pay for primary-care doctor visits.

The Bazelon Center for Mental Health Care has created a worksheet to help consumers select the right Medicare drug plan for them. You can find it at www.bazelon.org/issues/drugs/drugplandirections.htm.

Coverage under Medicare and Medicaid is very complex. Don't hesitate to contact your local Social Security office to ask for help.

The Medicare Rights Center (www.medicarerights.org) can be an invaluable resource. The Center provides free counseling services for people with Medicare problems and maintains a consumer hot line at 800-333-4114 to answer questions about choices, the appeals process, or complaints about care or treatment.

You can find some additional information on Medicare in *Eldercare For Dummies,* by Rachelle Zukerman, PhD (Wiley).

College mental healthcare

If your loved one has a first break while at college, find out whether a student health service fee has been included as part of her tuition. Many colleges encourage students to pay for health insurance, and some insist on it, offering a time-limited health insurance policy, at the time of enrollment and each subsequent year, that often includes mental healthcare for uninsured students.

Many colleges offer counseling that may not be especially helpful at the time of a serious break, but that may be *very* helpful for a student returning to school after treatment who's stabilized and doing well on medication.

Clinical studies and trials

Clinical studies and trials (see Chapter 10) are another option for obtaining high-quality care. In many areas (especially places that have academic medical institutions), your loved one may be able to participate in a clinical study designed to assess treatments for schizophrenia. Very often, during the course of a study, the costs of clinical assessment and tests are free, and there is reimbursement for associated travel expenses. In some cases, there's also a small stipend for time spent for longer or more-frequent-than-usual evaluations.

The quality of care received during the research is usually quite good. In any study, a participant is allowed to withdraw from participation at any time, and withdrawal from the study cannot adversely affect their treatment afterwards.

To find out if there are any studies going on where you live, go to `www.clinicaltrials.gov` and search by the diagnosis *schizophrenia.*

You and your loved one need to be fully informed about the study and possible risks and benefits.

If your loved one is considering enrolling in a clinical trial, discuss the pros and cons with the clinician currently responsible for your loved one's psychiatric care or even with your family doctor.

Working with Schizophrenia: Your Legal Rights on the Job

When your loved one is diagnosed with a serious and stigmatizing illness, like schizophrenia, she may be reluctant to tell her employer or colleagues. In the meantime, she may endure various challenges connected with the disease and its treatment. Medications may make her drowsy or impair her ability to concentrate. She may have self-doubts about her own ability to perform and may worry what her supervisor and colleagues will think of her or say. Should she tell them about her diagnosis, or should she keep it a secret?

If she missed time at work and was on sick leave, she doesn't necessarily have to tell anyone in her workplace what happened. The decision is hers to make. If she has no problem performing her job, she'll probably be more reluctant to reveal the diagnosis. But if she's having problems returning to work, she's less likely to find support in the workplace and she may find it uncomfortable if she provides no explanation for what others may see as laziness or inefficiency. Depending on her limitations, she may even risk her job by not saying anything.

Your loved one needs to find out about her rights under the American with Disabilities Act (ADA) and the Family Medical Leave Act (FMLA). Depending on the type of place where she works, she may or may not be covered by these pieces of federal legislation. Interpreting these laws is complicated. You or your loved one may need to talk to an attorney.

The Americans with Disabilities Act

The ADA, enacted in 1990, makes it unlawful for private employers with 15 or more employers, state and local governments, employment agencies, labor organizations, and management committees to discriminate in employment against a qualified individual with a disability that substantially limits one or more life activities.

Disability is broadly defined to include neurological symptoms, mental disorders, or psychological disorders.

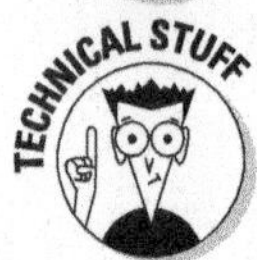

The ADA does not apply to discrimination in federal employment, which is prohibited under Title V of the Rehabilitation Act of 1973.

Under the ADA, an employer cannot discriminate in hiring individuals with disabilities who are capable of performing a job. If your loved one is applying for a new job, an employer cannot ask him about a disability, nor can he be required to take a medical exam before a job offer.

After your loved one has been hired, his employer can't ask him questions about his disability unless they pertain to the functions of the job. And if your loved one has a mental disability that substantially limits a major life activity, his employer may have responsibilities under the ADA to provide reasonable accommodations so he can perform his job. Reasonable accommodations may include flex time, leave for outpatient appointments or hospitalization, assignment of a supportive supervisor, and more feedback about job performance.

Of course, if your loved one doesn't disclose his disability, it may be more difficult for his employer to understand what's going on and to come up with a reasonable accommodation — which may be an argument for your loved one telling his employer about his schizophrenia.

If your loved one does decide to disclose his schizophrenia to his employer, he has several options:

- He can merely state that he has a medical condition.
- He can say he has a brain or emotional disorder, or a chemical imbalance.
- He can tell his employer his specific diagnosis.

For more information about your loved one's employment rights as an individual with a disability, go to www.eeoc.gov/facts/ada18.html. To find information on how to file a complaint with the U.S. Department of Justice, call 800-541-0301.

The Family and Medical Leave Act

Under The Family and Medical Leave Act (FMLA), an employee covered by the act is entitled to 12 weeks of unpaid leave during a 12-month period for certain family and medical reasons. Plus, it's against the law for an employer to use a person's decision to take leave as a factor in firing her or denying promotions. To find more information about FMLA, go to www.dol.gov/esa/whd/fmla.

Your loved one's psychiatrist, case manager, or job counselor may be able to offer guidance on making some tricky decisions. They can help your loved one assess her illness and its possible impact on her work. Another key advisor may be the human resources department; they can help advise your loved one about the employer's sick leave policies and whether she has options such as part-time or flex-time employment.

In a supportive work setting, disclosing as much as your loved one feels comfortable disclosing to her supervisor and colleagues can help her better meet the demands of her job. Also, if an emergency occurs, the employer will be in a position to respond appropriately. But it's always prudent to be selective in whom you tell, what you say, and when you say it. Your loved one will have to trust her instincts, and the advice of others when it comes to deciding whether or not to disclose schizophrenia to an employer.

If your loved one tells her employer, she should remind them that any health information she provides is confidential.

Planning for Your Loved One's Care after You're Gone

If you're caring for someone with schizophrenia, you may worry about what will happen to her if you die or can no longer take care of him. Planning for the future is fraught with emotional and logistical complexities.

The goal of future-care planning is to minimize current stress, concern, and worry for caregivers and to minimize disruption and problems for their loved ones in the future. Families generally want to provide their loved one with as much independence as possible and with sufficient resources, within realistic limits.

Some of the issues that you may need to plan for include the following:

- Where will your loved one live?
- Who will bear financial responsibility for his care?
- What types of insurance will be in place?
- Who will make treatment decisions if your loved one is unable to make them on his own?
- How will healthcare emergencies be handled and by whom?
- Who will oversee or help manage your loved one's financial and legal affairs? Will she need someone to handle her entitlements (known as a *representative payee*)?

Everyone involved needs to be in on the planning and decisions necessary to identify and resolve all the issues related to future care:

- Your loved one should have a large say in his own future.
- Caregivers and providers will need to weigh in and help identify whether those preferences are realistic and appropriate, and how they can best be achieved.
- Families often find that they also need to involve lawyers or other professionals because planning for the future often involves wills, inheritances, and property issues. Consult with an attorney who specializes in estate planning for families with a person with a disability.

For example, under ordinary circumstances a disabled adult cannot have assets that exceed $2,000, excluding his home or car. However, families can get around this rule if they set up a *special needs trust* (also called a *supplemental needs trust*). Instead of leaving an inheritance directly to a loved one with schizophrenia (or any other disability) and potentially jeopardizing her continued eligibility for SSI and Medicaid benefits, the law enables you to establish a trust. A trustee named by the family is able to hold and manage the inheritance for the person with schizophrenia while the person continues to receive SSI and Medicaid.

To simplify some of these challenges, NAMI has helped establish a national, nonprofit Planned Lifetime Assistance Network comprised of more than 23 programs in 18 states across the country to serve as a safety net for the future and also to help parents who can't handle the current burden of care on their own. At a minimum, each program tries to resolve three key service issues for families and their relatives:

- The development of a care plan
- Identification of resources to support the care plan
- A person to carry out the plan

You can find a list of state PLAN programs with contact information at `www.nationalplanalliance.org`. You can also call 518-587-3372 or e-mail npa@nycap.rr.com for more information.

Part III
Treating Schizophrenia

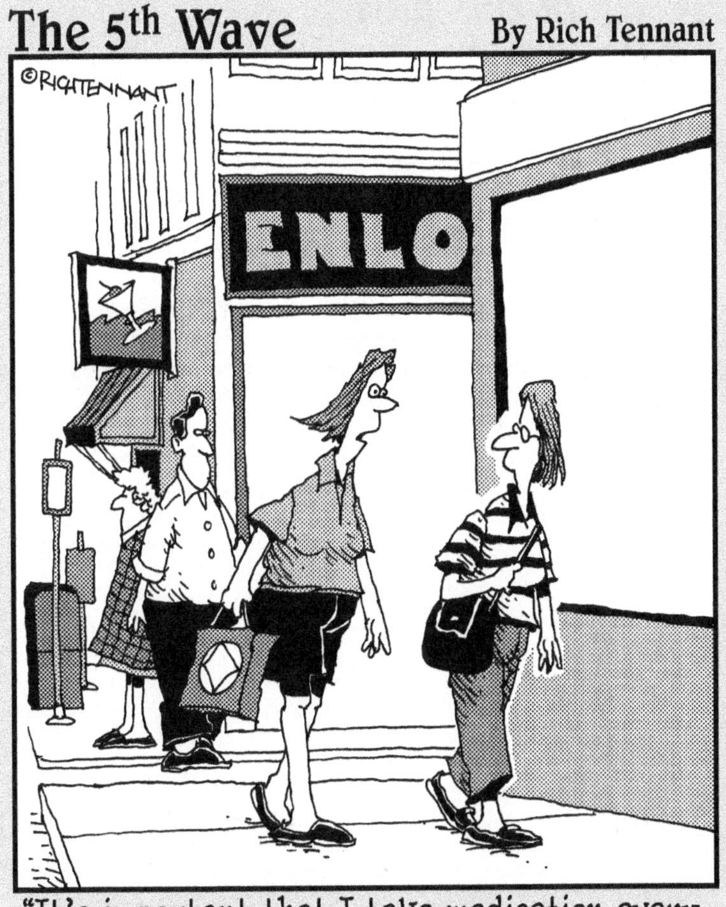

"It's important that I take medication every day to stabilize my condition. But the most important thing I have to remember to take is the good with the bad."

In this part . . .

Here we fill you in on the different types of treatment available for schizophrenia. Medication is the mainstay of schizophrenia treatment, but medications only control symptoms and aren't a cure. Finding the right medication with minimal side effects for any individual is still a process of informed trial and error. In this part, we explain the benefits and common side effects of antipsychotic medications and other drugs used to treat the symptoms of schizophrenia. We also describe the range of psychosocial and psychological treatments that can improve the odds of better treatment outcomes. Despite the best doctors and best treatments, some people with schizophrenia have symptoms that remain resistant to current treatments. Because research provides hope for the future, we explain what you need to know about research, identify promising new approaches, and provide cautions about untested treatments that provide false hope.

Chapter 8

Medication and Other Medical Approaches

In This Chapter

- Understanding how medications work
- Looking at commonly prescribed medications
- Finding the right medication
- Minimizing serious side effects
- Enhancing medication compliance

One of the most important advances in the treatment of schizophrenia over the last half-century has been the discovery of antipsychotic medications — medications that reduce the troubling symptoms of schizophrenia and give people with schizophrenia the chance to live normal lives. Today, medication is considered the mainstay of schizophrenia treatment.

In this chapter, we look at the different types of medications available and their common side effects. We also cover the importance of compliance, the family's role in helping ensure that their loved one stays on medications, and some of the difficulties you and your psychiatrist may experience in finding a medication that works. We also look at other medical therapies such as electroshock treatment and review the pros and cons of their use in conjunction with medication. (For information on psychosocial and other psychological treatments, turn to Chapter 9.)

Antipsychotic Medications

Antipsychotic medications have revolutionized the treatment of mental illness, including schizophrenia. In the following sections, we look at how and why they work, explain the difference between first- and second-generation drugs, and delve into treatment guidelines and what they mean for you. (If you're interested in the history of these medications, check out the nearby sidebar, "The first antipsychotic medications," for more information.)

The first antipsychotic medications

Before the discovery that certain medications could effectively reduce the symptoms of schizophrenia, most people with schizophrenia spent their time locked away from society in institutions. Various attempts were made to "treat" the disturbing symptoms of psychosis — hallucinations, delusions, suspiciousness, agitation, and disorganized thinking — but no tested treatments existed that were proven to be safe and effective.

There were some early efforts to use medications, along with other therapies, but the medications used at the time were mainly sedatives. And sedatives had to be given in such large doses that they were more likely to put people to sleep, cause confusion, or make people unable to react than they were to tame the symptoms associated with the disorder.

Then, in France, in 1952, a new medication, chlorpromazine (brand name: Thorazine) was developed for an entirely different purpose — to reduce the chance of cardiovascular shock during surgery. Serendipitously, when the medication was tried in agitated psychotic patients, doctors found that it calmed them without causing the sedation or drowsiness associated with sedatives. This was a watershed moment in the treatment of schizophrenia. It eventually led to the release of patients from institutions, a reduction in the number of psychiatric beds needed, and a new ability to treat people with schizophrenia in less restrictive settings.

Pharmaceutical companies were eager to make their own version of this new "tranquilizer," clinicians were excited that they finally had a promising tool in their medicine bags, and researchers wanted to find out how the drug worked, because they knew it might offer clues about what was wrong with the brains of people with schizophrenia.

Understanding how medications work on the brain

In order to understand how antipsychotics work on the brain, you need to understand how the brain is organized and how it works. The brain is an organ, and all organs of the body can be thought of as having a structure, a function, and a resultant action.

The *structure* of the brain (shown in Figure 8-1) is more complicated than most other organs. It has four lobes — the frontal lobe, the parietal lobe, the temporal lobe, and the occipital lobe. Within these structures, there is gray matter (made up of cells) and white matter (which is more like insulated electrical wires).

There are some 100 billion cells in the brain, although the actual number mainly decreases over the course of a person's lifetime. Because the cells are very close to each other, they can communicate over the very small spaces between them; these spaces are called *synapses.* The way in which the cells communicate is both electrical and chemical. If a cell is stimulated, it produces a very small amount of a chemical, called a *neurotransmitter,* for a very short period of time (literally fractions of a second). This chemical stimulates the receptor on the next cell — if that cell has the matching neurotransmitter receptors. This chemical stimulation leads to a miniscule increase in electrical voltage inside the cell (brought about by opening of sodium ion channels) compared to the cell's environment.

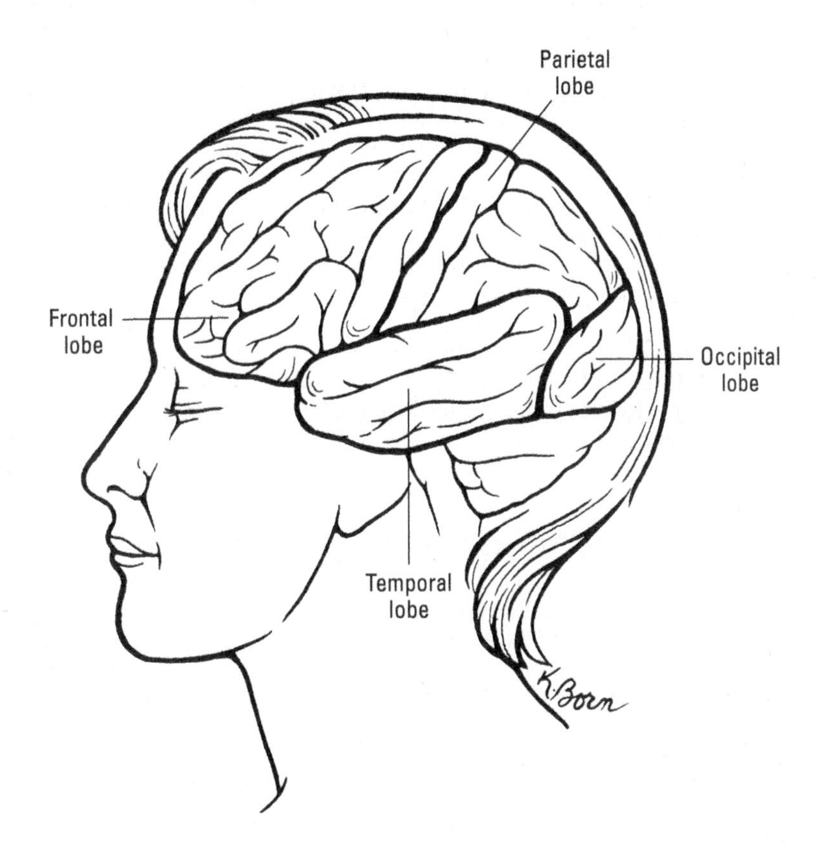

Figure 8-1: The brain is divided into four lobes, making the brain one of the more complicated organs in the human body.

Based on how often the cells stimulate one another and their locations in the brain, they become organized into circuits. You can think of these circuits as "wires" that "connect" one part of the brain to another. Some of the circuits are specialized for the senses (such as sight and sound), some are specialized for thinking, and some are specialized for different moods. All these structures give rise to the *function* of the brain called the *mind,* which refers to all the conscious and automatic (unconscious) activities of thinking, feeling, sensing, and integrating (or organizing). The *resultant action* of the mind is *behavior,* what a person does (such as eating, sleeping, loving, and so on).

Through the use of precise electrical, chemical, and imaging techniques, scientists now know that medications that affect behavior work, to a large extent, by raising or lowering the amount of neurotransmitters (or the sensitivity of the transmitters) found in the different areas of the brain. In this way, a medication influences the important cell connections in the brain. If a neurotransmitter is involved with thinking, mood, or perception, it can affect the symptoms seen in schizophrenia.

Of course, the brain isn't quite that simple. There are multiple neurotransmitters that can all influence each other and the cells they stimulate. Some of the major neurotransmitters are dopamine, glutamine, serotonin, norepinephrine, and gamma-aminobutyric acid (GABA).

The earliest antipsychotic medications, which resulted in a tranquilizing effect, and all the similar antipsychotic medications that have since been developed influence the *dopamine system,* which is involved with the positive symptoms of schizophrenia. (See Chapter 3 for more on positive symptoms.)

Introducing first-generation medications

After the introduction of the first antipsychotic drug, chlorpromazine (brand name: Thorazine), in the early 1950s, other pharmaceutical companies marketed similar medications, which are now collectively referred to as *first-generation antipsychotics.* Table 8-1 identifies the most commonly prescribed first-generation antipsychotic medications.

First-generation antipsychotics are also sometimes called *typical antipsychotics* or *conventional antipsychotics.*

All the first-generation medications are equally effective (on average) in controlling the symptoms of schizophrenia. However, for reasons still unknown, some people seem to respond better to one antipsychotic medication than they do to another.

Table 8-1 Commonly Prescribed First-Generation Antipsychotic Medications

Generic Name	*Brand Name*
Chlorpromazine	Largactil, Thorazine
Fluphenazine	Permitil, Proloxin
Haloperidol	Haldol
Loxapine	Loxitane
Molindone	Moban
Perphenazine	Trilafon
Thioridazine	Mellaril
Thiothixene	Navane
Trifluoperazine	Stelazine

Among people treated with these first-generation antipsychotic agents, about 35 percent do not have a good therapeutic response (defined as still having *positive symptoms* after trying two or more different medications for the recommended period of time). This condition is referred to as *treatment resistance* and, until about 1990 and the development of second-generation medications, few other proven alternatives were available to patients or their doctors.

Moving on to a second generation of meds

In 1990, clozapine (brand name: Clozaril), an antipsychotic medication marketed outside the United States, proved to be successful in a large clinical study that looked at treatment-resistant patients (see the preceding section). Remarkably, researchers found that about one out of three previously treatment-resistant patients significantly improved after taking clozapine.

However, clozapine had a serious drawback. In about 1 percent of people, it caused a marked and sudden decrease in white blood cells — a condition that can be fatal. So, in order to prevent this problem, anyone taking clozapine had to have weekly white blood cell counts before their prescriptions could be renewed. After some time, the blood draw could be reduced to every two weeks, and then monthly. As you can probably predict, many potential users of clozapine weren't happy with the idea of having to get their blood drawn so often, just to stay on this medication.

After clozapine was marketed in the United States, other pharmaceutical companies rushed to develop medications that would be as effective as clozapine without the effect of decreasing the white blood cell count. In 1994, risperidone (brand name: Risperdal) was the first of a new group of antipsychotic medications to hit the market. Collectively, these new antipsychotics are referred to as *second-generation antipsychotics.* Table 8-2 lists the most commonly prescribed second-generation antipsychotic medications.

Second-generation antipsychotic medications are also sometimes called *novel antipsychotics* or *atypical antipsychotics.*

Table 8-2 Commonly Prescribed Second-Generation Antipsychotic Medications

Generic Name	*Brand Name*
Aripiprazole	Abilify
Clozapine	Clozaril
Olanzapine	Zyprexa
Paliperidone	Invega
Quetiapine	Seroquel
Risperidone	Risperdal, Consta
Ziprasidone	Geodon

Unfortunately, other second-generation medications haven't proven to be as effective as clozapine in treatment-resistant schizophrenia, but they offer one important advantage over first-generation antipsychotics: They're far less likely to cause adverse motor side effects (such as stiffness, tremors, or Parkinsonian-like abnormal involuntary movements).

In part, as a result of the aggressive marketing of these new medications, they're now much more widely prescribed than first-generation antipsychotics in spite of their significantly higher costs.

Following treatment guidelines

Given the large number of antipsychotic medications available, it's not surprising that a variety of professional associations and government agencies have published treatment guidelines (also called *practice guidelines*).

Being the first to receive new drugs

When new medications come to market (whether for schizophrenia or any other physical or mental disorder), it's not necessarily a good idea to be first in line to try them. There are several reasons for this:

- **The proof for efficacy required by the U.S. Food and Drug Administration (FDA) is only that a new medication is more effective than a placebo, not more effective than other medications already on the market.** A *placebo* is what used to be called a sugar pill — it looks just like the real thing, but it doesn't have any medication in it. So, in other words, the drug just has to be better than nothing.
- **Because new medications have, on average, only been given to about 3,000 people before a drug is on the market, it's not uncommon for new and possibly dangerous side effects to be discovered only after the medication has been given to hundreds of thousands of people or for longer periods of time than when the drug was being studied.**
- **The new medication almost always costs significantly more than the older medication, especially if a *generic* (non-brand-name) equivalent of the older medication exists.**

If your loved one is not doing well and all the older medications have been tried and failed, you may welcome the opportunity to try a new medication. Be sure to ask your psychiatrist if the new medication represents a truly new approach or is more likely a "me, too" variation of an older product. "Me, too" drugs are generally more expensive (so they're heavily promoted by pharmaceutical manufacturers) and tend to have more unknown risks because there's less experience using them on large numbers of people.

Treatment guidelines provide recommendations, either based on research or expert consensus, to guide practitioners on how to assess and treat various psychiatric disorders. Although these guidelines differ in detail, they consistently recommend the following for antipsychotic treatment of schizophrenia:

1. **Start with a single antipsychotic medication (usually a second-generation medication), and evaluate the efficacy of that medication in four to six weeks.**
2. **If the first medication has not reduced the patient's symptoms, try another antipsychotic medication — either first- or second-generation.**
3. **If there still is no good response to treatment, try clozapine (brand name: Clozaril).**

Many guidelines are also written specifically for consumers and their families. The federal government maintains an online clearinghouse of these documents at the National Guideline Clearinghouse (`www.guideline.gov`). Reading through practice guidelines can't make you a doctor, but it can inform you about various treatment decisions your loved one will be making with her doctor, and it can help you raise the right questions.

Starting on an Antipsychotic Medication

Medication decisions can be complicated and frustrating. Medications for schizophrenia may have to be changed, increased, decreased, and tinkered with to obtain optimal results. This situation can be frustrating for both patients and families, not to mention expensive, if new medications need to be bought before the old ones are used up. In this section, we look at the different factors that go into finding the right medication for each patient.

Recognizing the reason for trial and error

Deciding on the perfect drug for a particular patient isn't an easy task. Although many studies have been conducted to find the "right drug for the right patient," trial and error is still the only way to find the drug that works best with fewest side effects for a given individual. Usually, medication decisions are made on the basis of the potential side effects associated with different medications (for example, drowsiness, abnormal movements, drop in blood pressure, or weight gain), as well as the physical and mental state of the patient.

If the patient has ever been treated with an antipsychotic medication before, it helps the doctor to know what medications were used, whether they were successful in controlling symptoms, and whether they produced any uncomfortable side effects. This is where family and friends (or the person with schizophrenia) can be extremely helpful in working with the doctor to choose an antipsychotic medication.

Patients and their families should always keep a summary of the medication someone has taken, with the information listed in more detail in Chapter 14, so they have it available when it is needed.

Selecting the proper dose

Every FDA-approved medication has a *recommended dose,* which is the result of studies carried out before a drug goes on the market. However, with increased experience with the drug (both by your psychiatrist and others), the dosage found to be most beneficial may change even though the labeling does not.

For example, after risperidone (the first of the second-generation medications after clozapine) was marketed, it was found that the 8-milligram dose was higher than needed in most patients, and 4 to 6 milligrams rather than 8 to 16 milligrams became the dosage commonly used. Conversely, with other second-generation drugs such as ziprasidone (trade name, Geodon) and quetiapine (trade name, Seroquel) the initial doses recommended were found to be too low. The point is that sometimes the dose the psychiatrist prescribes may be different from what the package insert says is the recommended dose.

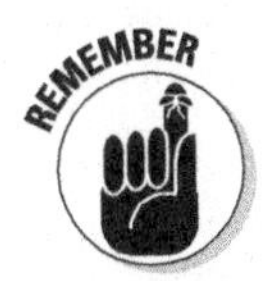

Finding a doctor who is familiar with the most up-to-date research on dosing, and who has experience gleaned from treating a large number or people with schizophrenia, is essential to receiving the correct dose of medication for your loved one, guided by what it says on the package insert.

The characteristics of the person receiving the medication are another important factor that influences dosing. For example, on average, heavier people will be prescribed higher doses than lighter people. Older people, children, and people with other health problems (heart, liver, or kidney problems, for example) will also receive lower doses.

Most pharmacies now provide printed information about the medications they're dispensing. It's a good idea to read this information, especially when a new medication is prescribed. The U.S. National Library of Medicine has a Web site (`http://druginfo.nlm.nih.gov`), where you can find consumer-friendly and trustworthy information about most medications; you can access it by entering either the generic or brand name of the drug. Many other sites provide information about drugs, but you need to assess the quality of the site (see Chapter 10).

Looking toward personalized medicine

A psychiatrist isn't able to use a crystal ball to consistently select the right drug for a patient. Instead, psychiatrists have to resort to a regimen of trial and error. This is frustrating to patients who sometimes say they're being used as human guinea pigs, and it's also frustrating to doctors who want to get it right the first time. But it isn't all that different from treatment for many other medical disorders (such as high blood pressure, arthritis, and so on).

In both general medicine and psychiatry, there's reason to hope that this may soon change. As more knowledge is gained about the human genome, it appears that small differences in genes may lead to differences in response to different medications. As research proceeds, it may become possible to analyze a person's individual genome and select the right drug from the get-go. This approach has been called *personalized medicine.*

Choosing the form of medication: Tablets, pills, liquids, or injections

The form and route of administration is another decision to be made with some medications. Many antipsychotic medications not only come in different oral forms, but also may be given by injection in slow-release and rapid-acting forms.

Swallowing tablets, pills, or liquids

Many medications are taken orally (by mouth), but there can be difficulties using oral medications. Some people have a hard time swallowing pills, and others avoid taking their medications by only pretending to swallow pills and later spitting them out (known as *cheeking*).

Although tablets and capsules are the most common oral forms for antipsychotic medications, there are also liquid preparations (useful for older adults and children), which can be added to some juices or squirted into the mouth. There are also quick-dissolving tablets, which when placed under the tongue, dissolve and are absorbed quickly; these are useful when people have difficulty swallowing or if they're cheeking the medication.

Cheeking sometimes leads to a diagnosis of "treatment-resistant schizophrenia" when, in fact, the medication never had a chance to have a therapeutic effect. If cheeking is suspected (although it is sometimes very difficult to detect), blood samples can be taken to see if medication is, in fact, in the person's system.

Injectable medications

Injection, usually into muscle (either the shoulder or buttocks) is another route of administration, but one that is not very popular in the United States. Not all first- or second-generation antipsychotics are available in injectable form, and there are two very different kinds of injectable medications that are given for different purposes: rapid-acting and slow-release *(depot).*

Rapid-acting forms

A rapid-acting form of injection (such as haloperidol, chlorpromazine, olanzapine, or zyprasidone) is usually given when a psychotic person is very agitated, aggressive, and uncooperative, either at a doctor's office or in a clinic or hospital. Although no one likes injections, the purpose of doing this is to rapidly calm the patient so that he will be more cooperative in taking oral medication and more amenable to verbal or behavioral therapies.

These injections are not given as a punishment (as is sometime portrayed in movies or books); instead, they should be thought of in the same way that an injection is given to someone who can't breathe after a bee sting. It is a temporary measure to get a potentially dangerous or out-of-control situation under control, and assure the patient's safety until he's amenable to other treatment.

Slow-release forms

Another type of injectable antipsychotic medication is purposely designed as a slow-release form. (These are *depot* (extended-release) forms of some first- and second-generation antipsychotics that can be given by mouth.) The advantage of the injections is that they can be taken roughly once or twice a month, avoiding the daily medication hassles that often occur when people have schizophrenia (see the "Why people refuse to take or stop taking medication" section, later in this chapter).

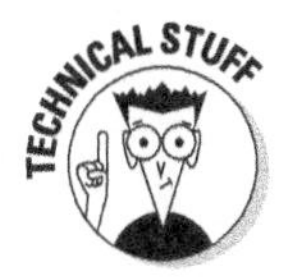

Slow-release antipsychotic injections are known as *depot* medications in the medical community. You may hear members of your loved one's medical team refer to the medication by this term.

One distinct advantage to slow-release injections is that if a person taking a slow-release antipsychotic starts showing *more* symptoms, a clinician can rule out noncompliance as the cause.

There are two slow-release first-generation antipsychotics available in the United States: haloperidol (brand name: Haldol) and fluphenazine (brand name: Prolixin). A slow-release form of the second-generation antipsychotic risperidone (brand name: Consta) is also available.

As of this writing, slow-release forms of olanzapine and a risperidone metabolite (paliperidone) are currently under review at the FDA for possible marketing.

Another advantage to slow-release injections is that if your loved one is not doing well, the oral form of the medication can be given (increasing the dose) without the person having to take an entirely new medication. Also, when someone moves from an inpatient to outpatient setting and it may take some time before the person gets appointment see her doctor, a long-acting medication can smooth the transition until she's seen.

Deciding on dosing schedules

Some medications are taken only once a day, while others are taken every few hours. This is partly based on a medication's *pharmacology* (how long its effect lasts), sometimes how large a dose needs to be given, and whether the treatment is just being started or has been taken for some time.

Certain antipsychotic medications have a long *half-life* (the time it takes for half the medication to leave the body) and even if they're given only once a day, they can have an effect for a full 24 hours. Others have a shorter half-life and must be given two or more times a day to have their continued desired effect.

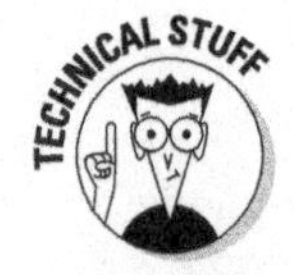

The measure *half-life* is used because it allows a comparison of the duration of effect (action) of similar medications and, therefore, how often during the day the medication has to be taken.

Obviously, if a person with schizophrenia objects to taking medication or is forgetful, or if no one is around to be sure he takes his medication, a medication with a longer half-life is better. If this situation applies to your loved one, you may want to raise the issue with his doctor.

Missing a single dose of a medication given only once a day is more significant than missing a single dose of a medication given several times a day. Making up for missed doses of medication by giving a larger amount at the next dose is usually not possible — in fact, doing so can actually cause an overdose. If your loved one misses a dose, continue with the next regular dose, and don't try to make up for missed doses.

Very often, when medication is first started, it will be prescribed in smaller doses several times a day. Then, as blood levels build up and if there are no serious adverse effects (such as drowsiness, dizziness, fainting, and so on), the frequency of administration can be reduced. Usually the dose to be given once a day is increased and is preferably taken just before bedtime.

Tying the time of administration to a daily activity (especially waking up in the morning or before going to bed in the evening) is helpful as a reminder to take medication. It's also helpful (and sometimes necessary) to take the medication at the same time(s) every day so blood levels never get too high or too low.

Some medications need to be taken with food in order to be fully absorbed; others need to be taken on an empty stomach. In addition, some medications need to be taken alone — taking them with other pills at the same time could reduce the effectiveness of the drugs. Be sure your loved one follows the doctor's instructions on how to take medications. If you and your loved one aren't sure, ask. When and how someone takes medication can make a big difference.

Managing Medication Adjustments

Taking antipsychotic medications often isn't as straightforward for people with schizophrenia as it is for someone with a physical condition.

Medications may need to be changed, doses may need adjusting, and keeping a list of when to take multiple medications can be daunting for anyone, especially a patient struggling with mental-health issues.

There are some general rules for managing a regimen of antipsychotic medications, however, that apply in most cases. After your loved one starts on medication, it's important that she does the following:

- **Take it as prescribed — the correct number of pills or capsules, the prescribed number of times per day, and with the prescribed time intervals in between.** For example, a medicine taken twice a day usually should be taken 12 hours apart unless the doctor gives other directions (for example, take with meals).
- **Tell the psychiatrist how she's been doing since the last time she was seen.** Are her symptoms better, the same, or worse?
- **Tell the psychiatrist if she's having any new or different symptoms or health problems.** These may be related to the medication, and the doctor will want to make that determination.

Switching and adding medications

Even when your loved one follows doctor's orders and does everything he's supposed to do, the first medication he takes may not work right away. Let's say he's been taking a prescribed medication for four to six weeks and the symptoms that brought him to the doctor aren't that much better or some others symptoms (possibly related to the medication) are giving him problems. It's possible that the medication may not be the right one for him. In that case, your loved one, his doctor, and you have a variety of alternatives to choose from in terms of deciding on the next steps. These include

- Raising or lowering the dose of the current medication
- Switching to another medication
- Adding another medication from a different class of drugs (discussed later in this chapter)
- Adding another medication from the same class of drugs

Good reasons for switching include:

- When the symptoms for which the medicine was prescribed don't improve or even get worse
- When the medication is giving your loved one other symptoms (for example, drowsiness, sleeplessness, weight gain, or dizziness) that are making her life more difficult

- When you or your loved one wants the doctor to consider whether another medication may be better for her (either a medication that's more effective or one with fewer side effects)

When everyone has decided that you should make a switch and there's a clear rationale for doing so, the question always arises of how long it'll take and how you'll know if it was a good idea. Some of the questions you'll want to discuss with the doctor, if you all agree to switch medications, include the following:

- **Are you switching my loved one to a drug for the same indication as the one she was taking before, within the same class of drugs?**

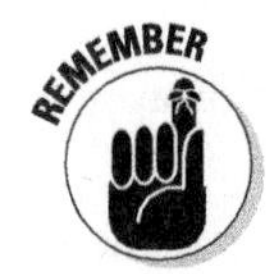

  The term *indication* is used to identify a diagnosis or symptom that a drug is designed to treat. When pharmaceutical manufacturers go to the FDA, they provide evidence of the safety and effectiveness of a drug for a specific indication. When a drug is used for indications other than the one or ones for which it was approved, a practice that is legal, the use is considered *off-label.*

- **Will you be adding a new medication to her older one — but for the same indication?**
- **How is the switch going to be made?** Will it be abrupt or will there be a gradual reduction of the original medication as the new one is gradually increased?
- **Are there any side effects we should be aware of or report to you if they occur?**
- **When and how (in person, by phone) should we talk again?**

  When medications are being changed, doctors will generally want to see patients more often or communicate with them by phone. If this isn't arranged, be assertive and ask for an appointment if you have any concerns.

For a real-life story about a patient who switched medications several times before landing on the right combination, check out the "Brett's story" sidebar in this chapter. ***Note:*** At one point when Brett was switching medications, his doctor recommended hospitalization so that he could be monitored more closely. It's worth pointing out that most switching of medications only rarely requires a move to an inpatient setting. Various factors — medical, psychiatric, and logistical — are used to determine whether hospitalization is necessary.

Combining medications

People with schizophrenia (or any other chronic condition for that matter) very commonly take multiple medications. There are different reasons why multiple medications are prescribed, but when two medications from the same treatment class (in this situation, antipsychotics) are given together, this is called *co-prescribing* or *polypharmacy*. It's important for patients and their families to understand the basics of polypharmacy.

The most common situations in which antipsychotic polypharmacy make sense include the following:

- When schizophrenia is treatment-resistant, or doesn't respond to the usual antipsychotic therapy
- When some of the symptoms of schizophrenia respond to treatment but others do not
- When there are significant side effects that make it impossible for the person to take a higher dose but where a higher dose is needed to control some symptoms of the disorder

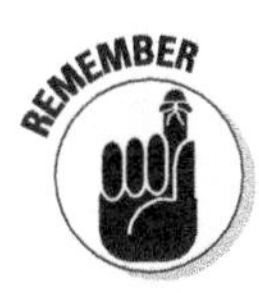

Distinguishing between *rational polypharmacy* and *irrational polypharmacy* is important. Although *polypharmacy* has gotten a bad rap, if done for the right reasons and carried out in a logical way, it can be beneficial (refer to the nearby sidebar, "Brett's story," for an example). Logically enough, this is called *rational polypharmacy.*

An example of *irrational polypharmacy* would be a doctor concurrently starting a person with schizophrenia on two different antipsychotic medications at the same time, without trying one alone and with no prior history suggesting that this practice would be safe and beneficial to the person.

If a psychiatrist starts two medications at the same time, it is impossible to determine which one is causing problems or desired effects.

Another problem may occur if a second medication is added without fully stopping the first (called an *incomplete taper*). In this case, if the person improves, it may be believed that it is the "combination" that is working when, in fact, it may just be the second medication, and using one medication would be just as effective, less likely to cause side effects, and considerably less expensive!

Brett's story

Brett's treatment experience provides an example of how and why rational polypharmacy takes place. A 20-year-old honors student and standout athlete, Brett had never experienced any psychiatric symptoms before. During his junior year, he started hearing threatening voices and believed that he was being followed by aliens. He bought a gun to "protect himself."

Brett became so fearful that he started placing phone calls to the police asking them for protection. His fraternity brothers were worried about him and got him to see the psychiatrist on campus, who diagnosed Brett with schizophreniform disorder (because his symptoms were of less than six months' duration — see Chapter 4). Brett was hospitalized on the psychiatric ward and treated with a second-generation antipsychotic agent, olanzapine (brand name: Zyprexa).

Within two weeks, the voices stopped, and Brett no longer felt threatened by aliens. He was discharged from the hospital to outpatient care and continued to take his antipsychotic. He seemed to be doing well — except he gained about 25 pounds over a relatively short period of time, and he was having trouble concentrating on his studies.

As midterms approached, both Brett and his psychiatrist noticed that his symptoms were worsening. He couldn't sleep, couldn't study, and started feeling like someone was messing with his mind. The psychiatrist and Brett both thought that the stress of midterms was too great and, after a meeting among Brett, his parents, and the doctor, everyone agreed that the most prudent thing would be for Brett to take a temporary leave of absence from school and return home.

With the reduced stress at home, Brett felt better — his sleep improved, and he no longer had thoughts of anyone controlling his mind. However, his weight continued to increase and within a month, he gained another 15 pounds. He was also becoming more sluggish.

When Brett started to think about returning to school the next semester, he began to have doubts. His memory wasn't as good as it used to be, and he was very self-conscious about his weight gain. He didn't know how his fraternity brothers would react to him. His thoughts about aliens began to crop up again.

His psychiatrist didn't want to increase his dosage, because of the substantial weight gain it had caused in the past. Instead, he suggested switching to another second-generation medicine that was less likely to exacerbate the problem. The dose of olanzapine was reduced as the new medication, ziprasidone (brand name: Geodon), was increased, until the olanzapine was stopped entirely. Brett's weight dropped, but he became increasingly suspicious and reported that the voices were commanding him to protect the human race from danger.

The psychiatrist tried Brett on another second-generation antipsychotic, aripiprazole (brand name: Abilify). Although Brett did not gain weight on aripiprazole, the voices and delusions became so severe that the psychiatrist suggested another voluntary hospitalization to adjust the medication in a safe and secure setting where he could be observed medically. The psychiatrist gradually stopped the aripiprazole and gradually restarted olanzapine but at a lower dose than before. When Brett started to improve, the psychiatrist didn't raise his olanzapine dose any further (to avoid any additional weight gain), but he added a first-generation antipsychotic, haloperidol (brand name: Haldol) in a small dose because it's known to be good for controlling hallucinations and delusions and doesn't cause significant weight gain.

On this regimen of antipsychotic polypharmacy, Brett continued to improve so that he was well enough to return to school the following semester.

Coping with Common Side Effects

In order to be effective, a medication interacts with body systems to bring about *therapeutic* (desired) effects. Because medications rarely have an effect on just one single biological system in the body, along with the therapeutic effect comes other unwanted or side effects.

When these side effects are undesirable, they're called *adverse effects.* Adverse effects can be mild or severe, and from a medical point of view they're either not serious or serious (for example, requiring hospitalization or causing lasting disability). Regardless of whether a side effect is serious from a medical point of view, and regardless of the reason your loved one is taking a medication, no one likes to put up with annoying side effects — these side effects are often one of the reasons for noncompliance (see "Why people refuse to take or stop taking medication," later in this chapter).

Some side effects only become a problem when the person has another physical or mental disorder. For example, a medication can cause urinary blockage in a man who has an enlarged prostate, but the same drug poses no problem in a woman or a young man with a normal prostate. Such side effects are more of an unknown when a drug is brand new and is less likely to have been used by a large number of people.

Side effects vary from medication to medication. The most common side effects are usually mild, not serious, and transient — but they can still be annoying enough to discourage people with schizophrenia from continuing to take the medication. Because every individual is biologically unique, people vary widely in the side effects that affect them and how bothersome they feel (regardless of whether the side effects are medically serious).

Even side effects that are not medically serious (for example, dry mouth, blurred vision, drowsiness, or drooling) can lead to noncompliance with medication regimens and should be taken seriously by everyone involved in a patient's care.

When your doctor prescribes an antipsychotic medication, he should tell your loved one what side effects she may experience and which of them are serious enough that she should call or visit the doctor if they occur. Your loved one should tell the doctor about all new or worsening physical symptoms she's experiencing because they could be medication-related.

Three kinds of side effects associated with antipsychotic medications are serious enough to have a doctor consider a change in treatment: movement disorders, weight gain, and metabolic problems. These side effects vary widely between first- and second-generation antipsychotics and among the different medications within these two different generations.

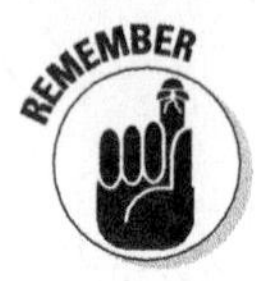

Antipsychotic medications are potent and effective treatments for schizophrenia. It may take some time to find the right drug(s) at the right dose(s). Careful vigilance, monitoring, and management to reduce side effects are essential to improve compliance and maximize medication effectiveness.

Movement disorders

Movement disorders occur as a side effect especially of first-generation antipsychotic medications — most often those that are called *high-potency drugs* (drugs that are very strong in small doses) or drugs that are given in high doses.

Among the most commonly used first-generation antipsychotics, haloperidol (brand name: Haldol) and fluphenazine (brand name: Prolixin) are two that often give rise to these side effects. The side effects are caused by the drugs interfering with the central nervous system structures in the brain that play a role in controlling motor functions.

Sometimes the side effects come on suddenly at the beginning of treatment and cause the patient to feel jittery and unable to stay still. This condition is called *akathisia.* Although it can be extremely frightening, it usually can be controlled rather quickly by reducing the dose or adding a counteracting medication. Other dramatic motor symptoms (such as back stiffness, the eyes rolling up in the head, or the neck turning to one side), called *dystonias,* can occur when medication is first started.

Although these symptoms usually aren't life-threatening, they should be attended to immediately because they're uncomfortable and frightening. No person should have to put up with these controllable side effects.

With continued treatment, some people develop a group of symptoms termed *pseudoparkinsonian* symptoms, because they look like, but aren't really due to Parkinson's disease. These symptoms include tremors (frequently of the fingers, but sometimes of the tongue and/or head); stiffness of the body, face, and limbs; and difficulty initiating movements. Again, dose reduction or the use of counteracting medications, called antiparkinsonian agents — such as benztropine (brand name: Cogentin) or diphenhydramine hydrochloride (brand name: Benadryl) — is usually very helpful.

After prolonged use of a medication, some patients may develop a neurologic syndrome called *tardive dyskinesia* (meaning, late occurring abnormal movements). If not diagnosed early, this condition can become chronic and occasionally is irreversible. With this syndrome, arms, legs, mouth, tongue, and even the body trunk may begin to move slowly and uncontrollably causing abnormal involuntary movements. Usually the person with the disorder is not particularly troubled by it, but it's very noticeable to others. Needless to say, this condition can be very stigmatizing to the person with the movements. The first time you notice any sign of these movements, report them immediately to your loved one's clinician, who will likely prescribe another medication.

Although tardive dyskinesia tends to occur in people who have used first-generation medications, in some rare instances it has been diagnosed in people using second-generation medications. It is not clear whether this is due to their having used first-generation medications in the past. Elderly people, women, and people with mood symptoms are more likely to develop tardive dyskinesia.

Weight gain

Although not immediately recognized as a problem when second-generation antipsychotic medications first came into use, weight gain has turned out to be a significant adverse side effect, especially for some of these medications. In particular, clozapine (brand name: Clozaril) and olanzapine (brand name: Zyprexa) have been associated with rapid and profound weight gain in many patients taking these medications.

Before weight gain was recognized as a problem, patients weren't advised to monitor their diets or encouraged to exercise. Doctors also made no attempt to switch drugs or avoid other medications that also may cause weight gain, compounding the problem. Many patients gained significant amounts of weight on these medications, which put them at risk for cardiac and other physical problems.

Today if weight gain starts to be a problem and is recognized, patients can be tried on other second-generation antipsychotic drugs that are less likely to cause weight gain (such as ziprasidone or aripiprazole). If a medication is working particularly well and your doctor doesn't want to change medications, she may prescribe medication to counteract weight gain instead of changing medications.

When families aren't aware of the properties of these medications, they simply blame the weight gain on the person's eating habits (for example, too much junk food) or lack of exercise, which creates conflicts between patients and families. Watching a relative become free of positive symptoms but gain so much weight that his physical health and appearance are severely compromised is very painful. Worsening this problem, negative symptoms can interfere with a person's motivation to exercise or take care of himself.

You may want to suggest to your loved one that he get help for what's a very difficult problem to solve on his own. Suggest that your loved one discuss his weight problem openly with his psychiatrist and internist, and perhaps a nutritionist. By adjusting your loved one's medications, they may be able to make weight loss easier (although there is no magic bullet for weight loss, and he'll still need to watch his diet and get regular exercise). You may want to suggest that the person join a health club or take part in an exercise program at a mental-health program.

Try to be as supportive as possible in a situation that's largely not under your loved one's control. Don't inadvertently sabotage your loved one's efforts at treating his illness or controlling his weight.

Metabolic problems

Along with the problem of weight gain, doctors noticed that some people on antipsychotic medications developed elevated blood sugar, which led to a diagnosis of Type 2 (non-insulin-dependent) diabetes. Occasionally, this came on suddenly, and the patients had such severe problems with sugar metabolism that they had to be hospitalized due to a life-threatening metabolic situation.

Much more frequent has been the need to medically treat the diabetes with either oral antidiabetic drugs or with insulin, and to develop strategies to manage diet and exercise. In fact, wellness and fitness approaches have become much more frequent in the care of people with long-standing schizophrenia. These programs are offered by many psychosocial rehabilitation programs in the community.

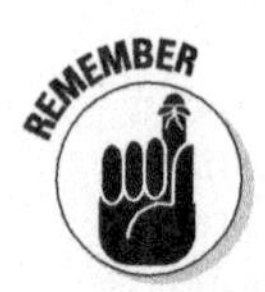

It's vital for doctors and families to encourage regular health checkups for people with schizophrenia. Be sure that the physician caring for a person with the disorder is aware of the potential physical health problems associated with the use of these medications. Be sure that your loved one follows up with periodic laboratory tests as recommended by her psychiatrist or other physician.

Although they're hard to find, some physicians specialize in the medical care of people with psychiatric illnesses. You might ask your loved one's psychiatrist to recommend an internist who is experienced working with people with schizophrenia.

Frequently associated with the sugar metabolism problem has been another dietary metabolic problem, namely lipid (fat) metabolism of the type seen with coronary artery disease. When elevated cholesterol and triglyceride levels occur, they can be treated with statin drugs (such as Lipitor) as well as with diet and exercise.

Other side effects

Other medication-induced problems can also occur. Most first-generation and some second-generation antipsychotic agents (including risperidone) cause a rise in the hormone prolactin. In some males, high prolactin levels can cause enlarged breasts (which can prove quite embarrassing, especially in adolescents and young adults) and may also be implicated in irregular or missed periods in females. Small hormone-producing but *benign* (not cancerous) pituitary tumors have also been associated with first-generation antipsychotic medications.

Finally, a life-threatening (but fortunately, very rare) side effect known as neuroleptic malignant syndrome (NMS), characterized by high fever, confusion and *hypotension* (low blood pressure), is a real medical emergency that must be treated immediately — otherwise, the patient may die. Patients and their families should be alerted to the remote possibility of NMS by their doctors and immediately call the psychiatrist (who may well suggest that the person with schizophrenia go to an emergency room right away).

Other Classes of Medications Used to Treat Symptoms

Although schizophrenia is most commonly associated with symptoms such as hallucinations, delusions, and disorganized thinking, symptoms such as depression, anxiety, or sleep disorders also can occur during the course of this chronic illness.

Different classes of drugs are used as additional treatments: Mood symptoms often require antidepressants or mood stabilizers to control them, while problems with anxiety, nervousness, and sleep problems can be treated (usually for short periods of time) with anti-anxiety agents or sleeping pills (also called *hypnotics*).

Negative symptoms and cognitive impairments are two other categories of symptoms that need to be addressed in treatment, but because there aren't any FDA-approved medications for their treatment, we discuss them in Chapter 10, on research.

Antidepressants

Symptoms of depression (such as feeling blue or hopeless, lack of interest in people or things, changes in appetite or sleeping patterns) may occur during the course of schizophrenia, but they're not the primary or most prominent symptoms. Nonetheless, they can be quite disabling to the person with the disorder and discouraging to loved ones and caregivers as well.

That's why it's fairly common for doctors to prescribe antidepressant medications (such as Elavil or Zoloft) along with antipsychotics to control the symptoms of depression. Care must be taken when antidepressants are used — the uplifting effects of these drugs can worsen the positive symptoms of schizophrenia, particularly when the antidepressant is initially prescribed or when the dose is raised.

Suicide rates are markedly elevated in people with schizophrenia so identifying and treating depression can be life-saving. Although the person in the throes of depression may not believe it, depression *is* a treatable illness.

Knowing just how much antidepressant is needed can be a bit of a balancing act. Providing good feedback to the physician about how your loved one is dong (for example, sleeping better or sleeping worse; becoming more or less aggressive; becoming more or less interested in news, TV, and the world around her) can really help the doctor adjust medication appropriately. Depression at times can become so severe that a person feels suicidal. (See Chapter 14 for more about the risk of suicide in schizophrenia.)

Sometimes when positive symptoms are treated and people with schizophrenia have a better grip on reality, the awareness of the very real setbacks and losses they have encountered as a result of their illness can lead to depression. Whenever someone feels depressed, it's important that he tell his clinician and family. However, it's also important for family members to be aware of the possibility of depression, watch for its symptoms, and if it is severe, encourage their loved one to tell his doctor.

Mood stabilizers

For some people with schizophrenia, mood symptoms of *elation* (excessive energy and activity) may occur along with, or independent of, symptoms of depression. The elation may become edgy (sarcastic and aggressive) and border on *hypomania* (which is characterized by not needing sleep, as well as rapid and continuous talking).

If these symptoms occur or cycle with depression, medication known as *mood stabilizers* (medications that are used to even out moods) can be helpful. One of the most widely used mood stabilizers is lithium. Although there is some question about whether lithium relieves depression, it is a virtual godsend in preventing, shortening, and controlling elated or manic behavior.

The dosage of lithium must be monitored carefully (by laboratory testing of lithium levels in the blood), because there is a very small difference between an effective therapeutic level and one that is toxic. When the levels are adjusted, however, the medication can be taken over prolonged periods of time with only occasional blood monitoring unless the person develops diarrhea, vomiting, or profuse sweating and fluid loss or dehydration. Under these circumstances, lithium administration must be suspended and the dosage adjusted again.

Besides lithium, other mood stabilizers that are regularly used as anticonvulsant drugs are also in common use. These medications are, for the most part, being used *off label* (meaning, they haven't been approved for the treatment of schizophrenia — although several have been approved for the treatment of bipolar disorder). The most common mood stabilizers in this class are valproate (brand name: Depakote) and lamotrigine (brand name: Lamictil). These medications are not without their own side effects (such as weight gain or a severe and life-threatening rash called *Stevens-Johnson syndrome*), and they should be used only when there is an established need and when prescribed by experienced clinicians.

Because of its propensity for weight gain, some patients call Depakote "Depa-bloat." The same cautions we provide earlier pertaining to excessive weight gain need to be considered when using this medication as well.

Antianxiety medications

It's not unusual for people with schizophrenia to feel nervous, jittery, or tense. Generally, antipsychotic medications reduce or take the edge off these symptoms. In fact, some antipsychotic drugs are used for the treatment of anxiety (without schizophrenia). Sometimes however, something more specific or potent may need to be used to address these uncomfortable symptoms.

The most common class of antianxiety agents are the benzodiazepines (such as Librium, Valium, Xanax, and Clonapin), which are prescribed medications. However, these medications have a dependence/addiction potential and should be used only for short periods of time with good monitoring.

This same class of drugs contains some compounds that are sold and used as sleeping pills. Frequently anxiety can be accompanied by the inability to fall asleep and, thus, antianxiety benzodiazepines may be given at night to help induce sleep. There are, of course, other hypnotic medications (for example, Ambien or Lunesta), but it's better to avoid using too many medications, especially when they may produce physical or mental dependence.

Anxiety may sometimes be experienced as a result of *akathisia* (feelings of inner restless) that are a side effect of certain antipsychotic medications (especially first-generation ones). The proper treatment is either to reduce the dose of antipsychotic medication or to switch to another, perhaps second-generation, antipsychotic agent. ***Remember:*** Using an antianxiety medication instead of removing the cause of the anxiety is *not* the best course of action — it's better to figure out the root cause of the anxiety and solve that problem rather than relying on medications.

In many people with schizophrenia, one of the first symptoms of worsening or relapse is difficulty sleeping. If this is the case, increasing the dose of the antipsychotic agent is generally preferable to taking a sleep medication. Don't hesitate to ask a doctor what he thinks is the cause of your loved one's sleeplessness before asking for a prescription for a sleep medication.

Adhering to Medications

Studies show that most people don't take prescribed medication properly. Many families are frustrated by relatives who are unwilling to take medication at all or who are unwilling or unable to take it consistently. Others find that their loved ones go off medication as soon as it begins working and they start to feel better. This doesn't only hold true for psychiatric medications. Many other chronic physical illnesses, such as diabetes or hypertension, demand long-term *compliance* (sticking to a prescribed treatment regimen), and people aren't always willing to comply with a doctor's orders over the long haul.

Large studies of compliance to all types of medications prove that people are less likely to recognize the importance of taking medications for chronic conditions like Type 2 diabetes (where compliance rates are estimated at only 20 percent) or high cholesterol than they are for disorders that have noticeable physical symptoms. Families and doctors need to reinforce the importance of taking these medications regularly.

Taking any medication can be a catch-22; almost every medication that works has potentially undesirable side effects. The worse the side effects, the less likely it is that a person will take the medication prescribed as ordered. But when schizophrenia is inadequately or inappropriately treated, the effects on a person's quality of life and that of the people around him can be devastating. The person is more likely to be hospitalized, abuse alcohol and/or drugs, be jailed, or become homeless. With no proper treatment in sight, families feel a sense of hopelessness and despair.

Because medications are the most important tool in the psychiatrist's arsenal, doctors need to maintain an open dialogue with reluctant patients and their families to fully explain the risks and benefits of these medications. Every effort needs to be made to find a medication that's not only effective, but acceptable to the patient and her family.

Why people refuse to take or stop taking medication

Although the reasons why people refuse to take or stop taking antibiotics or cholesterol-lowering medications are similar to the reasons why they don't adhere to antipsychotic drug regimens, psychiatric symptoms add some additional barriers, including uncomfortable side effects, lack of insight into the illness, disorganized thinking, the high costs of medication, and attitudes toward psychiatric medications. We cover all of these in the following sections.

Uncomfortable side effects

Antipsychotic drugs have many side effects, ranging from annoying to potentially serious health concerns. Although the symptoms vary from drug to drug, many patients report that antipsychotic drugs make them feel drowsy, stiff (sometimes patients report feeling like zombies), confused, unclear, or not like themselves. Sometimes symptoms of the illness become confused with side effects of the medication.

Many times, these side effects become more tolerable over time, but often they're uncomfortable enough that they cause a person with schizophrenia to stop taking her medication before the side effects subside.

Side effects (described in the "Coping with Common Side Effects" section, earlier in this chapter) must be viewed as valid concerns that need to be addressed to see how they can be prevented or avoided.

Lack of insight into the illness

When schizophrenia first appears, you may be baffled and frustrated by the fact that your loved one doesn't seem to realize that anything is wrong with him. One study estimated that approximately half of all individuals with schizophrenia and 40 percent of those with bipolar disorder don't recognize their symptoms. The degree of insight a person has can vary over the course of the illness but, in most cases, it is most impaired when the disease first appears.

Why insight is so compromised remains an area of controversy. It could involve some denial, with the patient unwilling to admit that she's sick. But more likely it's a deficit in *cognition* (thinking) in the brain. Regardless of the cause, lack of insight often becomes a source of misunderstanding and conflict between patients and their relatives. The relatives just wish they could shake the person and make her understand. The patient feels like her relative is trying to control her behavior (which is true, to some degree, but for good reason).

One family member told us a story about her husband who had been ill during most of their marriage but refused to take medication for more than two decades. He never accepted his diagnosis, even though he was becoming progressively more psychotic and dysfunctional — and the couple was at the brink of financial ruin. He would substitute aspirin for his prescribed medication (saying that all pills looked the same) and often refused to take medication at all. Only after multiple hospitalizations, including a ten-month inpatient stay, did he come to terms with his illness and his need for medication.

Disorganized thinking

When thinking is disorganized, understanding or following any rules or regimens — including how and when to take a complex mix of medications — is difficult. Drug regimens can be extremely complicated for people with schizophrenia, who often need to take multiple pills to effectively control different symptoms. Not only does it require remembering which pills to take at which times, with or without food, but also which prescription needs to be refilled when.

Written aids like schedule charts or graphs, or physical aids such as pill boxes, which separate pills not only by day of the week but also by time of day can be very helpful to those struggling with disordered thinking. Help from others in keeping scheduling straight may also be necessary.

High costs of prescription meds

The costs of prescription medication can be financially crushing especially for individuals who live on fixed or limited incomes, and those whose health insurance doesn't cover the cost of medications. According to the Kaiser Health Foundation, the wholesale prices for the 50 most often prescribed brand-name medications increased by nearly 8 percent in 2007. Many of the second-generation (atypical) antipsychotics that psychiatrists are likely to prescribe either are still under patent or are toward the end of their patents, which means they will soon become available in generic form. The pharmaceutical industry tries to encourage patients to switch to similar, but newer, "me-too" drugs that are higher priced.

If patients are enrolled in Medicaid or Medicare, they may have outpatient prescription drug coverage, but state policies differ regarding copayments, the number of prescriptions that can be filled, and the specific drugs that are covered.

Some patients try to save money by taking pills less often than prescribed, or by dividing prescriptions in half to make them last longer. This can make treatment seem ineffective and can lead to the doctor "tinkering" with medications, when in reality the patient isn't taking the dose prescribed. Chapter 7 provides information about some of the prescription assistance programs that help provide support for people on limited incomes.

Attitudes toward psychiatric medications

There's still a great deal of stigma attached to taking medications for a mental disorder as compared to taking them for physical problems. Sometimes, patients see taking medication as a constant reminder that they have an illness they don't want to have, so they either won't start medications or suddenly stop. Other times, people go off their medications as soon as they feel better, not realizing that stopping the medication will result in relapse. Some patients and their families believe that the more medication you take, the sicker it means you are — which is simply not true.

It's a common tendency for patients to feel that they want to try going off medication to see if everything will be all right. Usually people are feeling good because the medication is working. Many times, doctors want to try to reduce dosages or eliminate one or another medication, and this may be possible, but it needs to be done under the close supervision of the prescribing physician to prevent relapse.

Another common complaint made by patients and families, and mentioned earlier in this chapter, is that they're being used as "guinea pigs" because their doctors have to depend on trial and error. To some extent, this is true — but patients (and their families) need to understand that medication regimens must be individualized for the person, because what works for one person may not work for another and what once worked for your loved one may not work for him now. This is often hard to accept, because it makes it evident the very real limitations of what the medical profession knows and doesn't know about schizophrenia and its treatment.

What you can do to ensure your loved one takes his medications

As much as possible, try to get your loved to take her medications at the same time each day. Here are some ways she can remember to do that:

- Associate taking medication with a daily routine (brushing her teeth or eating breakfast, for example) or a visual cue (for example, a kitchen counter).
- Use a divided pill container to help your loved one keep track of her medicines that have already been taken and those that haven't.

- Make sure that your loved one's doctor explains — and you and your loved one understand — the reason she's taking each medication and the risks of not taking them. If your loved one knows why she's taking the medication, she may be more likely to stay on track.
- Ask your loved one's psychiatrist to minimize the number of daily doses whenever practical (remembering that short-acting drugs may require more doses).
- Don't let running out of pills serve as an excuse for not taking them. Remind your loved one not to wait until the last day to refill a prescription; retail pharmacies aren't required to keep every type of medication in stock, so you want to make sure your loved one renews her prescriptions about a week before they'll run out. If she uses a mail-order pharmacy, make allowances for the time it will take for the medications to get to her door.

People often stop taking their medications because they are experiencing annoying side effects. Remind your loved one to report any uncomfortable side effects to her doctor before she stops. A change in dose, change in the medication, or change in the time they are taken may remedy the problem.

When Medication Doesn't Seem to Work

There are times when the best attempts at finding a workable medication or combination of medications fails. Even after trying several antipsychotic medications at different doses, in different combinations, and with various other medications alongside — and with use of non-medication treatments (such as psychotherapy, peer support, psychosocial rehabilitation, and so on) — an individual's symptoms may remain severe and unresponsive to treatment. Even after obtaining a second opinion (see Chapter 5), you and the doctor may come to the conclusion that there are no other options available at the moment.

In situations like these (which, fortunately, are relatively infrequent), if a person is in continued psychic and possibly physical distress either electroconvulsive therapy (ECT) or other physical treatments (see Chapter 10) may be worth trying.

Few treatments have been so misunderstood and vilified as electroconvulsive therapy (ECT), commonly referred to as *electroshock therapy.* Sometimes ECT is even confused with the controversial approaches that use powerful shocks to modify behavior — they have nothing in common except that they both use electrical energy. Although certainly not a first-line treatment for schizophrenia, several studies have demonstrated the effectiveness of ECT when used in difficult cases — and even when used as a long-term follow-up treatment for treatment-resistant schizophrenia.

ECT is given in a humane and precisely measured way, using general anesthesia and muscle relaxants to avert any pain or physical fractures, which could be caused by the seizures that are induced by passing an electrical current through the brain. The team (usually comprised of an anesthesiologist, psychiatrist, and nursing personnel) that administers ECT should be carefully trained and experienced, and should use one of the electronic devices that can deliver very programmed amounts and types of electrical current waves. Under these circumstances, ECT is generally safe — although, like all physical treatments, it can have side effects. The most common side effect of ECT is temporary memory loss, which infrequently can be more prolonged.

ECT can be a life-saving treatment for patients with agitation associated with schizophrenia that can't be controlled (called *intractable agitation*) or with treatment-resistant catatonic schizophrenia (see Chapter 4). When a person with schizophrenia hasn't responded to other treatments, ECT can also make the difference between a person being hospitalized indefinitely or becoming an outpatient.

Before rejecting ECT or a suggested therapy, you and your loved one should talk to the doctor about the ins and outs of the procedure. Don't rely on negative media portrayals such as those you may have seen in *One Flew over the Cuckoo's Nest* as your source of information. Those movies also show insulin shock treatment, a procedure that is no longer used.

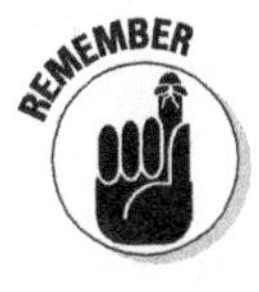

Although no one can say for sure precisely how or why ECT works (which is also true for many other treatments in medicine), there is clear clinical evidence that is it both safe and effective when given under proper medical supervision under the proper circumstances.

Looking back at previous medical therapies

In the past, many treatments that seem completely senseless or terribly inhumane in hindsight were tried in an effort to control the symptoms of schizophrenia. These treatments ranged from uncomfortable but harmless treatments (such as cold baths) to potentially medically dangerous treatments (such as injections of insulin to induce low blood sugar and coma), as well as permanently damaging treatments (such as lobotomies). There is little evidence that any of these now-abandoned treatments were generally effective, especially in treatment-resistant cases.

Chapter 9

Psychosocial Approaches

In This Chapter

- Looking beyond medication alone
- Identifying the goals of psychosocial treatments
- Understanding new developments in individual, group, and family therapies
- Addressing the vocational, social, and thinking skills deficits associated with schizophrenia
- Recognizing the roles of self-help and family psychoeducation

It would be wonderful if all the symptoms and signs of schizophrenia could be whisked away by merely swallowing a pill. Unfortunately, even the best medications alone aren't a cure-all. While medication is essential to treat and control acute positive symptoms (see Chapter 8), medication alone falls short in helping the person with schizophrenia regain his sense of self-worth and his ability to function in society after a first psychotic break or a recurrent psychotic episode.

The losses associated with an acute episode of schizophrenia can be devastating. Medication — although it can usually help stabilize symptoms so life is more "normal" — can't erase the pain of feeling stigmatized, left out, and unable to cope with tasks that seem to come easily to peers, such as living independently or holding down a job.

In this chapter, we identify and explain the array of psychosocial treatments, therapies, and approaches — beyond medication — that should be available as part of a comprehensive system of care for people with schizophrenia. These include psychological, rehabilitative, and cognitive therapies, along with self-help and family approaches, that lessen positive symptoms, improve thinking and social skills, reduce the risk of relapse, and improve quality of life.

Although any one individual may not need or use all these approaches, every community should have them available for those who need them.

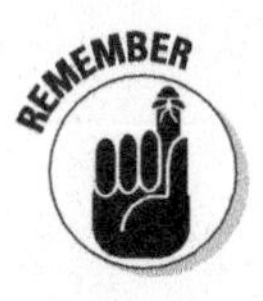

Unfortunately, many psychosocial therapies are not available in every community. One of the best ways to get a handle on what exists in your community is by asking a case manager or social worker. You or your loved one can also contact your state or local mental-health authority (see the appendix) and find out about the availability of programs in your geographic area.

Because of the complexity of the mental-health service system, many private practitioners aren't likely to know about the full range of psychosocial rehabilitation services available in their own communities.

Understanding Psychosocial Therapies

We use the term *psychosocial treatments* to describe the psychological, social, and combined psychosocial approaches (usually used in conjunction with medication) that aim to help people improve their current level of functioning so it is the best that it can be — so they can feel productive and good about themselves (see Chapter 15).

Psychosocial treatments are aimed at:

- Lessening the symptoms and impairments caused by the disorder
- Helping people better manage their illness, which includes teaching them how to:
    - Recognize and cope with persistent symptoms of the illness (such as hearing voices or being unable to concentrate)
    - Maintain a consistent medication regimen
    - Monitor and cope with the potential side effects of treatment
    - Prepare for and prevent (to the extent possible) recurring episodes
- Helping people achieve social, academic, training, or vocational goals
- Helping people learn or relearn practical life skills, such as:
    - Managing money
    - Housekeeping
    - Shopping
    - Doing laundry

- Keeping up with basic hygiene and maintaining their personal appearance
- Navigating public transportation

- Teaching people ways to decrease stress, avoid conflict, and manage anger
- Helping people reconnect with others
- Helping people understand and cope with their diagnosis as they move toward recovery (see Chapter 15)

Evidence shows that adding psychosocial treatments to medication therapy results in better outcomes than either medication alone or psychosocial therapy alone. For example, people who are treated with a combination of medication, social skills training, and family therapy have only a 5 percent chance of relapse, compared to a 40 percent chance of relapse among those treated with medications alone (see Figure 9-1).

Taking advantage of various psychosocial approaches isn't a matter of choosing one over another, or using them as substitutes for medication. For the practical and optimal treatment of schizophrenia, it's advantageous to combine medication and psychosocial approaches that enhance once another.

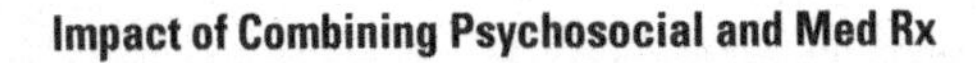

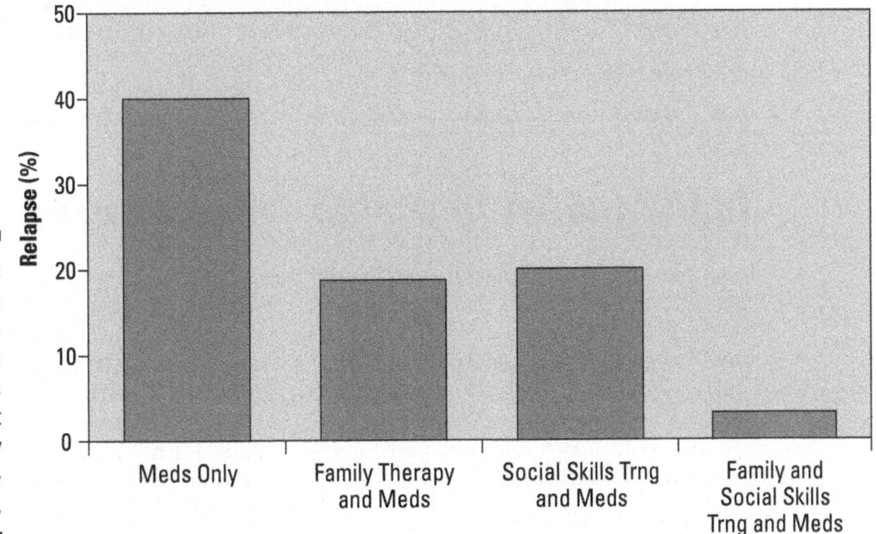

Figure 9-1: Relapse rates are lower when people aren't treated only with medications.

When talk was king

Psychotherapy (talk therapy) is what most people think of when they picture treatment for mental illness: the patient lying on the couch, recounting everything she can remember happening to her since she was an infant or toddler, while the psychiatrist sits, stone-faced and silent, listening until the patient finally reaches some *catharsis* (emotional cleansing) of feelings and insight into her behavior. About half a century ago, before the widespread use of *psychopharmacology* (medications), psychotherapy was the prominent, dominant, and almost universally accepted treatment for all psychiatric illnesses, including schizophrenia.

Then medications appeared that, at least in many people, seemed to work like magic. Talk therapy was outdated; the remedy was in the tablet. Medications *can* have near miraculous results in reducing psychosis. However, the person affected still has to pick up the pieces of his life and try to put them back together. This is something medication can't help with. It takes another person — or a group of people — to help the person with schizophrenia find ways to become a functioning member of society again.

Today a combined approach is seen as what's needed: keeping psychotic symptoms under control with medications, supportive therapy that is focused on problem-solving, psychosocial approaches to help the patient regain independence, and self-help to enable an individual to regain his confidence, sense of self-esteem, and hope for the future. When talk therapy is used today, it takes a different form: It's usually briefer, more practical and supportive, and focused on specific goals.

It's worth noting, too, that the past half-century has seen significant advances in psychological therapies. The psychoanalytic theory monopoly was broken, and different kinds of therapies surfaced. In general, the newer therapies centered more on practical rehabilitation of the individual, in much the same way that someone is rehabilitated after a physical injury (such as a broken arm or a stroke), instead of trying to solve the puzzle of finding the root causes of someone's illness in her history.

Individualizing a plan for treatment

Each person with schizophrenia has different needs, and the same person has different needs at different points in her illness. Treatment planning needs to be flexible enough to adapt to these changes. For example, right after hospital discharge, your loved one's major challenges may be to cope with positive symptoms — and a combination of cognitive behavioral therapy and family psychoeducation may be very helpful. When those challenges are met, your loved one may be ready to prepare for a job and be in a position to benefit from social skills training and vocational rehabilitation.

One important purpose of an individualized plan is to identify ways to monitor and reduce stress so the person with schizophrenia doesn't take on too much too soon. Typically, schizophrenia occurs at a phase of life when people are building their lives and careers, so they may feel a sense of urgency to resume school full-time to make up the courses they missed or to go back to work before they lose their job or housing. Like medicine, psychosocial rehabilitation needs to be sensitively and intelligently dosed and monitored.

As with most things in life, timing is everything, and it certainly is an important consideration in determining the phasing of treatments for patients with schizophrenia. When someone is severely psychotic (with symptoms that may include hallucinations, delusions, disorganized thinking, and agitation), it makes no sense to try to teach social skills or to try to decrease denial and improve insight with psychotherapy. Likewise, when acute positive symptoms are largely controlled and a person with schizophrenia is feeling lonely and would like to have a job and a fuller life, it won't do much good to merely adjust one or more medications. Together, the individual, the clinician, and the family need to decide on the timing and selection of the correct mix of interventions to meet their mutual goals.

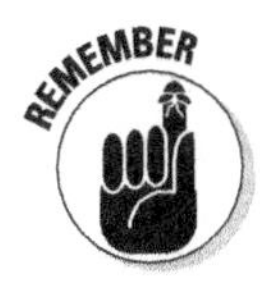

Schizophrenia is a persistent (chronic) illness that periodically worsens (a condition called *relapse*) and then improves (a condition called *remission*). Thus, the treatment needed varies with the phase of illness, the nature of the problems, and the individual's stage of recovery (see Chapter 15). Each person with schizophrenia faces unique difficulties and changing circumstances that require different approaches at different times.

Both clinicians and case managers play an important role in coordinating the participation of everyone who needs to be involved in the design of an individualized plan that assesses your loved one's needs and helps identify resources for its implementation. It doesn't stop there. The plan needs to be modified, as appropriate, over time as circumstances change.

The staff of local psychosocial rehabilitation programs — which are often funded by government, the private sector (usually nonprofit), or multiple sources of funding — can also take the lead in developing individualized plans for consumers that take advantage of the various resources available in the community.

After a psychotic break, many patients and their families want to plunge right back into normal life and make up for lost time. Others may be so devastated by the illness that they've lost all hope and think there's no way out. In either situation, a solid psychosocial evaluation and development of a comprehensive plan for treatment can help individuals and their families control symptoms — and simultaneously identify and set realistic goals for treatment and recovery.

Clearly, research shows that combining psychosocial treatments with medication improves outcomes compared to medication or other biological treatments used alone. One of the limitations of research on psychosocial treatments, which is common to treatments in general medicine as well as psychiatry, is that scientists still don't know what approaches work best, for which individuals, at various phases of the illness.

Certainly, we can say that the field has evolved greatly over the past two decades with a greater range of approaches being implemented and studied in local communities. We're better able to identify the full range of deficits associated with schizophrenia and to evaluate which deficits and skills are compromised for a particular individual.

The choice of psychosocial treatments should be linked to the individual needs of the patient. Not too far in the future, the hope is that we will minimize deficits through early recognition and treatment and that people with schizophrenia will be able to take advantage of treatments that are individualized and personalized for them.

Understanding what psychosocial rehabilitation can do

People with schizophrenia face many challenges after an acute episode has subsided and they are psychiatrically stable. Psychosocial rehabilitative interventions can be instrumental in providing the tools, training, and experience people with schizophrenia need to solve problems, manage their illness and its treatment, and create and nurture social and vocational skills, with coordinated planning by professionals, family members, and consumers.

For example, although antipsychotic medications are essential in bringing the acute symptoms of schizophrenia (such as hallucinations and delusions) under control — for many, these drugs may not completely eliminate symptoms. This means that some people may need to learn how to live with persistent voices in their heads, find ways to express themselves more coherently, learn how to distinguish between seeing things that are real and those that aren't, and learn how to contend with the real losses they've endured as a consequence of their illness.

Also, the side effects of taking medications can add a new set of problems. The same drugs that provide hope for recovery may leave patients with uncomfortable, potentially unhealthy and/or disabling side effects — such as dry mouth, drowsiness, weight gain, diabetes, tremors, loss of sexual desire, or insomnia — which may then need to be dealt with.

Many people with schizophrenia have lost some or all the roles that define them in society. They may no longer have a socially acceptable answer to the common question, "What do you do?" Rehabilitative therapies are designed to build a bridge between a person being sick (and doing very little) and being able to return to homemaking, school, training, employment, or some other meaningful activity — activities that are vital to a sense of satisfaction and self-worth.

Building or rebuilding vocational/occupational skills

Even when a person with schizophrenia is eager to work, time off for hospitalizations or acute episodes at home not only creates holes in a résumé, but also can lead to deficits in a person's skills and job performance. Because the onset of the disorder commonly occurs in adolescence or young adulthood, the individual may not have had the opportunity to acquire technical or other work skills and may have had little or no experience with the rigors of maintaining a 9-to-5 job.

A person with schizophrenia can face many vocational challenges:

- Not having a driver's license, not having a car, or having a hard time learning the bus route to work.
- Not having marketable job skills or training. (One patient we knew had learned how to do complex math algorithms in college, which were no longer used because the work could be done more quickly by computer.)
- Having his education interrupted or halted prematurely in high school or college because of the illness.
- Having little or no work experience, unexplained gaps in employment, or no references.
- Not knowing how to go about looking for a job.
- Not knowing how to prepare a résumé.
- Not being able to interview well because of limited social skills.
- Having a hard time adjusting to the rigors of an office or other workplace setting (for example, getting there on time, punching a time clock, working at a sustained pace, following instructions, working a full shift).
- Worries about potential loss of Social Security benefits (which are based on the inability to hold a competitive job).

There are ways to protect benefits during trial work periods (see Chapter 15).

Transitional or supported employment programs are generally time-limited efforts to help restore the skills and confidence people need to return to productive employment. The beauty of these programs is that the person with schizophrenia gets support from the program and from an employer who understands the nature of her new employee's history and/or limitations and who has an expressed desire to provide support and help.

Many of these programs employ job developers who work with industry to create employment slots for people with disabilities. These may be full-time jobs or part-time opportunities that can help people ease their way back into the workplace. Sometimes, programs even provide a coach who will accompany the individual on-site to train individuals and monitor their work.

Through the Rehabilitation Services Administration (RSA) of the U.S. Department of Education, every state receives funds to provide employment-related services — such as counseling, job training, education, supported employment, and so on — to assist individuals with physical or mental disabilities. Although waiting lists may be long and the programs aren't specifically geared to people with mental disorders, these resources shouldn't be overlooked because they can provide invaluable support. To find the agency in your own state, do an online search for *vocational rehabilitation* and the name of your state.

Participation as an unpaid volunteer in the community is another low-pressure way to ease back into the world of work and give your loved one the feeling that she's able to contribute to others.

Easing the loneliness and social isolation of schizophrenia

One common problem for people with schizophrenia that can be addressed through psychosocial therapies is loneliness. It's a human instinct to want to connect with other people, and families and friends experience great pain when they witness the isolation of a loved one with schizophrenia. Both the disease and the treatment of schizophrenia make it more difficult to make and keep friendships.

Being in and out of hospitals, in and out of schools, or in and out of work can lead people with schizophrenia to be out of sync or to lose contact with their peers. A student may have dropped out of college because of the illness and lost contact with roommates and classmates, or a person may have lost his job because of the illness and be too embarrassed to reconnect with former coworkers or supervisors.

Additionally, the positive and negative symptoms of the disease (see Chapter 3) itself may make it uncomfortable to be around people. It's not uncommon for people with schizophrenia to:

- **Hear voices while someone else is to talking to them.** This can be confusing for them, making it hard to focus on what the other person is saying and causing them to be slow in responding.
- **Feel suspicious, be wary of new people, and inaccurately perceive that people they know are thinking or reacting negatively to them.**
- **Be highly distractible because of their inability to focus (due to voices, hallucination, depression, or anxiety).**
- **Have no motivation or low energy (because of negative symptoms).** This can result in the person with schizophrenia having no interest in forming or maintaining social ties.
- **Be too irritable, anxious, or depressed.** This makes it uncomfortable for them to be around others and for others to be around them

- **Have low self-esteem because of their diagnosis and its stigma or be embarrassed by the side effects of medications (such as significant weight gain or tremors).**
- **Act inappropriately because of cognitive and social deficits, which cause people to rebuff their efforts or feel frightened of them.** For example, a person with schizophrenia may stand too close to people, be unable to discern what to say or what not to say, ask invasive questions, be unresponsive, have an unkempt appearance, or exhibit other odd behaviors.
- **Have a hard time adapting to large-group situations and find them stressful.**
- **Feel discomfort and guilt about not knowing who to tell or not to tell about their illness.** For example, should you tell a date? An old classmate? (For more on breaking the news, see Chapter 11.)

Because of these residual symptoms, some people with schizophrenia have a hard time being around other people with the same illness (because they serve as constant reminders of their own illness), have *social anxiety* (an out-of-proportion fear of being evaluated by people around them), or just don't feel like they fit in with other more "normal" people who don't understand their challenges. (On the other end of the spectrum, some people feel more comfortable socializing with others who are experiencing and overcoming similar challenges; see "Self-help groups," later in this chapter.)

In either case, even on a practical level (because of the impact of the illness on their finances) they may not have the pocket change they need to pay for dinners out, going to a movie, public transportation, the supplies needed for a hobby (like painting or photography), or the membership fees to join a health or fitness club.

Family relationships, especially sibling ones, may be strained because either the family hovers over the ill individual too much in an effort to encourage the person to be more social or excludes him from family functions to avoid discomfort for the individual and everyone else. Cumulatively, all these factors leave a person with the illness feeling detached and lonely, which can be ameliorated by various psychosocial interventions.

Learning new skills and relearning forgotten ones

Psychosocial skills training is a structured educational approach that usually takes place in groups that are focused on specific objectives for a set number of sessions. The skills are ones that are relevant to helping a person with schizophrenia better function as a member of her community. Training may cover:

- Activities of daily living
- Assertiveness

- Social skills and basic conversation skills
- Use of leisure time
- Money management
- Symptom and medication management
- Accessing Social Security and other benefits

The training is usually preceded by an evaluation, either one that's done by a trained observer or by *self-report* (for example, the consumer is asked to fill out a questionnaire describing his own limitations). Larger tasks are broken down into smaller ones and various behavioral approaches are used including role playing, modeling, and positive reinforcement (often in the form of food or drink). For example, if someone were learning how to present himself for a job interview, the training might focus on how to shake hands, how to make eye contact, what to say, what to ask, and how to dress.

Research suggests that skills training improves social skills, assertiveness, and readies people to leave hospitals sooner after a prolonged hospitalization.

For almost three decades, the U.S. government — first through the National Institute of Mental Health (NIMH) and then through the Center for Mental Health Services (CMHS) — jointly with the National Institute on Disability and Rehabilitation Research (NIDRR) of the Department of Education, has supported the growth of the Center for Psychiatric Rehabilitation at Boston University (`www.bu.edu/cpr`). This national center supports research, training, and services that are focused on helping people achieve "a decent place to live, suitable work, social activities, and friends to whom they can turn in times of crisis." The Center's Web site has a wealth of resources suitable for consumers, families, and professionals.

The National Research and Training Center on Psychiatric Disability, located in the Department of Psychiatry at the University of Illinois in Chicago (`www.cmhsrp.uic.edu/nrtc`) is a sister center, funded by the same federal agencies as the NIDRR. Its Web site offers free online workshops, Webcasts, and online continuing education courses.

Centers targeting the needs of children and adolescents with psychiatric disability are located at the University of South Florida (`http://rtckids.fmhi.usf.edu`) and Portland State University (`www.rtc.pdx.edu/index.php`).

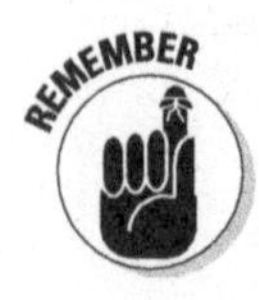

One of the more successful approaches to psychosocial rehabilitation is the assertive community treatment (ACT) program (see Chapter 5). ACT programs provide intensive outreach and care to help people live independently in their own homes. Trained professionals are available 24/7 to help individuals gain the practical skills they may have lost or never learned. They also oversee medication, making sure that medical and psychosocial care is coordinated for severely ill people in the community.

Looking at Individual Therapies

Individual therapies are one-on-one approaches with a clinician working directly with a client. Three of the most common therapies practiced one-on-one are psychodynamic therapy, supportive therapy, and cognitive behavioral therapy. We cover each of these in the following sections.

Psychodynamic therapy

Although *psychodynamic therapy* (meeting with a therapist on a regular basis over a long period of time to get to the root of a problem) was the dominant therapy for the first 50 years of the 20th century — think Woody Allen— these treatments weren't scientifically evaluated during their heyday. In fact, there's still no credible evidence that they're specifically beneficial in treating the symptoms or impairments associated with schizophrenia.

One problem is that the cognitive and memory deficits associated with schizophrenia can interfere with the ability of the person to benefit from this kind of therapy. (In fact, all psychosocial treatments must overcome this hurdle to be effective. People with schizophrenia must be able to understand and actively participate for any treatment to be helpful.) Thus, psychodynamic therapy is usually used for people with psychiatric disorders whose thinking remains intact.

Supportive therapy

People with schizophrenia, contending with many real-life problems, need someone experienced to talk to. *Supportive therapy* (therapy conducted by a professional trained to work with people with serious mental illnesses) is an important complement to medication and other psychosocial treatments. In these days of managed care, the time allowed for patients and their psychiatrists to spend with each other is often rationed by insurers and other third-party payers.

Therefore, it is important that your loved one has a trained professional as part of his team, with whom he can openly discuss his problems and find ways to overcome them. For example, if a person with schizophrenia was having problems making friends, the therapist might help her find ways to meet people and make the first overture.

Having such a safe, supportive relationship to learn new ways of coping is vital to recovery. This can be especially valuable for people who have trouble opening up to a group. Even though family and friends may be supportive, they aren't trained for and are usually too emotionally involved to play this role.

Psychologists, social workers, or other counselors who work with people with schizophrenia can help them cope with stressors in their lives, encourage adherence to treatment, help patients determine other needed treatments and supports, and serve in the role of a coach — providing encouragement and support. Psychotherapy can also be useful to overstressed loved ones who are unable to cope with the impact of the diagnosis on their own lives.

Cognitive behavioral therapy

Cognitive behavioral therapy (CBT) is usually conducted on a one-on-one basis in an outpatient setting, usually by a trained therapist, but it also can be practiced in groups. Like any individual therapy, CBT requires close collaboration between a patient and therapist. Therefore, it's important to interview the therapist before your loved one starts treatment, to make sure your loved one feels comfortable working with that individual (see Chapter 5).

When selecting a therapist for individual therapy, it's always prudent to ask for referrals from people you trust and to consider the first few sessions as an interview to get a good sense of the individual, whether your loved one connects with him, and whether it seems like talking with this person will be helpful.

CBT was originally developed in the late 1970s for the treatment of people with depression and anxiety disorders. At that time, it was the most proven psychosocial intervention, and even though it was not originally used for treating schizophrenia, there's now convincing evidence for its effectiveness, especially in reducing positive symptoms that remain in spite of adequate antipsychotic treatment.

During treatment, the patient describes her symptoms, and those that are most troublesome are targeted for attention. The goal is to change thought patterns in order to help the patient solve problems. This is sometimes called *cognitive-restructuring.* For example, a patient can be taught ways to ignore the voices she's hearing.

Some of the specific elements of CBT may include:

- **Belief modification or validity testing:** Challenging delusional thinking
- **Focusing/reattribution:** Explaining the meaning of stressors behind auditory hallucinations
- **Normalizing psychotic experiences:** Helping the patient see that her experiences are responses to stressful events
- **Cognitive rehearsal:** Practicing how to better handle a future situation similar to one that was challenging in the past

- **Journal writing:** Keeping notes to encourage insight, learning, and self-discovery

In essence, the CBT therapist challenges faulty thinking patterns (such as delusions and hallucinations) in an attempt to modify thoughts and behaviors. The reductions in positive symptoms seen with CBT continue after the course of treatment has been completed.

Unfortunately, CBT doesn't seem to affect rates of relapse and rehospitalization. Some studies report that CBT helps with compliance in taking medication and, in fact, a specific variant of CBT emphasizes this particular behavioral goal. Another limitation to CBT is that it doesn't seem to improve social functioning as well as supportive therapy. Also, because CBT requires a level of fairly organized thinking, it's less useful for individuals who have cognitive deficits or who are still acutely psychotic. Nevertheless, for persons who have persistent psychotic symptoms even with antipsychotic medication, CBT offers another tested and proven method of getting symptomatic relief.

Getting Involved in Group Therapies

Group therapies can be led by professionals, consumers, family members, or some combination of one or more of them. They may include psychotherapy groups or various forms of self-help groups (also called mutual support or peer support groups) and family groups.

Group psychotherapy

Psychotherapy groups typically include 6 to 12 patients who meet with one or two therapists (who facilitate the discussion). From each other, patients learn how to cope with the illness and its symptoms. Group therapy provides a perfect forum to meet new people and learn how to get along with others.

For some, group therapy offers a number of advantages over individual therapy, including

- **Opportunities to meet people and improve social skills:** This may be particularly beneficial to people who are extremely shy or have social anxiety.
- **Lower cost as compared to individual treatments.**
- **Opportunities to provide and obtain peer support:** People generally feel better about themselves when they're able to help other people with their problems.

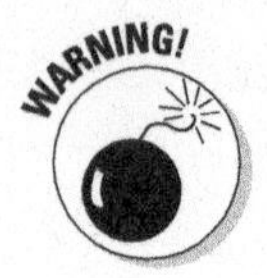

Group therapies are generally more appropriate after acute symptoms have subsided. They may be particularly difficult for people who still remain suspicious and paranoid.

Self-help groups

Self-help groups have a long history. An estimated 2 percent to 3 percent of the U.S. population is involved in some form of self-help group at any given time. These groups, often led by people with an illness or disorder (or by their family members), provide mutual support and practical help to others in similar circumstances. These groups are empowering for consumers because it allows them to see their peers as role models and they take advantage of what can be learned from people who have experienced an illness first-hand.

Self-help groups range from informal gatherings at someone's kitchen table or a local coffee shop to more formal ones run by local organizations or national programs. Some of the more well-known self-help groups include Alcoholics Anonymous (AA) and Mothers Against Drunk Driving (MADD). Many of these groups are also very effective advocacy organizations because of their commitment, tenacity, and credibility to their causes.

Because a substantial portion of people with schizophrenia (estimated at 50 percent over the course of their lifetime) have co-occurring substance use disorders, AA programs can potentially play an important role in recovery. However, some of these programs, in an effort to help their members remain substance free, discourage members from taking their antipsychotic medications — which can be very risky for someone with schizophrenia. Your loved one should be cautious about joining AA if the leader of the group isn't familiar with co-occurring disorders.

Some "double-trouble" groups are developed specifically for people with co-occurring disorders. Seek one of these out — your loved one can benefit from approaches that treat both disorders simultaneously. (See Chapter 6 for more information on co-occurring disorders.)

Research on self-help for people with schizophrenia suggests that these groups increase knowledge about the illness, enhance coping, improve vocational involvement, and provide realistic hope for the future. The groups can take many forms including consumer-operated mental-health programs run by consumers (such as case management, crisis, or peer support programs); more informal clubhouse models and drop-in centers; or peer support programs, to name just a few. Some of the characteristics these programs share in common include

- Mentorship (opportunities to interact with positive role models)
- The sharing of coping strategies

- Support of other people in similar circumstances
- Exchange of information and resources
- Enhanced self-esteem
- Formation of friendships and socialization in low-stress situations
- Free or low-cost assistance

You can access a searchable database of self-help programs for a variety of disorders, including schizophrenia, at www.mentalhelp.net/selfhelp.

In the following sections, we cover some examples of self-help groups, but because these programs generally evolve at the local level, they tend to vary considerably from community to community, except in the case of several national programs Most self-help programs, in fact, are one-of-a-kind efforts sparked by recovering individuals who want to give back to their peers.

One example of a national program is Recovery, Inc. (www.recovery-inc.org), which was one of the first mental health self-help groups. It was founded in 1937 and is still alive and growing today. Recovery groups, of which there are now more than 700 chapters across the United States, bring together people with a variety of diagnosed and undiagnosed mental and emotional problems, including schizophrenia. Members meet regularly in their local communities (usually in a house of worship although there is no association with or discussion of religion) to learn techniques for handling the stress and the daily hassles people encounter in their lives. The approach is somewhat reminiscent of cognitive behavioral therapy (CBT) because it focuses on learning to change the thoughts and behaviors caused by psychiatric symptoms.

In a controlled study of Recovery, leaders and members reported fewer symptoms and fewer re-hospitalizations. Other studies of mental-health self-help groups have found improvement on psychological, interpersonal, and community adjustment measures; improved member self-confidence and self-esteem; fewer hospitalizations; more hopefulness about the future; and a greater sense of well-being.

Recovery meetings are intended to augment, not substitute for, psychiatric treatment.

Another example of a national model is the NAMI Peer-to-Peer program, which consists of nine two-hour courses that are taught by three trained mentors, individuals who are living with mental illnesses. To learn more about this program and find out whether courses are being given in your community, go to www.nami.org, and from the Find Support drop-down list, choose Consumer Support. Then click the Peer-to-Peer link. (Or just go to www.nami.org/template.cfm?section=Peer-to-Peer.)

Because schizophrenia is a brain disorder, society often uses the term *patient* to describe individuals with schizophrenia, as they would refer to anyone with a physical disorder. However, there's considerable controversy in the field of mental health about language, because some of it can be very stigmatizing. So in this section, we use the word *consumer* or *peer* to describe the patient or recipient of services.

Grass-roots consumer-run programs include, but aren't limited to, clubhouse models, drop-in centers, case-management programs, outreach programs, crisis services, employment and housing programs.

Clubhouse models

Psychosocial clubhouses, whose numbers are growing across the United States, provide peer support in an informal setting, and often provide help in locating other services. Participants, called *members,* often share responsibility with paid staff for the upkeep of the clubhouse. The clubhouses serve as training grounds to provide people with schizophrenia with skills they can use in the workplace and with the opportunity to forge social bonds. They also promote a sense of belonging as one may feel as a member of any other type of club. Some, but not all, provide residential care until a person can get permanently housed in the community.

The first such clubhouse, Fountain House (`www.fountainhouse.org`), opened in New York City in 1948. Today, the program has served more than 16,000 members. At Fountain House and many other clubhouses, members and staff learn to work together closely to enrich the environment for all their members. Thresholds (`www.thresholds.org`), in Chicago, is another well-known example of a clubhouse model.

The International Center for Clubhouse Development (`www.iccd.org`) has identified the defining characteristics of clubhouse programs:

- An emphasis on working roles within the clubhouse
- Opportunities for returning to competitive employment through transitional and independent employment programs
- Recreational programming for evenings, weekends, and holidays
- Access to community services, benefits, and supports
- Outreach efforts when members are absent
- Educational opportunities
- Access to or provision of housing, which is viewed as a fundamental right of all members
- Shared decision-making and governance of the clubhouse

The same Web site (`www.iccd.org`) provides a Clubhouse Directory under the About the ICCD tab.

One self-help approach that incorporates self-assessment and self-monitoring, and is now being used in many states, is the Wellness Recovery Action Program (WRAP) developed by Mary Ellen Copeland, PhD (`www.mentalhealthrecovery.com`). It is a self-management program that provides consumers with the tools they need to pursue their own wellness — teaching them, for example, what to do when they get stressed, how to maintain a healthy lifestyle, and how to identify early warning signs of relapse. WRAP is unique because its focus is on prevention and recovery as opposed to control of symptoms. Several large-scale studies of the program are now ongoing.

Drop-in centers

Funded by county or city mental-health authorities and various other private mental-health programs, drop-in groups are informal places for people with schizophrenia to meet. People are free to come and go as they please, and there generally aren't any professionals involved in these operations. These programs sometimes appeal to consumers who are uncomfortable using traditional services.

Drop-in centers (as well as clubhouses) for homeless persons with serious mental illness are sometimes called *safe havens*. These programs are voluntary, welcoming, and try to avoid instituting unnecessary rules and requirements that would inadvertently discourage their use.

Volunteer programs

A number of programs make use of volunteers (from the community) or peers (recovering individuals) to provide supportive friendships, information, and assistance to people with serious mental illness, including those with schizophrenia. One of the best known of these programs is Compeer, Inc. (`www.compeer.org`), an international nonprofit organization that has more than 80 chapters serving more than 65,000 adults and children worldwide. Compeer programs offer one-on-one mentoring relationships, skill-building, and interim telephone support, all of which are intended as a complement to professional treatment.

To find out about the drop-in centers, clubhouses, or volunteer programs in your own community, contact your local city or county mental-health department. The appendix lists national consumer clearinghouses and technical assistance centers, funded by the federal government, that can help your loved one become involved in self-help programs.

Internet chat rooms and social media

With the growth of Internet chat rooms and new forms of social media, there are a multitude of opportunities for individuals with schizophrenia to talk with one another and participate as they choose. For example, there are more than 47,000 active members on the schizophrenia-focused discussion forums at `www.schizophrenia.com`. There are also groups on Facebook (www.facebook.com) and MySpace (www.myspace.com) that may be interesting to people with schizophrenia. For example, the Facebook Mental Health Awareness group has more than 5,000 members, many of them consumers.

You can think of these sites as the virtual equivalent of a drop-in center. They can provide useful information and opportunities for social connections.

Several caveats for your loved one with regard to chatting or posting on forums on the Internet:

- Be careful about revealing your identity or providing personal information online.
- Make sure your loved one uses good judgment in selecting an appropriate e-mail address and doesn't reveal his true name or identity.
- Remember that these chat rooms are generally unsupervised, and people can get nasty in any chat room.
- Be skeptical of advice if you know little about its source.
- Online chats can complement face-to-face ones, but they shouldn't be used as a substitute.
- Be careful what you write on a Facebook or MySpace profile. You never know who'll be reading it or whether it'll come back to haunt you.

Chapter 10 provides additional caveats for evaluating information you find on the Internet.

Supporting the Whole Family

The use of family therapies in the treatment of schizophrenia began soon after World War II, when the prevailing theory for mental illness was that families of people with schizophrenia communicate in disturbed ways. (This was the blame-the-family era.) The goal of treatment was to repair the family system instead of focusing on the treatment of any one individual, even the person with schizophrenia.

Traditional family therapy focused on treating family pathology and dysfunction rather than providing families with the coping skills to help them support their relatives with schizophrenia. The most unfortunate consequence was that families were often viewed as part of the problem rather than people whose help and support could be fundamental to recovery (see Chapter 2). This often set up a schism between patients, their families, and doctors — and it made parents, especially, feel guilty and ashamed.

Now, family therapy is generally focused on helping families better cope by helping them understand schizophrenia, improving communication patterns among family members, and identifying solutions to help them and their loved one's illness. Because of the strain having a relative with schizophrenia can place on a marriage, some families also benefit from couples therapy.

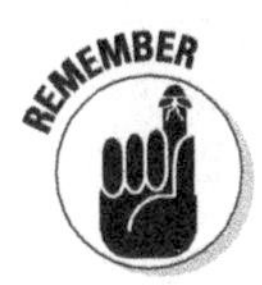

Not every person with schizophrenia has a family — and some patients refuse to have contact with their families or have alienated them by their behaviors. Support can come from many places, and for some individuals, friends, roommates, volunteer organizations, and religious organizations comprise "family."

Family psychoeducation

Family psychoeducational groups educate families by giving them the information and skills they need to support their relatives' recovery. The groups are led by mental-health professionals or trained group leaders and focus on improving patient rather than family outcomes. As the patient improves, the family's quality of life typically improves as well.

The groups augment, but do not substitute for treatment, including medication.

Although the various models of family psychoeducation share many characteristics in common, they differ in several ways:

- Participation of one family versus multiple families
- Participation of family members exclusively versus family members and people with schizophrenia
- Varying lengths of duration, ranging from ten weeks to more than five years
- A focus on different illnesses and different phases of the illnesses

These programs have been shown to reduce relapse among consumers and to lower rates of hospitalization. In addition, they lead to increased participation in vocational programs and employment, improved family satisfaction, and decreased overall costs of care. To increase the number of these programs, efforts have been made to integrate them with ACT programs (see Chapter 5).

One of the largest psychoeducation programs for families, sponsored by NAMI, is called the Family-to-Family Educational Program. When patients leave hospitals, the most common scenario is for them to return to their families. This makes it essential for families or close friends to understand everything they can about the illness and its treatment. Moreover, the families and/or friends need to accept the diagnosis and to have realistic expectations for treatment and recovery.

This free, 12-week course for family caregivers of people with severe mental illness is taught by trained family volunteers and provides information that can help them find the right resources and ask the right questions, ultimately leading to better care for their relative and less stress for the rest of the family. Every family member should take this course soon after a loved one has been diagnosed with schizophrenia.

We think it's useful for as many members of a single family as possible to participate in family psychoeducational programs. This gives more people the opportunity to understand the disorder and sets the stage for spreading caregiving responsibilities among various family members.

Family support organizations

One of the most significant forces for advancing the treatment of schizophrenia has been the development of family support organizations, most notably the National Alliance on Mental Illness (NAMI).

Family support groups generally serve three functions: Mutual support; information; and advocacy for improved mental-health services, increased funding for mental-health research, and improved public awareness to reduce stigma and discrimination.

Founded in 1979, the grassroots organization has affiliates in every state and in more than 1,100 local communities across the United States. NAMI state and local affiliates sponsor self-help groups for families who meet together to better understand mental illness and to better cope with the challenges the illness poses for themselves and their relative. Families who once felt isolated and helpless now realize that they aren't alone and can depend on one another for support.

To find a NAMI affiliate in your community, go to `www.nami.org` and select the Find Support tab.

You may hear about programs offering art, music, drama, or other creative therapies for people with schizophrenia. There is scant empirical research supporting the effectiveness of these therapies for schizophrenia. But apart from their use as a treatment per se, the creative arts are life-affirming pursuits that bring pleasure and provide a way for people to relax, enjoy, and create. If your loved one demonstrates a proficiency or interest in the arts, encourage him!

Considering Cognitive Remediation

One of the most important recent advances in the field of psychosocial rehabilitation has been the emphasis on cognitive remediation (CR). The term *cognition* refers to the way a person thinks. Needless to say, the way a person thinks affects the way he approaches and performs many tasks in his daily life.

Neuropsychological testing has shown that the vast majority of people diagnosed with schizophrenia have a variety of cognitive impairments thought to be related to abnormal brain function, including

- Difficulty sustaining attention
- Impaired memory
- Difficulties with verbal learning
- Problems making decisions
- Delays in the speed of thought processing

The severity of the disability can be marked; over 85 percent of individuals with schizophrenia score more poorly on cognitive functioning than 90 percent of healthy individuals.

Only recently have the severe consequences of these cognitive impairments — in preventing social and vocational recovery from schizophrenia, as well as interfering with the therapeutic benefits of other psychological inteventions — been recognized. As a result, treatment of cognitive impairment has become a therapeutic goal using biologic (see Chapter 8) and/or psychosocial approaches. Through a variety of techniques, CR — not to be confused with cognitive behavior therapy (CBT) — attempts to do one of the following:

- Restore or improve thinking skills in either all or some deficit areas
- Teach the person with schizophrenia ways of compensating for cognitive impairment
- Modify the environment in which the person with schizophrenia functions to reduce her dependence on cognitive success in order to succeed

Although attempts at cognitive rehabilitation began almost 40 years ago (in a more limited way), there is still no one commonly accepted or preferred way to carry out the training. Increasingly, *repetitive skills training* (learning through repeated use) is done on the computer, while other forms still use paper and pencil. Part of teaching consumers to compensate for their disabilities stresses organizing information instead of having to remember individual things. For example, CR encourages the use of lists and other aids placed in the environment to help the person with schizophrenia to remember what needs to be done and to keep organized.

Despite the fact that CR training varies from program to program, it's clear that improvements in cognitive functioning do occur. Not enough studies have been conducted to determine how long the improvements last after training stops, or whether cognitive improvement also improves psychosocial functioning.

Combining other forms of psychiatric rehabilitation, such as social skills training and coaching, with specific cognitive remediation training seems to bring about greater changes in psychosocial functioning than CR alone. Rehabilitation programs often combine pure CR training along with other rehabilitation methods. Some of these combined programs include cognitive remediation therapy (CRT), neuropsychological educational approach to rehabilitation (NEAR), cognitive adaptation training (CAT), and cognitive enhancement therapy (CET). (You don't need to know detailed information about these various programs, but it's useful to be familiar with these names so when you hear the terms used, you can identify them as an approach to cognitive remediation.)

This is a time when many new methods are being tried to enhance cognitive functioning. We believe that when more widely standardized and tested psychosocial and biological (medication) approaches become available, combining them may lead to vast improvements in treatment. Better success may also be found by devising treatments that are more specific to a person's individual impairments.

One of the biggest drawbacks to the use of CR today is the lack of programs and practitioners trained to provide CR. Some researchers are developing methods for families to be able to apply these methods on their own. For example, having family members remind the person with schizophrenia to compensate for memory problems by diligently writing things down and keeping lists or having someone who is highly distractible only undertake one task at a time (as opposed to multitasking).

The New York State Office of Mental Health has produced a handbook for friends and family members titled *Dealing with Cognitive Dysfunction Associated with Psychiatric Disabilities*. You can download for free at `www.omh.state.ny.us/omhweb/cogdys_manual/CogDysHndbk.pdf`.

Expanding Psychosocial Options

Consumer choice should be a major factor in selecting treatments. For choices to be informed, your loved one needs to know more about the risks and benefits of various treatments and be able to compare each of them in terms of their cost and effectiveness. This may be a tall order until your loved one reaches a certain point in the process of recovery.

Moreover, in the real world, most communities do not provide the full range of psychosocial, individual, group, self-help, and cognitive remediation treatments that are necessary to facilitate optimal treatment. The growth of the patient and family advocacy movement holds much hope for stimulating more interest and funding in these types of treatments.

The bottom line: Working together, consumers, families, and professionals need to:

- Identify an individual's particular strengths and deficits.
- Find out about the availability of psychosocial rehabilitation practitioners and programs in the community.
- Develop an individualized plan to minimize, remediate, or adapt to deficits created by the illness.
- Become advocates to ensure that there are effective and self-affirming choices available to maintain and/or restore the dignity, self-worth, and productivity for people with schizophrenia.

Chapter 10

Finding Help and Hope through Research

In This Chapter

- Identifying what families and friends need to know about research
- Examining new approaches to drug discovery and newly emerging technologies
- Looking into the brain
- Finding out about complementary and alternative treatments for schizophrenia
- Determining whether participating in a clinical trial is right for your loved one
- Keeping abreast of new research on the Internet

Almost every day, there's a news report on television, on the radio, or in a newspaper or magazine announcing some fantastic new health breakthrough. These breakthroughs sound so promising that consumers often rush to their doctor for the "latest treatment," only to find out that the marvelous results reported are from preliminary studies, conducted with small numbers of people, and that they haven't been verified by other researchers. It may be years before the reported treatments or drugs are available to the general public. Yet, if your loved one is suffering from a disorder such as schizophrenia, these reports provide a glimmer of hope for the future. In fact, some of these reports turn out to herald real advances.

Although having all the answers necessary to prevent and cure schizophrenia would be wonderful, research is generally a slow, incremental process, where one scientist's findings build upon another's. Clinical trials take considerable time to complete, and many don't live up to their original promise.

In this chapter, we look at the most current research on treatments for schizophrenia — its promises and pitfalls. We also answer the question of why new drugs take so long to get into pharmacies and how doctors know that certain drugs work. Finally, we take you behind the scenes of research, giving you insight into how clinical trials are done, and help you decide whether your loved one should participate in a clinical trial.

Understanding the Process of Research

Research is technically defined as "the systematic collection of data which is intended to be used beyond the place where it is collected." Without continued research, medical knowledge would stagnate. Early medical advances sometimes involved accidental discoveries of new medications or treatments, but today's advances are more likely to be the result of years of medical research. And research today is generally no accident.

Although much has been learned about diseases of the brain over the last few decades, leading to improved treatment, care, and quality of life, much more remains to be learned. Fortunately, a growing number of interdisciplinary researchers (in psychiatry, biology, chemistry, neuroscience, psychology, and medicine) are working diligently to answer the still unanswered questions about the causes of schizophrenia, with an eye toward prevention, early intervention, and better treatment and services. Because they share these same goals, people with schizophrenia, their friends and family members, and mental-health professionals have led the charge for increased research.

Aside from the human costs, the financial costs of mental illness in the United States are estimated at more than $150 billion annually, with the largest portion of that cost due to the lost productivity associated with mental disorders. Yet, research on mental illness has traditionally been underfunded compared to research on chronic physical problems like cancer, diabetes, and heart disease. This is due, in no small part, to the social stigma associated with schizophrenia.

The 2008 funding for the National Institute of Mental Health (NIMH) was about $1.4 billion, an increase of about 0.1 percent over the year before. This marks the fifth consecutive year that the NIMH budget grew at a rate less than biomedical research inflation, which is estimated at 3.5 percent per year. This makes for a highly competitive research environment, with many research projects competing for the same funding.

Recently, there has been a greater emphasis on the importance of *translational research,* which takes findings from the laboratory bench to the proverbial bedside. This research is conducted at the basic laboratory level with the clear expectation that it will be applied to a clinically relevant problem. For example, instead of studying hearing for its own sake, investigators focus their work on the role of hearing in relation to the auditory hallucinations prominent in schizophrenia.

Making sense of the mental-health research enterprise: The major players

A number of public and private sources support mental-health research. One of the most important is the National Institute of Mental Health (NIMH): At the federal level, the NIMH, a part of the National Institutes of Health (NIH), is the focal point for the funding of mental-health research on brain, mind, and behavior — ranging from basic science to clinical practice.

With overall funding caps and growing inflation, NIMH is expected to place greater emphasis on funding schizophrenia research, particularly around the first signs of the illness before diagnosis, around genetics, and around cognitive deficits (see Chapter 3).

NIH maintains a search engine called CRISP (`www.crisp.cit.nih.gov`) that enables anyone to look at the current portfolio of mental-health research grants funded by the federal government.

Other important players in mental-health research include

- **The Substance Abuse and Mental Health Services Administration (SAMHSA):** SAMHSA, which includes the Center for Mental Health Services (CMHS), funds studies on the implementation, cost, and effectiveness of mental-health and substance-abuse services. The agency has led the charge in pioneering studies of peer and consumer-run services, identification and treatment of co-occurring mental-health and substance-abuse disorders, and mental-health initiatives focused on special populations.
- **The Agency for Healthcare Research and Quality (AHRQ):** AHRQ focuses on developing information tools to assist health (including mental health) policymakers to improve the way care is organized, financed, paid for, and regulated.
- **National Alliance for Research on Schizophrenia and Depression (NARSAD):** The donor-supported NARSAD is the world's leading charity dedicated to mental-health research. As of March 2008, NARSAD has awarded a total of $219 million through 3,243 research grants to scientists in 418 institutions in the United States and 26 other countries. The organization raises and distributes funding for promising psychiatric research in order to develop new preventive measures, better diagnoses, and improved treatments for these conditions. NARSAD also educates the public about the value of psychiatric research.

  NARSAD recently collaborated with the NIMH to create the Schizophrenia Research Forum (`www.schizophreniaforum.org`), a unique online resource for scientists and the public. One portion of the site highlights new and significant research findings.
- **Other private foundations:** The Stanley Research Foundation, the Robert Wood Johnson Foundation, the van Ameringen Foundation, the John D. and Catherine T. MacArthur Foundation, and many others are instrumental in funding psychiatric research. Additionally, private industry, particularly pharmaceutical and biotechnology companies, provide funding support for additional studies of new compounds, drugs, devices, and technologies.

Looking at Clinical Trials and How They Work

Much of what is known in medicine, including which medications work best, is determined by medical research done through *clinical trials* (experimental studies designed to determine whether there is a cause-and-effect relationship between an *intervention* (treatment) and an *outcome* (symptom) — for example, is a drug effective in controlling positive symptoms of schizophrenia?). *Controlled clinical trials* are considered the gold standard for research. In these studies, the new treatment (called an *intervention*) is compared to an ineffective treatment or to an already existing treatment in a fair, unbiased way.

Seeing how clinical trials are conducted

In a controlled clinical trial, one group of people (called the *experimental group*) is given a drug, and another group of people (called the *control group*) is given a *placebo* (an inert substance, like a sugar pill) or a known standard medication. The *investigator* (the person conducting the research) compares the effects seen in these two groups. If there's a *statistically significant difference* (a difference not likely to be due to chance) between the two groups in terms of reducing the symptoms (called the *outcome measure*), the medication is determined to be effective.

Each person going into the trial has an equal chance of getting the active medication or the placebo; this is known as *randomization.* By assigning people to the different treatment groups randomly, it's more likely that the groups will be equal and that any differences seen will be due to the treatments they receive. Another way of preventing bias in a trial is called *double-blinding.* This means that neither the person receiving the medication nor the person evaluating the response knows whether an active or inactive medication has been given. If they did know, they might unintentionally be more enthusiastic if they knew they were receiving or judging the active rather than the inactive medication.

In some circumstances, experimental research can't be conducted. For example, a researcher wouldn't give an ill person a drug that makes his condition permanently worse. So in cases like this, researchers use *correlational* methods, which look at the relationships between two variables to see if they're related. Correlational methods are unable to definitively establish cause and effect.

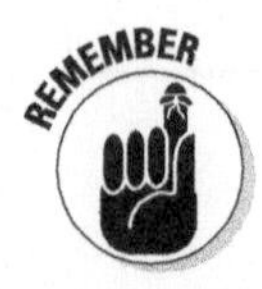

In the case of medications, the first clinical trials (called Phase I trials) are conducted using healthy volunteers, to make sure the drug has no serious side effects.

Clinical trials are easier to evaluate when interventions or outcomes can be precisely measured. Some clinical trials related to schizophrenia test psychosocial approaches. Although the principles of experimental design are similar, it's more difficult to accurately measure the dose, quality, or purity of a complex psychosocial intervention as compared to measuring, for example, the dose of a medication.

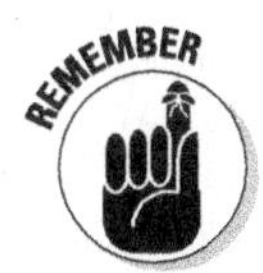

No one study, however well designed and executed it may be, is ever considered as absolute proof that something is beneficial. Studies are repeated by other investigators to be sure they get the same results and that the findings are reliable.

Evidence-based treatment is a term often used to identify interventions that have been tested and have been proven effective. In the case of medications, the Food and Drug Administration (FDA) must find the treatment safe and effective and that the benefits of the medication outweigh its risks before the drug can be sold.

Deciding whether to participate in clinical trials

In all areas of medical science, clinical research depends on the participation of volunteers. If your loved one with schizophrenia doesn't respond to various existing treatments, her doctor may suggest that she consider enrolling in a clinical trial that will compare a promising new treatment (which may not be available elsewhere) to one or more treatments that are already used and approved. Being asked to participate in a clinical trial can be both exciting and a little frightening.

People participate in clinical trials for a variety of reasons, including the following:

- To advance science and help save lives
- To take advantage of new treatments and be at the forefront of therapeutic breakthroughs
- To try something different when their illness is treatment-resistant
- To receive high-quality medical care with close monitoring for little or no cost

At the conclusion of a study, researchers have a responsibility to disseminate their findings to other researchers, clinicians, the general public, and to policymakers.

What is informed consent?

Informed consent refers to the process of fully explaining to the person participating in research what the study entails, including potential benefits and risks, and then obtaining her voluntary agreement (or consent).

Informed consent is so important in research that no human participants can be involved in any way until after informed consent has been obtained. Informed consent presents special problems when subjects may not be deemed legally capable of understanding what's involved with a study. But having a mental disorder doesn't necessarily mean that a person is unable to understand or evaluate the benefits and risks of participating in clinical research. Many people with schizophrenia can provide informed consent.

When an individual is not able to provide informed consent because she lacks the capacity to understand the proposed research, she often has the capacity to name a surrogate or substitute who can make the decision for her. Safeguards exist so that consent is obtained both from the participant and a legally authorized representative, such as a parent, a guardian, or a spouse.

Deciding whether to participate in a clinical trial requires some thought and investigation. When your loved one is considering whether participating in a clinical trial makes sense, here are some things you'll want to do:

- **Using the Internet or visiting the library, find out whatever information you can about the available treatments for your loved one's condition.** The National Library of Medicine (NLM; `www.nlm.nih.gov`) provides current information on various conditions and their treatment. You may also be able to get information from some of the mental-health research and advocacy organizations we list in the appendix. The more you learn, the better prepare you'll be to ask questions about the trial and what it can do for your loved one.
- **Discuss treatment options with your loved one's psychiatrist or another health professional whom you know and trust.** They can help you weigh the respective risks, outcomes, and benefits of participation in a trial.
- **Involve a trusted friend or family member in the decision.** Bring them with you when you go to learn about the trial. They may hear things you don't hear or see things differently.

Most clinical trials cover the cost of evaluation, treatment, and transportation. What is paid for and what is not should be spelled out in the informed consent form (see the nearby sidebar, "What is informed consent?"). The study director will also help your loved one transition into some appropriate type of follow-up care after your participation in the study is completed.

Finding the right trial for your loved one

Sometimes your doctor will know about a trial going on that may be just right for your situation. But don't be limited by recommendations from one doctor or a particular institution that advertises in the newspaper or on the radio. Here are some tips for finding the right trial for your loved one with schizophrenia:

- **Find out the trials for which your loved one may be eligible.** The National Institutes of Health (NIH) maintains a registry of clinical trials (www.clinicaltrials.gov) to provide patients and family members with information about governmental and privately sponsored trials. The site includes general information about each trial's purpose, who may participate, location, and a phone number to call for more information.

  The information at www.clinicaltrials.gov is intended to be used in conjunction with advice from healthcare professionals.

  Eligibility for clinical trials is usually based on very specific study criteria. For example, your loved one may be too old or too young, have other complicating emotional problems, or have health problems that preclude participation. Don't take rejection personally. Instead, recognize that it's intended to protect your loved one and make sure that the trial provides the precise answers for which it is designed.

- **Speak to the study director or other investigators at the site.** If your loved one participates in a trial, the research will likely be conducted at a physician's office, clinic, hospital, or other healthcare setting. Be sure to meet with the staff at the site beforehand so you and your loved one feel comfortable there and understand the procedures.

- **Learn about the process of informed consent.** Carefully read the informed consent form that outlines key facts about the clinical trial — including procedures, risks, benefits, and expected outcomes. The form should be user-friendly and easy to read. If it isn't, be sure to ask questions. Even after enrollment, you have the right to raise any concerns you have with the director of the study or the director of the institutional review board (IRB; see the sidebar "Institutional review boards: They've got your back," in this chapter).

  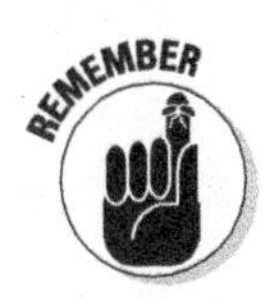

  Informed consent is not a one-time event but a continuing process. You also have the right to withdraw from a study at any time for any reason.

Although participating in a clinical trial may not be the right choice for every person, every condition, or in every situation, it does offer possible benefits for some patients — and trials provide information and hope for others who will benefit from the results.

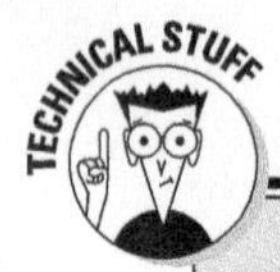

Institutional review boards: They've got your back

An institutional review board (IRB) is a committee established under federal and state regulations to protect the rights and welfare of people who participate in research. IRBs review all proposed research involving human subjects. They approve only studies that meet strict criteria for the protection of people who participate in them. IRBs are comprised of health professionals, scientists, lay people, consumers, family members, community members, quality assurance representatives, statisticians, and ethicists; this broad range of expertise allows the IRB to consider the burdens potentially placed on participants.

If you're participating in a trial being conducted by a hospital or other large institution, that institution may have its own internal IRB that reviews and approves all their clinical trials. Studies done through physicians' offices are overseen by a central IRB, which looks at research done at a number of different clinical sites.

Any IRB, whether specific to an institution or centralized, looks to make sure safeguards are in place to protect participants. When research studies are discussed, approval is made only if the following criteria are met:

- Risks to subjects are minimized.
- Risks are reasonable in relation to anticipated benefits.
- Selection of subjects is equitable.
- Informed consent will be sought and documented from each subject or the subject's legally authorized representative.
- Appropriate monitoring will take place.
- Adequate provisions will be in place to protect the privacy of individuals and the confidentiality of their data.
- Useful information will likely result from the study.

Many family members volunteer to participate as healthy volunteers in non-interventional studies where they may have MRIs taken or provide blood for genetic studies. This is one way friends or family members of persons with schizophrenia can help advance research on their loved ones' illnesses.

New and Promising Directions in Research

There has never been a more exciting or productive time in the history of schizophrenia research than the present. New techniques in the basic sciences (molecular biology and genetics) have allowed scientists to better study the neurobiology of the brain and its relationship to schizophrenia.

New pharmacologic and clinical imaging techniques allow scientists to study the brain as well as follow the course of the disorder and examine the impact of treatment.

More attention is being focused on public attitudes and the harmful effects of the negative stigma associated with schizophrenia, and on the importance of both peer support and recovery (see Chapter 15). Psychosocial treatment and health services research is aimed at studying a broad range of interventions to improve functioning and quality of life, as well as the best ways to deliver these treatments (see Chapters 9 and 15).

So, with all this research and discovery, why don't scientists yet have all the answers? Simply put, this type of complex, *biopsychosocial research* (research that combines biological, psychological, and social approaches) does not progress in a simple straight line from point A to point B, like constructing a building from a plan. It's more like painting a picture, where each scientific article is a little dab of paint on a different part of the canvas. We can't recognize the picture until enough paint has filled up the blank spots on the portrait. Sometimes we can't even be sure of what is background and what is foreground without repeating studies and determining their relevance to the other dabs of color on the canvas.

In the following sections, we fill you in on new drugs and other treatments and technologies that are on the horizon, which may prove successful in treating schizophrenia.

New directions in drug discovery

One area of development involves the creation of new classes of medications — which may work along with the current antipsychotics or possibly one day replace them.

Current antipsychotic medications are good at controlling the positive symptoms (hallucinations, delusions, and agitation) seen in schizophrenia. Because they're so good, we've come to recognize that, after the positive symptoms clear, people with schizophrenia still have underlying and very profound problems with cognition (memory, verbal ability, decision-making) and so-called negative symptoms (such as lack of motivation, problems socializing, and the inability to experience pleasure).

Very precise neuropsychological tests have been developed that can measure cognitive performance in people with schizophrenia. Not only have deficits been noted, but some deterioration in cognitive abilities has been found even *before* these individuals were diagnosed with schizophrenia. And perhaps even more important, the severity of cognitive impairment has been found to be related to the person's inability to function even *after* their positive symptoms are treated with antipsychotic medications.

Therefore, a great deal of focused effort is now underway to develop medications that specifically target the cognitive impairments of schizophrenia. Because antipsychotic medications are thought to work primarily by blocking dopamine receptors in the brain and these medications control positive symptoms, researchers are searching for medications that will affect other neurotransmitters and correct or lessen cognitive deficits.

In the following sections, we cover three new approaches that offer hope for treating some of the cognitive symptoms of schizophrenia that have long eluded prior therapeutic efforts.

Although it's somewhat hard to understand how all these different systems in the brain could be responsible for some of the symptoms of schizophrenia, these systems are linked to one another. If researchers can identify and correct the crucial malfunctioning system, the other "upstream" and/or "downstream" systems may also be corrected with significant therapeutic benefit.

Glutaminergic approaches

One clue about what system to study came about by the clinical observation that phencyclidine (PCP, commonly called angel dust), a drug of abuse, causes a variety of symptoms (including cognitive deficits) that look like schizophrenia. Using this drug, pharmacologists and biochemists were able to show that it had the effect of blocking a receptor in the brain (called NMDA), which was stimulated by the neurotransmitter glutamine.

Drugs other than PCP, which also block glutamine neurotransmission, were found to cause cognitive problems, too. Glutamine receptors are found widely distributed in the brain, and the glutamate system interacts with the dopamine system (as well as other neurotransmitters systems — for example, GABA).

With this understanding — in other words, that blocking glutamate receptors causes cognitive problems — the hypothesis emerged that cognitive problems in schizophrenia may be due to insufficient glutamine activity in the brain. In order to test this hypothesis (and see whether increasing or stimulating glutaminergic activity could reverse cognitive problems), a search has begun for medications that may have this biological effect.

Currently three substances that are relatively simple amino acids (glycine, serine, and sarcosine), all of which increase glutaminergic transmission, have been studied both in the laboratory and in human clinical trials. Some small clinical trials have had relatively positive results, but the largest trial using glycine called into question the effectiveness and practicality of using it as a treatment. In order to be effective, glycine has to be given in large quantities (usually as a citrus-like drink), and this has been found to be too difficult for many patients to tolerate and has caused to some gastrointestinal side effects. Studies with serine are ongoing in the United States and Israel, but sarcosine is not currently approved for study in the United States.

With this foundation, ways of facilitating glutaminergic transmission other than using the amino acid approach are underway. One fairly large clinical trial has been reported by Eli Lilly and Company using a *metabotropic* (a different type of receptor function) glutamate approach that reportedly affects both positive and cognitive symptoms favorably. Other companies are using so-called glutamine transporter inhibitor compounds to enhance glutaminergic transmission, but clinical results have not yet been reported.

So, although there is great research activity and drug discovery effort pointed in new directions, there hasn't yet been any proven success, either in terms of *efficacy* (producing a desired effect) or safety, in developing a new class of cognition-restoring or cognition-enhancing medications based on facilitating glutaminergic function.

Noradrenergic approaches

A second approach to treating cognitive deficits in schizophrenia is related to the *noradrenergic neurotransmitter receptor system* located specifically in the prefrontal cortex of the brain, which is known to be important for cognition. Studies of humans with schizophrenia and memory/cognition studies of animals both show the association of this system with some of the cognitive deficits found in people with schizophrenia.

Two types of medications have potential for correcting these deficits. One is called an *alpha 2a selective agonist,* and a medication with this activity named guanfacine has actually been tried as an add-on treatment in persons already receiving second-generation antipsychotics (see Chapter 8). Improvements in both memory and reaction time were noted in preliminary studies, but confirmatory studies need to be carried out over longer periods of time to see if meaningful clinical improvement is seen.

The other approach to correcting noradrenergic problems is with the use of so-called specific norepinephrine reuptake inhibitors. Medications with this activity (for example, atomoxetine [brand name, Strattera]) are already in use to treat attention deficit/hyperactivity disorder (ADHD). Results of controlled clinical trials testing this therapeutic possibility have not yet been reported.

Cholinergic approaches

The cholinergic system is another system that plays an important role in relation to cognitive functioning. Its major neurotransmitter is called *acetylcholine,* and it attaches to a nicotinic receptor and a so-called muscarinic receptor. Both types of receptors have been shown to be implicated in neurophysiologic malfunctions in some people with schizophrenia.

Some 80 percent of people with schizophrenia are heavy smokers, and it's thought that the nicotine in cigarettes may actually reverse some of the neurophysiological (nervous system) deficits associated with schizophrenia. It's been suggested that medications that directly stimulate these receptors — so-called *nicotinic agonists* — might be useful therapeutic agents. However, so far there are no significant clinical trial results available.

Other new technologies

Recent advances in technology have led to the development of new techniques that once could never have even been imagined. Two such techniques that are currently being studied in multiple sites include deep brain stimulation and repetitive transcranial magnetic stimulation.

Deep brain stimulation

Deep brain stimulation (DBS) — which sounds a little like science-fiction — involves implanting a battery-powered, high-frequency pulse generator, either in the region of the collarbone or in the abdomen, and running a wire under the skin up the neck, behind the ear, and to the head. Tiny electrodes are placed at specific sites in the brain, and electrical signals are sent to interfere with brain activity at these preselected sites. The type and strength of pulses sent can be varied by a computer controlling the battery-operated stimulator.

DBS was developed and has been proven useful for treating various types of movement disorders (such as Parkinson's disease); in fact, it's estimated that some 35,000 people around the world have had DBS electrodes placed. Its use for the treatment of mental disorders is at a very preliminary stage — more studies have been done on the effects of DBS on depression and obsessive-compulsive disorder than on schizophrenia.

Repetitive transcranial magnetic stimulation

Transcranial magnetic stimulation (TMS) is a noninvasive way to cause an electrical activation of the brain, using a magnetic field (which easily passes through the skull). This electromagnetic stimulation can be precisely varied in its strength, location, duration, and frequency and is a tool for studying the brain and as well as a potential treatment.

Repetitive transcranial magnetic stimulation (rTMS) is the use of grouped pulses of stimulation, which causes a continuous activation over brief periods (minutes) of a treatment session. rTMS has been more intensely studied as a treatment for depression, but a number of experimental treatment studies have been carried out in people with schizophrenia.

Attempts have been made to use rTMS to treat both the positive and negative symptoms of schizophrenia. People with persistent treatment-resistant auditory hallucinations have had the hallucinations markedly reduced in some studies, but this improvement has not been lasting, and no follow-up studies have been conducted. Some studies have not shown beneficial effects, but these differences may be accounted for by both patient differences and differences in the way the rTMS was administered (for example, duration and frequency).

Studies attempting to treat negative symptoms have also shown mixed success. Different frequencies of stimulation at a different location (in the prefrontal cortex) from the auditory hallucinations studies were used. The most promising results seem to occur when the frequency of stimulation used is matched to the alpha (brain wave) frequency seen in each individual, rather than just using the same frequency for everyone.

In general, then, rTMS looks like a potentially promising noninvasive treatment, but the correct "dosing" (duration, frequency, location) is not well enough studied or understood to consider it a viable treatment alternative.

Opening New Windows into the Brain

Opportunities to study the brain, especially the living brain, have increased dramatically over the past 35 years. Before the advent of newer imaging techniques — such as magnetic resonance image (MRI) and positron emission tomography (PET) — the ways to directly study the brain were limited. These included X-rays and *brain biopsies* (removing a piece of brain during neurosurgery).

Surgically placing electrodes in the brain permitted direct examination of the electrical functioning of the living brain. Indirect measures such as electrical recordings from the scalp (called *EEG* and *evoked potentials*) and measuring chemicals in the spinal fluid that bathes the brain were other techniques that were used with some success. Postmortem studies of the brain could be carried out, but brain composition changes with death and no measurement of ongoing mind function was possible.

With the discovery and refinement of MRI, however, it became possible, without touching the brain directly, to image the structure (the physical configuration), the function (activity), and the composition (chemistry) of the brain. No radioactivity is involved — only magnetism — so imaging can be done as often as necessary with no physical risk to the person being imaged.

You may also hear an MRI referred to as an fMRI (short for *functional MRI*) and MRS (the *S* stands for *spectroscopy*) studies.

PET imaging and a related technique known as single photon emission computed tomography (SPECT) were also developed about 35 years ago. Both of these techniques require the administration of a small amount of a radioactive substance to the person being imaged. Although very useful for studies of brain receptors and specific drug actions, frequently repeated examinations using this technique are not possible because of the radioactivity involved. Nonetheless, PET and SPECT give rise to some types of information not available through MRI study. Thus, MRI and PET are considered complementary imaging methods.

Both MRI and fMRI studies have shown differences in the structure and function of the brain between groups of people with and without schizophrenia. These differences have pointed at areas and functions where something has gone wrong.

No new treatments, either biological or psychological, have yet directly resulted from MRI studies. But imaging has been important in learning more about schizophrenia and the brain, and it offers hope for the future. By investigating the biology of what has gone wrong, researchers are likely to find ways to "fix" the broken areas.

Another potential use for MRI is to help test whether treatments are actually having an effect. If scientists know that one area of the brain in people with schizophrenia has to work harder to solve a cognitive task and they give the person a medication, they can use the MRI to see if the brain doesn't have to work as hard to solve that task with medication. (The technology may actually be able to see improvement in brain function prior to any changes in the behavior of the person.) If the medication doesn't work on the brain function, then researchers don't need to conduct long and expensive clinical trials. Testing in this way is sometimes called *proof of concept.*

Another way to use the MRI to study the brain is a technique called diffusion tensor imaging (DTI). With this method, we can see the white matter of the brain and know whether it's intact or damaged. In the brains of people with schizophrenia, white matter pathways that connect different areas of the brain have been found to be damaged. This means that vital communication between one part of the brain and another, which must be closely synchronized to function appropriately may be out of sync — something like what you experience when the sound and picture of someone talking on TV or in the movies doesn't match. Imagine if that happened to your thinking!

Very precise studies, presenting sounds (tones of differing pitches) and pictures (with areas missing) have been demonstrated to be seen differently by people with and without schizophrenia. These differences in sensory abilities may make it hard for people with schizophrenia to interpret the voices or facial expressions of individuals talking to them. Correction of these basic biological defects — either with medication or with computer training — could have a potentially important therapeutic impact.

Psychosocial and Other Treatment Research

Psychosocial therapies (also called *psychosocial rehabilitation* and *psychiatric rehabilitation*) are essential to the treatment of schizophrenia. These include a variety of interventions aimed at restoring a person's ability to function at home and in the community.

Psychosocial treatments that occur in real-world settings are infinitely more complex and costly to study than more specific interventions that can be studied in a laboratory of other controlled conditions. They often have multiple outcome measures, some of which are more ephemeral to study such as the concept of *quality of life* (a person's sense of overall well-being). Sometimes, *ethnographic methods* (the systematic study of individuals in their own environments) are used to provide qualitative, observational findings to enhance more quantitative ones.

There aren't the same financial incentives to study psychosocial treatments that there are to study medical treatments. Pharmaceutical industry or other corporate stakeholders are invested in studying medications and devices that will ultimately be patented and profitable. For all these reasons, research on psychosocial treatments has lagged in comparison, and is generally funded exclusively by the federal government, state governments (to a lesser extent), and private philanthropy.

Increasingly the problem of better defining and measuring the "intervention" is being addressed by writing manuals to carefully describe how various psychosocial treatments are to be administered. This has made it possible to carry out credible clinical trials. Also, the goals of some of the newer psychosocial interventions (such as CBT) have become more focused (for example, on reduction of hallucinations or more logical thinking) and briefer rather than global attempts to "make over personality" that were more characteristic of older psychoanalytic approaches, which often took years.

The following psychosocial interventions have been studied extensively and have shown positive outcomes:

- **Family psychoeducation:** Classes and groups involving the person with schizophrenia and her family — or the family alone — to improve mental-health literacy, communication, and coping skills among family members and other caregivers
- **Supported employment:** Employment programs that provide education, training, and a sense of self-worth and productivity
- **Assertive community treatment:** Intensive case management programs that provide outreach and coordinate complex systems of care for individuals wherever they are living
- **Skills training:** Programs designed to help consumers relearn skills of daily living never learned or that they have forgotten because of the illness
- **Cognitive behavior therapy (CBT):** An individual therapy that focuses on changing behavior by changing negative thinking
- **Cognitive remediation:** Aimed at improving cognitive skills impaired by the illness by teaching compensatory strategies to overcome them, similar to that being done with victims of stroke and traumatic brain injuries

Just a few of the other treatment approaches being studied include: individual psychotherapy, family therapy, peer-support groups, self-help groups, consumer operated programs, drop-in centers, clubhouses, assisted and supportive housing programs, and creative therapies (such as art, music, and movement).

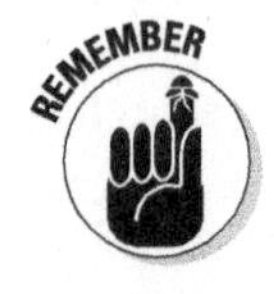

Based on the available current research, in order for psychosocial interventions to be effective they must be used along with antipsychotic medications. The two working *together* provide the most effective treatment, and although there are always exceptions, in general, psychosocial interventions used alone do not result in long-term favorable outcomes.

Evaluating Complementary and Alternative Treatments

Complementary treatments are ones used together with conventional medicine. *Alternative treatments* are ones used in place of conventional medicine. A variety of complementary and alternative treatments have been tried as treatments for schizophrenia. People seek these treatments because:

- They've found that other treatments haven't worked at all or only have addressed some symptoms.
- They suffer from uncomfortable side effects of their treatment.
- They can't afford the high cost of prescription medications and conventional psychotherapies.
- They strongly desire to use what they see as safer and more "natural" alternatives.
- They don't believe that schizophrenia is a brain disorder and attribute it to other causes (such as nutritional deficiencies).

In the following sections, we cover some of the complementary and alternative treatments that have been studied.

Omega-3 fatty acids

Studies have looked at the use of omega-3 fatty acids as a dietary supplement to reduce the positive symptoms of schizophrenia. These fatty acids aren't manufactured by the body, so they need to be consumed through foods or dietary supplements. A systematic review of studies by the Cochrane Collaboration (which publishes treatment reviews in all fields of health) found that the effects of essential fatty acid (EFA) supplementation may have some beneficial effects but that the results were inconclusive "due to the limited number of studies and lack of usable data."

Fish oils (a source of omega-3 fatty acids) cannot be used by people allergic to iodine or who are using blood thinners. Additionally, there is some speculation that EFA-supplements can precipitate *mania* (excitability).

Antioxidant vitamins

Some research suggests that antioxidant vitamins may be helpful in addressing the negative symptoms of schizophrenia. Foods containing antioxidants include blueberries, prunes, spinach, and strawberries. Although there probably is no inherent danger in eating these foods as part of a balanced diet, again, evidence is inconclusive.

Vitamin E

There is some anecdotal evidence that vitamin E has helped some individuals with *tardive dyskinesia* (involuntary, repetitive movements of the tongue, lips, face, trunk, and extremities associated with the long-term use of first-generation antipsychotic medications). However, a *meta-analysis* (a study of other studies) found that most of the trials that were conducted were too small or of too short duration to provide definitive results. A Cochrane review concluded that the benefits were minimal and might be limited to preventing further deterioration. A large study by the Veterans' Administration did not show vitamin E to be effective.

In a study conducted to evaluate long-term use of vitamin E to prevent cancer in men and women with vascular disease or diabetes, those taking the vitamin had a 13 percent increased risk of heart failure. An advisory posted on the Web site of the National Center for Complementary and Alternative Medicine (NCCAM) states: "These results emphasize the need to study vitamins and other natural products prior to making public health recommendations." This cautionary note reinforces that even something as simple as a vitamin may pose serious health risks for certain individuals. Consumers need to be aware of the risks of using yet unproven treatments. At the present time, neither the efficacy nor safety of vitamin E can be recommended as a treatment for schizophrenia.

N-methylglycine

A number of studies have suggested that N-methylglycine (sarcosine), another investigational compound that acts at the NMDA receptor site (see "Glutaminergic approaches," earlier in this chapter), may improve positive, negative, cognitive, and general psychiatric symptoms in schizophrenia. Because it is investigational, it is still not considered a recommended treatment. Besides, to our knowledge, pharmaceutical-grade sarcosine is not available in the United States.

Acupuncture

Acupuncture has been used as a treatment in China for more than 2,000 years with few adverse effects. A Cochrane review suggests that acupuncture is more socially acceptable, tolerable, and affordable than conventional drugs. However, a review of controlled clinical trials comparing acupuncture to antipsychotics, or using acupuncture as an adjunct to antipsychotics for people with schizophrenia, concluded that there isn't enough rigorous research to determine its efficacy and that better-designed studies are needed before it can be recommended as a treatment.

The Risks of Unproven Treatments

Eating a nutritionally balanced diet is important for people with schizophrenia — just as it is for everybody else. But many lay people erroneously believe that schizophrenia is caused by poor nutrition. Thus, a range of nutritional therapies — including niacin, vitamin B6, and megavitamins — have been promoted as treatments for schizophrenia, without a credible evidence base supporting their safety or efficacy. For example, flushing and rashes are associated with the use of niacin, and megadoses of vitamins have been implicated in causing health problems.

All food supplements are regulated as foods rather than drugs, so the rules for marketing them are much less restrictive than you may think. Neither safety nor effectiveness has to be proven in order for them to be marketed. In 2003, the FDA published proposed guidelines for supplements that would require accurate labeling and avoidance of contamination with other herbs, pesticides, heavy metals, or prescription drugs.

Bottom line: It's impossible to draw any positive conclusions about dietary supplements and vitamins as proven treatments for schizophrenia. In general, studies of alternative and complementary treatments for schizophrenia are conflicting, inconclusive, or methodologically weak. Some might even be dangerous.

As with research on conventional medicine, one small study is generally insufficient to prove whether something works. The same holds true for studies of alternative and complementary treatments. What is needed are controlled clinical trials with enough participants and rigorous methods that are repeated with the same results.

In addition to speaking to your medical team, Cochrane Reviews, peer-reviewed meta-analyses, and information from some of the following government agencies can be valuable resources to individuals and families considering use of unconventional treatment approaches:

- **The National Center for Complementary and Alternative Medicine (NCCAM),** a component of the National Institutes of Health (NIH), is the lead federal agency for research on complementary and alternative medicine. Its Web site (`http://nccam.nih.gov`) provides a searchable database of the scientific and medical literature on alternative healing practices.
- **The NIH Office of Dietary Supplements (ODS)** seeks to strengthen knowledge and understanding of dietary supplements by evaluating scientific information, supporting research, sharing research results, and educating the public. Its resources include publications and the International Bibliographic Information on Dietary Supplements database (`http://ods.od.nih.gov/Health_Information/IBIDs.aspx`).

- **The Center for Food Safety and Applied Nutrition** of the U.S. Food and Drug Administration (FDA) provides information for consumers such as "Tips for the Savvy Supplement User: Making Informed Decisions and Evaluating Information" (www.cfsan.fda.gov/~dms/ds-savvy.html) and updated safety information on supplements (www.cfsan.fda.gov/~dms/ds-warn.html). If you've experienced an adverse effect from a supplement, you can report it to the FDA's MedWatch program, which collects and monitors such information (800-332-1088 or www.fda.gov/medwatch).

Keeping Abreast of Research via the Internet — Wisely

Who can resist the siren call of the Internet when desperately looking for medical information? Open 24 hours a day, anonymous, free of charge, and always accurate — well, maybe not the last. Many people turn to the Internet to learn about medical research, but it's just as easy to find a quack as it is to find a cure if you believe everything you read. Anyone can start a Web site, and sometimes it seems that every snake-oil salesperson has.

On the other hand, the Internet is a good source of clinical trial reports and the latest research — if you know where to look. Your loved one's doctor should be keeping abreast of all the research developments in the field that may prove beneficial for her care, but the doctor probably isn't available 24/7. Just make sure to check out anything that seems exciting or promising with his office on Monday morning!

Social networking sites, user groups, *wikis* (Web sites that are edited by the public), and other Web sites can all provide useful and interesting information, but embarking on the information highway requires discretion, judgment, and caution.

Here are some things to think about when you're looking for accurate and unbiased information and trying to evaluate what you read:

- **Be critical of what you read.** Remember that many people post under false identities and that there's no way to verify what you read without doing more research.

- **Consider the source of all information.** Try to stick with sites sponsored by reputable organizations. The Web address can often help you identify the source of the information. If a Web address ends with `.gov`, it's a U.S. government site. If it ends in `.edu`, it's likely the site of an educational institution. If it's `.org`, it's a nonprofit. And if it's a `.com`, it's generally a for-profit business. ***Remember:*** These are just general guidelines — you may find a `.org` site that's not a nonprofit, for example.

  Be wary of commercial sites that are selling pharmaceuticals or other products. Make sure the information was derived from clinical trials and isn't just someone's opinion. Examine the credentials of the author and his references, usually listed at the end of the article. Find out who provided the funding for the trial and whether there might be any potential conflict of interest. Compare information on the same topic from different sites to see if they provide similar advice.

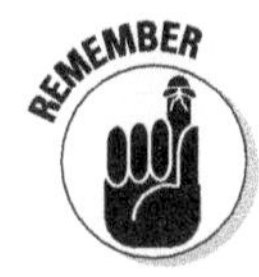

  Chat rooms and forums are rarely a source for solid clinical information.

- **Rely only on current information.** Every major page of a Web site should include the date that it was written or reviewed. Whenever possible, rely only on material that includes a date. On some sites, no one verifies whether information is still accurate or whether it became obsolete long ago.
- **Read only user-friendly material.** There are many, many sites to choose from, so be sure to use those that are easy to read and navigate. Don't waste your time trying to find information embedded in poorly designed Web sites.
- **Be cautious about sharing private information.** On the Internet, you can't be sure that information you divulge will remain private, so you need to be cautious. Before you fill out any forms or reveal any information about yourself or your family, make sure you review the site's privacy policy. When you post messages in chat rooms or on bulletin boards, consider using a pseudonym instead of your real name.

Remember that the Internet *cannot* substitute for medical advice. Given all these caveats, always be judicious in your use of the Internet as a source of definitive information concerning mental-health issues.

By exercising appropriate caution, the knowledge you get from the Web can help you become more literate about mental health, help you learn what questions to ask, and enable you to better communicate with professionals.

Part IV
Living with Schizophrenia

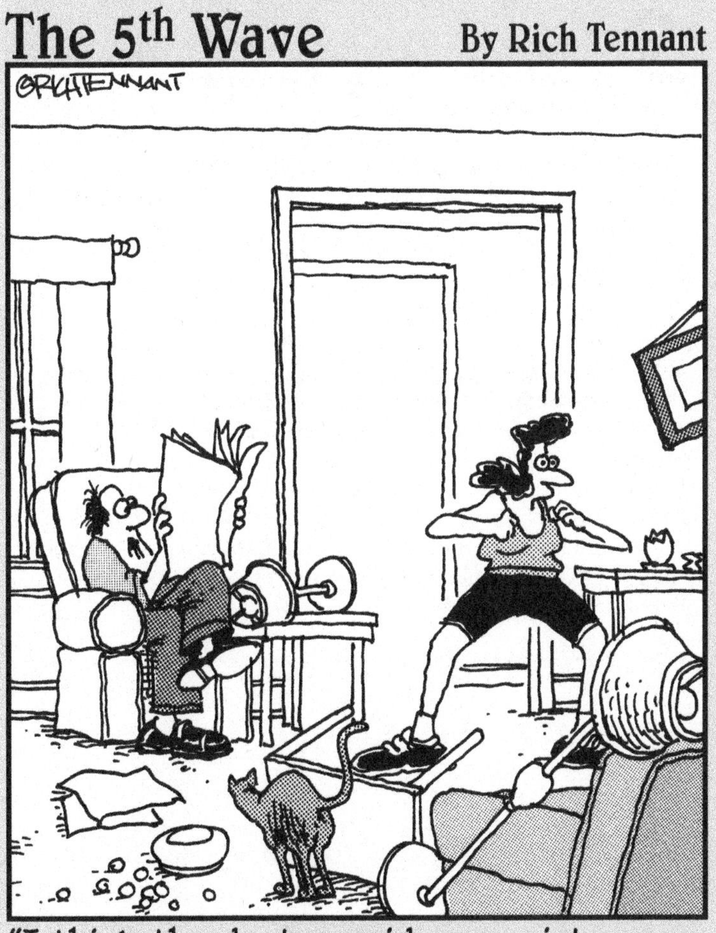

"I think the doctor said your sister may show signs of aggression when she comes home, not dominate your dojo."

In this part . . .

Schizophrenia doesn't just affect one individual — it affects an entire family. We offer concrete advice on how to break the news to others and how to cope with the challenges it poses to families. Caregiving has its demands and rewards, and we cover them in this part. To be an effective caregiver, you have to take care of yourself first and keep life as normal and balanced for those around you, and we show you how. We also offer advice about how to resolve conflicts, handle troublesome behaviors, and prevent and diffuse crises.

One of the most significant developments in the treatment of schizophrenia has been the development of advocacy organizations, such as the National Alliance for the Mentally Ill, a national organization of consumers and families providing education, support, and advocacy from those who have been there. With coordinated care and parity in insurance and other benefits, there is more hope than ever that people with schizophrenia will recover and live happy and productive lives.

Chapter 11

Schizophrenia and the Family

In This Chapter

- Adjusting to the diagnosis
- Breaking the news
- Coping with the challenges of caregiving
- Keeping the family safe and secure
- Planning for the future

When someone close to you has just been diagnosed with schizophrenia, you're likely to feel as though your world has come to an end. Many families have told us that the day they first heard the diagnosis divided their life into two discrete parts: before and after. Before, they may have only had vague feelings that something wasn't quite right. After, their worst fears were confirmed: Someone they loved was diagnosed with a serious mental disorder that they knew little about. They came face-to-face with the prospect that their loved one's strange or unusual behaviors were more than a small blip on the proverbial radar screen and weren't likely to go away anytime soon on their own.

One mother told us that, after diagnosis, "Things are never the same." You feel as though life — as you once knew it — has vanished and has been replaced by a strange new reality. You may worry about the impact of the diagnosis on the rest of your family: Will they be able to handle the changes this will bring? Will you ever be able to feel like a "normal" family again, to laugh and live like everyone else? You may also be concerned about what comes next in terms of treatment and think about the long-term consequences.

You may say, "Why me?" or "Why us?" — feeling that life has been unfair. You may look around you and be envious of those whose lives seem perfect in comparison (even though you never know what really lurks behind closed doors). Life is never fair and often throws unexpected curves — what counts most is how you cope with them.

In this chapter, we look at all the ways schizophrenia may impact your family and give you ways to cope with the challenges.

Adjusting to the Diagnosis

A diagnosis of schizophrenia is always frightening, but it doesn't mean that the future is bleak or hopeless for the person with the illness or for the rest of your family. Instead of thinking the worst, stop and take a deep breath. The good news is that you're finally able to attach a name and diagnosis to the same disturbing symptoms and behaviors that were worrying you before you knew what they were. Nameless fears are often far worse than a known reality.

Your initial reaction may be based on outdated and inaccurate information from years past. Perhaps you've heard stories of a relative who was diagnosed with a mental disorder decades ago and who, as a result of that diagnosis, spent much of his life locked away in a state mental hospital. Less than 50 years ago, people with serious mental disorders were routinely sent to institutions for long periods of time. "Out of mind" literally meant out of sight. Treatment options were limited, and the available medications had side effects that were hard to tolerate. A person being treated for schizophrenia may have looked peculiar, suffering from uncontrollable tics and movements that were common to an earlier generation of medications.

With the development of new treatments, new technologies, and changed social policies and attitudes toward the treatment of mental illnesses, many people with schizophrenia are able to live symptom-free or manage their symptoms. So instead of people being warehoused for long periods of time, hospitalizations (if they're necessary) tend to be brief and focused on stabilizing acute symptoms, with the goal of returning the individual to the community as soon as possible. With proper outpatient treatment and supports, people with schizophrenia can recover and lead meaningful lives.

By getting a diagnosis (see Chapter 4), you've taken the first step in getting help for your loved one and the rest of your family. Understandably, you won't be able to put all your concerns and fears behind you immediately; you need time to educate yourself and adjust. Initially, you may feel defensive, angry, ashamed, and/or bewildered. Friends and relatives may behave differently toward you, making you feel isolated and alone. All these reactions, while upsetting, are very normal and common. Initial negative reactions don't mean that your family members will never come to accept the new reality of your life. They need time, as you do, to go through the predictable stages associated with grieving.

When you're able to accept the diagnosis, you'll be able to modify your thinking about your loved one's annoying or vexing behaviors and view them through a new lens: as symptoms of a neurobiological brain disorder that can be treated and managed.

Staying positive and optimistic

For many years, it has been estimated that about one-third of those diagnosed with schizophrenia make a full recovery; another third get better but have intermittent (but treatable) repeat episodes; and the last third have persistent symptoms. As researchers learn more about the causes of and treatments for schizophrenia, there is every reason to be more optimistic about the future.

If your relative was recently diagnosed, the odds that her symptoms can be controlled are even better because of advances that have been made in mental-health treatment and research. Increasingly, relapses can be avoided (see Chapter 14), or recurrences can be managed quickly so that life can get back to normal; and early diagnosis and sustained intervention can help minimize damage to the brain, to self-esteem, and to relationships with family, friends, and neighbors.

Even if the symptoms of your loved one's illness seem to be persistent or are treatment-resistant now (see Chapter 8), the rapid pace of research and new technologies promise improved treatments. Finally, public awareness of mental illnesses has increased over the last decade, leading to greater acceptance and understanding.

Understanding the nature of the illness and its treatment will help you appreciate the small and large victories you will achieve as a caregiver and the improvements you will see in your loved one. You'll also learn how crucial it is to convey a sense of hope and optimism to your loved one, who may have experienced a string of losses before getting help. Most families learn that they're more resilient and resourceful, as individuals and as a family unit, than they could have ever imagined.

Avoiding the family blame game

When a person is diagnosed with any serious illness, it's natural for others to look for a cause or explanation. Why did she get lung cancer? Did she smoke? Why was she diagnosed with late-stage breast cancer? Didn't she get routine mammograms?

In the case of schizophrenia, if the person who is ill is someone's child, adolescent, or young-adult offspring, the tendency is for outsiders to erroneously blame his parents for something they did or did not do. Was his mother too controlling, too soft, or neglectful? Was her father too doting, too distant emotionally, or too involved with his work? Did both parents give mixed messages?

Even more unfortunately, it's extremely common for one parent to blame the other. Each thinks back about the family tree on the other spouse's side and invariably remembers someone who had one mental illness or another and pinpoints that as the source of all problems.

Don't be surprised if you find yourselves blaming each other for things that happened years before. Realize that pain and tension are to be expected, but you need to make every effort to support, rather than undermine, one another.

Schizophrenia is a neurobiologically-based brain disease. Even if there's a family history of mental illness, it doesn't mean that someone caused the mental illness.

Even if no one blames you, you may cast blame upon yourself. It's not uncommon for parents or partners to spend sleepless nights wondering what they did to cause this. Why didn't you realize what was happening sooner? Should you have divorced or not divorced your husband? Did you favor one child over another? Are you being punished for something you did long ago? If you're religious, you may find your faith wavering or disappearing completely under the weight of unrelenting guilt and anger.

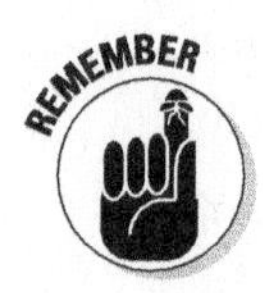

Heaping blame on yourself, the person with schizophrenia, or anyone else can only have negative effects. Schizophrenia is a no-fault disease. No one wants to have the illness and no one has the formula for creating the perfect mix of genetics and environment that prime another individual for getting it. There is no benefit in looking back — you need to look *forward.*

Breaking the News to the Family

After you hear a diagnosis, you need to decide who to tell, what to say, and when to tell them. This is generally the case with other physical health problems you or your family members encounter. But because of the myths and misunderstandings about mental illness, it's often difficult to tell even your closest friends, extended family, and neighbors, the people you ordinarily would lean on when you have a serious problem.

Just finding the right words to explain schizophrenia often presents a challenge. We hope that speaking with your doctor and reading this book will give you the information, tools, and words you need to feel comfortable explaining it to others.

Before you break the news to others, educate yourself by reading as much information as you can about the disorder. The National Institute of Mental Health (NIMH; `www.nimh.nih.gov`), the American Psychiatric Association

(APA; www.psych.org), the National Alliance on Mental Illness (NAMI; www.nami.org), and the National Association for Research on Schizophrenia and Depression (NARSAD; www.narsad.org) all offer easy-to-read booklets free of charge to the public. You can request them from any of these organizations, and many are available on the Internet or in public libraries (see the appendix).

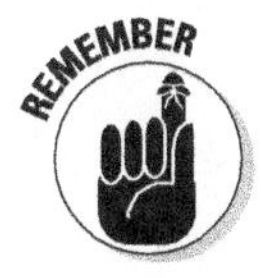

Because so many misunderstandings are associated with the diagnosis of schizophrenia, after you've had the chance to talk to them it often helps to provide written information to the people you decide to tell. If the news has taken someone by surprise, the person will be better able to comprehend what she has heard when she can read it more calmly, and see it in black-and-white.

Deciding who to tell

As difficult as it may be, except in rare circumstances, you need to tell your immediate family members about the diagnosis. They probably have some inkling about what's going on already — and you'll need to depend on them for their support. Your honesty in explaining what's happened and keeping the lines of communication open will make everyone feel like they're on the same team.

Don't be surprised if someone's initial reaction is negative, especially if they harbor misunderstanding about mental illness. Denial is common, as are several other misperceptions, such as:

- **The myth that schizophrenia is caused by bad parenting:** If people believe this myth, they may blame one or both parents of the person with schizophrenia.
- **The myth that people with schizophrenia are faking and are really just lazy and irresponsible:** If people buy into this myth, they may believe that the person has control over his symptoms and perhaps you've let your loved one "get away with it."
- **The myth that people with schizophrenia are messed up from alcohol and/or drugs:** If people believe this, they may think that the symptoms are solely caused by substance abuse, and that if the person stops abusing drugs or alcohol, the schizophrenia will go away.
- **The myth that schizophrenia isn't treatable:** If people think this, they may feel that the situation is hopeless.

When your family learns more about schizophrenia, they can become your most important allies.

Deciding whether to tell particular friends, neighbors, or employers depends on your own comfort level and whether you anticipate negative consequences. Though we strongly recommend telling your immediate family about your loved one's diagnosis, you don't have to tell *everyone* about your family's personal issues.

Here are some red flags that should make you more hesitant about telling someone about your loved one's mental illness:

- The person has previously shown a lack of sensitivity to people with mental illness or other disabilities.
- The person always asks invasive questions that make you feel worse.
- The person has loose lips and is likely to spread gossip for no good reason.
- Your loved one with mental illness would be embarrassed to tell the person herself.

Think through the possible outcomes before saying something you can't later retract. Although most friends and acquaintances will be supportive, it's possible that some may withdraw from you and your family. Conversely, some may feel very estranged and distant if they learn the truth long after the fact or from someone else other than you. Only you can gauge who you should tell and who you shouldn't.

Many people living with schizophrenia find it more comfortable and less stressful to be open about their disorder. It takes a lot of energy to keep a secret of any kind.

Make sure that the person with the illness is likely to be comfortable with the decisions you're making. This is another case where openness and honesty with your loved one is the best policy.

In the following sections, we cover the kinds of people you may decide to tell or not tell about your loved one's schizophrenia.

A spouse or partner

Sometimes the person with schizophrenia is a married adult wrestling with the issue of whether and when to tell his spouse or partner. This may seem like a no-brainer: How could someone conceal the fact that he has schizophrenia from a spouse? Sometimes a spouse has had a psychotic break in the past, met and married his spouse during a time when his symptoms were under control, and then has a recurrence during the marriage. Not only does the recurrence catch the well spouse by surprise, but it challenges the sense of trust between the two people.

There are no hard and fast answers about whether someone with schizophrenia should disclose her prior illness to her partner. In the best of circumstances, a spouse *should* be able to share information about any significant health condition with the person she's marrying, but fears about mental illness can be so great that it's sometimes simply too hard to do.

If a spouse finds out about the illness after the fact, he may initially be angry and will probably need to gather information and garner support to get over the trauma. The person with schizophrenia may feel remorseful, stressed, and fearful that the outing of the "secret" will signal the demise of the marriage. And it may. It can go either way.

We know one spouse of many years who never came to visit his wife when she was hospitalized for schizophrenia the first time during their marriage; it ultimately ended in a painful divorce. In another circumstance, we know a marriage of more than 30 years, where a caregiver hung in with her spouse because of her abiding love and ability to cope with the extra responsibilities she shoulders as the spouse of someone who is quite disabled and unable to work.

If someone you know who has schizophrenia, perhaps a daughter or cousin, asks your advice about whether she should tell her spouse or partner, the most helpful thing you can do is listen, so that the individual making the decision thinks through the consequences clearly and is confident in her decision. There are no rights and wrongs. In tough situations like this, people have to go with their gut and do what feels most comfortable to them.

Your kids

If you have young children in the family, try to explain what's happening around them, instead of assuming that they're too young to understand or to be affected by what's going on.

Keep your explanations very simple, give only as much detail as necessary to satisfy the child's curiosity, and be sure that he understands that this isn't a "closed" subject, but one he can feel free about discussing with you. You might say, for example, that Uncle Joe has a problem with the way his brain is working, and he's going to see a doctor to take medicine to straighten things out. You also want to reassure your kids about their safety, because they may have watched frightening TV shows or movies depicting mental illness.

If your children are older, they'll likely be able to handle more sophisticated explanations. For example, you might tell an adolescent that Uncle Joe has schizophrenia, which is a brain disorder, and that he is being treated with medication. You might discuss some of his symptoms and what it will mean in terms of his ability to get back to work.

The extended family

Deciding whether you should disclose the illness to more distant relatives depends on your relationship with them as well as your comfort level — and what you decide today isn't a decision that's set in stone. Many people living with mental illness find it less stressful to be open about their disorder with their entire family. Others feel that shielding Great-Aunt Mary, who lives a thousand miles away from the truth, may be best for everyone involved.

In all likelihood, close family members are already aware that something's wrong. The family grapevine is quite effective in most families, so even relatives you see only occasionally may know that your loved one has a problem. The truth may be easier to deal with than suppositions and gossip.

One mother confided to us that the hardest thing for her to do was to tell her elderly mother that her grandson had just been diagnosed with schizophrenia. She knew that her mother would never understand and would likely blame her daughter's permissive parenting style. As she anticipated, it wasn't easy but gradually, her mother came to understand the illness by attending support-group meetings with her daughter, and it made the relationship between mother, daughter, and grandson that much stronger.

Friends and neighbors

You may have friends or neighbors with whom you feel as close as — or even closer to than — your family. You may already have shared your concerns and fears with them. If you feel that they'll be able to provide you with support, you'll probably want to include them in your inner circle.

If you aren't sure or feel tentative about telling a particular individual, wait until you feel confident. It may simply be that the timing isn't right.

Employers

One of the most difficult decisions people face is deciding whether to tell an employer about the illness. If you're a caregiver of someone with schizophrenia, you may need to take time off from work to take your loved one to medical appointments, to provide transportation to programs, or to oversee care in your home.

Your loved one may want to tell her employer about her condition so she can benefit from accommodations under the Americans with Disabilities Act (ADA); see Chapter 12 for further guidance on handling these challenges.

Knowing what to say

As difficult as it is to break the news to someone else, you should expect that the people hearing it may feel uncomfortable, taken aback, or surprised. After all, you had time to prepare yourself for this talk and they didn't.

Don't be surprised at strange reactions. People often don't know what to say or don't make the kindest remarks when someone talks about illness, hardship or death. They may ask, "How did she get it? Does it run in your family? Is there any cure?" Recognize that they may need some time and information — just as you did — and that breaking the news may be a *process* rather than a one-time event.

Here are some guidelines that may make it easier for both you and the person who is first hearing about the illness:

- **Pick the right time and setting when you aren't rushed and you have privacy.** Blurting it out at Grandma's 80th birthday party probably isn't one of the best ways!
- **Explain that mental illnesses are no-fault brain disorders and that even scientists still can't pinpoint the specific causes of mental illness in a particular individual.**
- **Tell them that, in general, mental disorders are caused by a combination of genetic and environmental factors.**
- **Explain that no one is to blame, not your loved one or your family.** Explain that just as you wouldn't blame a person or his family for heart disease, diabetes, or asthma, you shouldn't blame a person with schizophrenia for his disease. The days of people blaming everything on someone's mother have gone out the window!
- **Use simple language that the other person can understand.** Try not to repeat or make use of unintelligible medical jargon you've read or heard from doctors or therapists.
- **Don't feel compelled to provide a specific label or diagnosis.** Deciding to reveal doesn't mean you have to reveal every single detail to every single person. Be judicious. (See the following section, "Deciding how much to tell," for more information.)
- **Explain that the disorder is treatable and that your loved one is being treated by a specialist.**
- **Because of the public misperception that people with mental illness are violent, you may want to add that your loved one doesn't pose any harm or threat to you or anyone else (if you believe this is so).**
- **Convey your hopefulness that the symptoms your loved one is experiencing will improve.**
- **Tell the person that you hope you can count on her confidentiality and support and that you've disclosed the information to her because you trust her.**

Deciding how much to tell

The Bazelon Center for Mental Health Law, an advocacy organization for people with mental disabilities, outlines four levels of specificity that people can use to explain mental disorders. Depending on how much you want to reveal and who you're talking to, these are some options for explaining schizophrenia:

- **Very general:** Say your loved one has a medical condition or an illness. This level of information may be appropriate for an employer.
- **A little more specific:** Say that your loved one has a biochemical imbalance, a neurobiological problem, a brain disorder, or difficulty with stress.
- **Specifically mentioning mental illness:** Say that your loved one has a mental illness, a psychiatric disorder, or a mental disability.
- **Giving the exact diagnosis:** Say that your loved one has schizophrenia.

When your family is unsupportive

In most families, there is always at least one relative — if not more than one — who simply "doesn't get it." They don't understand schizophrenia; don't want to learn about it; and blame the victim for either being lazy or defiant. Alternatively, they blame the family — either a parent or a spouse — for driving the person "mad." Or it may be a case of a grandparent or aunt who is in denial and tells you that your relative will "outgrow" whatever's wrong.

Most people don't full understand mental illnesses until they hit home. Their attitudes are usually driven by stigma, fear, or a lack of understanding. It may take time to engender support from your extended family. If your family isn't immediately supportive, you may be fortunate enough to have close friends who better understand.

Even when they disappoint you, never give up on the people who truly matter to you — family or friends. Make it your job to teach them about mental illness.

Often mothers say that even their husbands are in denial and refuse to believe that their child has a mental disorder. For that reason, if you look around the room at any NAMI support group, you're likely to see a preponderance of females over males. Perhaps, it's because women are traditionally the caregivers in our society and more willing to share intimacies with friends, colleagues, and outsiders than are men.

When everyone isn't onboard, this may make family gatherings awkward and dash expectations of having a "normal" family get-together, large holiday dinner or vacation. Here's some advice for getting over the hump of such social occasions:

- Keep the size of gatherings small.
- Try to limit parties or events to people who are known to the person with schizophrenia.
- Never force the person with schizophrenia to participate in social events; offer it as an option.
- Speak to the person with schizophrenia so she knows what to expect before she arrives.
- Be sensitive to the fact that other people may not know what to say.
- Ask the host to let the other guests know that your loved one is shy, withdrawn, whatever — and may have a hard time in a large gathering.
- Encourage other guests to act warm and friendly but to not ask too many questions.
- Realize that the event may not go perfectly, but that's okay. If you keep your expectations in check, you're less likely to be disappointed.

Considering the Challenges of Caregiving

Schizophrenia, like other major mental illnesses, affects not just an individual but his entire family — parents, spouses, siblings, children, and grandparents. Except for the person with the illness, however, its effect is probably most profound on those who assume the mantle of caregiver(s).

The challenges that caregivers encounter vary depending on the severity of the illness and its symptoms. But especially at the beginning, caregiving can be totally consuming — affecting your work, finances, health, relationships, and almost every other aspect of your life.

Many families say that the hardest part of caregiving is emotional: Setting aside the dreams and expectations they once had of the individual with mental illness, and re-orienting themselves to a new reality. For example, parents may have to live with the realization that their straight-A student or standout athlete not only is no longer is at the top of his game — instead, he's desperately in need of long-term psychiatric help.

When the caregivers are husband and wife, the tensions of living with a relative with schizophrenia can be so great that they challenge the marriage itself. Two parents may have different approaches to how the loved one's illness should be handled, or one may be in total denial while the other is trying to deal with the reality. It's estimated that one in five marriages become troubled (many leading to divorce) when a family member is diagnosed with a serious mental illness.

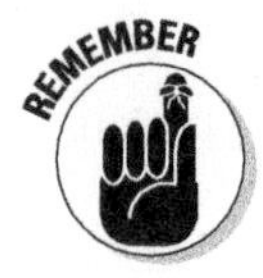

Mental illnesses, especially schizophrenia, are often accompanied by a loss of friendships for the person with schizophrenia. Your relative may come to rely on you for extra social support, either by phone or in-person. Provide it whenever you can while you encourage the individual to join peer groups, social clubs, and community organizations (see Chapter 12).

Accepting the job nobody wants

Whether your relative is your mother in mental decline with Alzheimer's disease, your child with Down syndrome, or your life partner with schizophrenia, no one signs up to be a caregiver for a person with special needs — it just happens. Family members assume the role of caregivers by default because society rarely provides any viable alternatives. The role is one that demands a tremendous investment of time and emotions.

When community supports are lacking, caregivers are thrust into the role of de facto case managers providing ongoing caregiving and oversight, as well as emotional and financial sustenance, for their loved ones. They may need to take time off from work to accompany their relative to medical appointments or to provide transportation to various social-service programs. They may need to suspend their own social lives as it becomes increasingly uncomfortable to entertain people at home or plan for dinners out because of the unpredictability of their lives. They may need to spend inordinate amounts of time talking to their relative on the phone, trying to dispel fears and misplaced anxieties. Or they may only be called upon to fill the void created by the loneliness common to people with schizophrenia who have trouble maintaining social relationships.

Professionals come and go over the years, but family members typically provide care that extends over decades — sometimes until death. Whether the ill person is a parent, a sibling, or a child, family members are always on call, literally and figuratively, whether their loved ones are living with them or living somewhere else. Consistently, family members describe the tension they feel each time the telephone rings. The call may come at work, while they're on vacation, or in the middle of the night. It may be a call from a hospital reporting a psychiatric emergency involving their relative, a call from a law enforcement official, or incoherent rambling from their loved one.

Family members also have cause to worry when they don't hear from their loved one. They wonder where the person is, whether she's adhering to treatment, and what she's doing. It's hard for caregivers to ever feel truly rested and relaxed because of the uncertainty of their lives and the unpredictability of the illness and its symptoms.

Staying home or coming home again

A person's home is a safe haven — a refuge from the world where you can retreat and feel safely taken care of — and this is true whether you have schizophrenia or not. So it's not surprising that a study by NAMI suggests that about four out of ten people with serious and persistent mental illnesses wind up living with their families. A study in New York State found that families provide more housing beds for people with mental illness than hospitals, adult homes, or nursing homes.

Often, you and your loved one with schizophrenia may have no viable alternatives but to live under the same roof for a substantial period of time. Sometimes people with mental illness never leave their parent's home; other times, they return from college or remain at home long after their peers are working and living independently. For families, it can mean that a once-empty nest is no longer empty. If the family has other young children who are still living at home, it can introduce conflict and chaos. A home that was once placid becomes filled with stress.

Chapter 12 provides some concrete strategies for minimizing stress in the home.

Remembering the demands and rewards of caregiving

The burdens of living with someone with schizophrenia can be overwhelming. When the illness hasn't yet been treated, hasn't been adequately treated, or is in its most acute stage, you may have to contend with a frightening constellation of unpredictable symptoms and behaviors.

One older mother told us of her terror, living with her son, a strapping young 24-year-old man who weighed more than 250 pounds and who consistently threatened her. She feared for her safety each night, moving a bureau in front of her door before she went to bed. Sometimes, family members are victims of assault and abuse. Another mother told us of a daughter who threw plates at her and destroyed many of the decorative items in her living room when she flew into one of her frequent rages.

Other caregivers are challenged by their loved one's illogical thoughts and behaviors. One mother told of her son who would take walks from one county to another until the soles of his shoes wore out. She was unable to convince him to curtail his travels and always worried that the phone would ring saying that he had been hit by a car or had gotten into trouble.

If someone is paranoid or suspicious, the tiniest comment can be misinterpreted as an insult and provoke anger and rage. Periods of psychotic behavior can be interspersed with periods of lucid thinking, making it hard to adjust to the ups and downs of daily existence.

In addition, the caregiver has to make sense of a mental-health system that's complex and often not user-friendly. With cuts in public funds at every level of government and pressure by private insurers to cut back on costs of medical care and medications, the system is trying to do more with less. This makes it difficult to access quality care, especially during crises.

Although the job may appear, at times, to be thankless, there are often rewards. With proper treatment, the acute symptoms are usually temporary. When caregivers see their loved one show signs of growing independence, clearer thinking, and diminished symptoms, the results are very gratifying. Many patients recover and exceed their family's and even their doctor's expectations.

Many times the relationship between the caregiver and the person with mental illness becomes reciprocal, with the person with schizophrenia helping around the house with routine chores and assisting in the care of their older parents.

Avoiding caregiver burnout

Because of the demands and stress of the job, caregivers are prime candidates for burnout. Some of the signs of burnout include

- Persistent feelings of exhaustion and fatigue
- Diminished interest in the things around you
- Free-floating anxiety
- Feelings of depression, isolation, and loss-of-control

When you get on an airplane, the safety instructions always suggest that parents put on their oxygen masks first before they do the same for their child. This also applies to caregiving. To perform adequately as a caregiver, you need to take care of yourself first if you want to be of any use to your relative. This requires, to the extent possible, that you find ways to identify and minimize stress.

Taking care of someone with schizophrenia, particularly when the individual is in the throes of psychosis (with disturbed, illogical or disorganized thinking) can be extremely draining. You may be tempted to drop everything around you and focus only on the illness, but you have to guard against this temptation. Find ways to pace yourself and set limits to how much you can or cannot do during the course of a day.

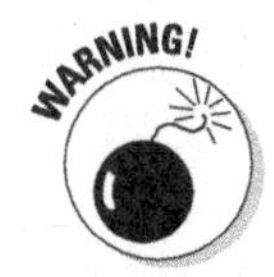

It never pays to be a martyr. Your resentment will seep out, even without your knowing. You'll also be shortchanging the rest of your family. Here are some tips to reduce the stress of caregiving:

- Get regular exercise.
- Keep to a balanced, healthy diet
- Don't shortchange yourself on sleep.
- Be prudent about maintaining your own physical health.
- Make time to nurture existing friendships.
- Build short breaks into your day and plan downtime over the course of the week.
- Plan respites or vacations from your caregiving responsibilities.
- Don't hesitate to ask for help from others when you feel overwhelmed.
- Above all, continue to do the things that normally give you pleasure: Pursue your hobbies, go to the movies or theater, take a walk on a sunny day.

One of the best ways to avoid burnout is to bond with a friend in a similar situation who can truly understand what you're going through. It's likely that your peaks and valleys won't occur simultaneously and that you'll be able to provide support for each other at various times.

Most important, always remain hopeful and remember that, as bad as things may seem today, the crisis you're experiencing now will eventually pass.

Keeping the Whole Family Safe

One of the myths associated with schizophrenia is that most people with schizophrenia are violent. This is far from the truth. In reality, people with schizophrenia tend to be the victims, rather than perpetrators, of violence. On the streets, they're often perceived as vulnerable, easy targets.

However, this doesn't mean that safety in the home should not be a concern or consideration. When someone with schizophrenia is actively psychotic — with unrealistic, delusional, or paranoid thoughts — she may pose a threat to other people in the family by her thought disorder. She may hear voices that tell her to harm someone around her or feel threatened for no valid reason and seek to retaliate.

The risks of violence increase:

- When mental illness remains untreated
- When the individual has a past history of violence and aggression
- When mental illness is complicated by use of alcohol and/or drugs
- When the person has hallucinations or delusions

You can, however, minimize the risk of violence in the home:

- Try to create predictable routines.
- Set up reasonable rules and limits for behaviors under your roof (for example, no loud music after 11 p.m., no use of drugs in the home, and so on).
- Set up appropriate and enforceable consequences when rules are broken.
- When an individual seems upset, try to diffuse rather than exacerbate his anger.
- Choose your battles; minimize confrontations on unimportant issues.
- Don't get so close to the individual that she feels physically threatened.
- Separate the person from the illness. Don't take offense from remarks that are clearly part of the illness.
- If you're worried enough, lock your bedroom door at night.
- Don't hesitate to get help when you need it in an emergency (see Chapter 14).

If you're physically threatened or you truly feel that you, your relative with mental illness, or someone else in your home is in immediate danger, call 911 and be sure to explain that the person has a serious mental illness.

Many times a written contract between you and your relative, agreed upon when the individual is stable, can help define boundaries and avoid arguments.

Many times a person with schizophrenia can appear menacing to an untrained or inexperienced police officer causing them to overreact with force. If you have any concerns that your relative may become dangerous, contact your local police department *before* an actual emergency. Explain that your loved one has a mental illness and is sometimes prone to odd or unusual behaviors. Explain that your relative isn't dangerous but you want to be able to call upon them in case you need their help.

Siblings and Schizophrenia

The sibling bond is one of the longest and closest of any familial relationship because siblings tend to be closer in age and generally outlive their parents. So when one sibling is diagnosed with schizophrenia, regardless of her age, it has a profound effect on the other.

Keeping other kids in the loop

When any child is affected by a serious illness — be it cancer, autism, diabetes, or schizophrenia — it's easy for parents to hover over that child and lose sight of the needs of the well siblings. This approach is problematic for the person with the illness, for the well sibling, and for the rest of the family. Families need to achieve balance in addressing everyone's emotional needs.

Of course, sometimes the person with schizophrenia will require extra attention — but parents need to make sure that other siblings don't feel neglected or ignored. Also, children are very perceptive when parents seem to be applying attention or even discipline unevenly. Being more attentive, or more lax, with one sibling than another can stir up resentment.

Young children, in particular, may feel jealous of the child or adolescent with the illness (who is the center of their parents' attention) and also may be confused about why their sibling is acting strangely. It's important for parents to find simple ways to explain that their sibling is having some problems and that they're seeking help from a counselor, doctor, or social worker to try to deal with them. Depending on the well sibling's age, the message can even be more explicit and say that something is wrong with her brother's brain (see the "Breaking the News to the Family" section, earlier in this chapter).

For example, the person with schizophrenia may be missing school, and the well sibling may feel jealous, resentful, or simply confused as to why the parents are allowing this to happen. Young children have an acute sense of fairness and are aware when they aren't being treated equally.

In cases like this, it's important for the parents to sit down with the well siblings and explain that not going to school is not acceptable, in general, but that their sibling is unable to go because he's sick. Also offer some words of encouragement — for example, saying that you hope that the child with mental illness will be feeling well enough to return to school after some weeks, months, or whatever and that you're happy that the well child is able to attend school regularly.

Don't saddle older siblings with more responsibility than they can handle. Although they may feel good about assisting their caregiver parents and may be very helpful, they shouldn't be overwhelmed with responsibilities beyond their years.

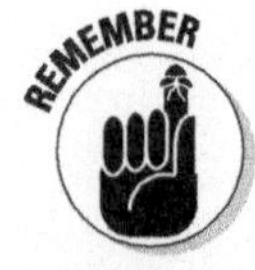

Children are likely to identify more closely with an ill sibling who is of the same sex and close in age. Some well siblings are more likely to be adversely affected than others because they're more sensitive, by temperament.

Sometimes well siblings are teased by other children because their ill sibling acts strangely or looks different. This can be very painful — but particularly during adolescence when there is so much emphasis on everyone conforming to their peers. Be alert to any signs of bullying or teasing of the ill or well siblings in your family so you can discuss or role-play strategies for handling them. Also be alert for any signs of depression.

Always be willing to answer questions and encourage your children to ask them.

Dealing with sibling fears

One of the most frightening fears of siblings is that the same thing will happen to them. Given that they share the same genetic pool and environment, their fears aren't totally unfounded (see Chapter 2 for information on the genetics of schizophrenia). The child or adolescent may also be reluctant to discuss such fears with an already overburdened parent. If this is the case, it often helps for the well child to see a mental health counselor for support and reassurance. Sometimes, this can be handled by a guidance counselor or school psychologist in the child's school. Before you take the chance, speak to the person yourself to make sure she's up to the job.

Because schizophrenia causes ripples throughout a family, share information with your child's teacher or school administration as appropriate and demand their assurance that it'll be kept confidential.

Older well siblings share some of the same concerns as older parents. They wonder what their roles and responsibilities will be — emotionally, financially, and so on — when their parents die. Will they always have to care for the person with schizophrenia? Parents shouldn't pressure or draft a well sibling into service for their ill relative. Each sibling needs to determine the extent of their involvement on their own.

As they embark upon careers and move to independence, some well siblings will follow the model set by their parents and become active caregivers of their siblings. In fact, many become healthcare professionals. Others may decide that they need to leave their sibling with mental illness behind. It's very common for well siblings to enter helping professions as a way to give back less directly. Open discussions, family meetings, or meetings with mental-health professionals can help siblings allay these anxieties — some of which may be valid and others of which aren't — and to make considered decisions about caregiving.

When a Spouse or Partner Has Schizophrenia

Any type of serious problem — medical, financial, legal — can create a wedge between spouses or life partners. This is especially true when one partner is diagnosed with a serious mental illness like schizophrenia. Although it's far more common for schizophrenia to surface in younger adults, the symptoms can become manifest when people are older, before or after they marry.

Because men with schizophrenia become ill earlier than women, they're less likely to marry than are women. In fact, only about one in four men with schizophrenia ever marries. Women are more likely to marry — some reports suggest that as many as 70 percent of them do. Unfortunately, separation and divorce rates are higher among people with schizophrenia than among the general population, for both sexes.

The impact of schizophrenia on a marriage depends on the severity of the illness, its duration, its responsiveness to treatment, and the ability of the two partners to communicate and cope.

Considering whether you can still be a couple

Schizophrenia can challenge many aspects of a partnership. Depending on the severity of the illness and whether the symptoms ebb and flow, a spouse or partner with the illness may have a hard time maintaining emotional intimacy, providing financial stability, or participating in social events. The well partner may feel shackled with responsibility as the primary caregiver and breadwinner for everyone in the family, including children, and may feel more like a parent than a spouse or partner.

Many spouses and partners, because of religious or spiritual reasons, or out of pure love and admiration, have met these challenges and provide ongoing support to their spouse. The relationship may be different than many more conventional ones, but both partners may say that they would never trade places with anyone else for a moment.

Well partners should make every effort to build upon the strengths of their mate, allowing the individual to handle any responsibilities the person is capable of. For example, if a wife is working full-time and her ill husband is left at home, he should pitch in with childcare and some of the household chores. The couple should also try to engage in some normal activities — going out to dinner together or going to a movie. The well partner should also make sure that children show equal respect for both parents.

Helping your kids understand what's happening

Children need to be given age-appropriate information about their parent's illness. They probably already realize that something is wrong with their parent; she may act differently than other mothers, or he may not go to work like other fathers. In some cases, there is an unusual role reversal where even very young children begin to "parent" their parents.

Other times, children don't realize that something is wrong because they think that everyone else's parents are "quirky" as theirs, because their experience outside the home is so limited. They may mistake symptoms for an unusual personality type (for example, a drama queen). Or they simply may be aware that something is wrong, but be unable to articulate their fears and concerns.

Younger children

When children approach school age, they may find that other kids tease them about their parent's odd behaviors or dress. As soon as children are old enough to understand, they need to be told that their parent has a problem with his thoughts, emotions, or behaviors; that their parent still loves them very much; that their parent is doing the best job possible; and that the well parent will make sure they're safe and well taken care of.

The well spouse also needs to make sure that the parent with schizophrenia is truly able to parent and manage the stresses that childcare entails. Another relative may have to step in to help with childcare, homework, grocery shopping, or carpooling when the illness is at its worst.

If you have any concerns about neglect, abuse, positive symptoms, or illicit substance use that are affecting a child, bring those concerns to the attention of your loved one's doctor immediately or to an appropriate social services agency if there is imminent danger.

Older kids

As children become adolescents and young adults, they may begin to feel angry or bitter about what they may have missed because of the illness. They may feel that they weren't properly parented, that the illness limited their interactions with other children, or that their family never had traditional celebrations or vacations like other families. They may have been cheated out of a part of their childhood or told lies that now lead them to mistrust.

They may also worry about whether the same thing — experiencing the symptoms of schizophrenia — will someday happen to them. Even before these signs become evident, and in the absence of adjustment problems, it's helpful to find a mental-health counselor to help the young person come to grips with the complex challenges of having a parent with schizophrenia.

Working Collaboratively with Professionals

Unfortunately, even some healthcare practitioners view families as part of the problem rather than part of the solution. Old theories die hard; they blame families for the illness or for exacerbating its symptoms. As a result, these doctors, psychologists, social workers, or other mental-health workers may limit communication with family members or fail to listen to them (which means they don't benefit from the information only families can provide).

It's extremely useful for professionals to receive feedback from family members (in addition to the person with schizophrenia) about how the person is functioning in real life, outside of the office setting where the individual is only seen for a relatively brief period of time. This will help a psychiatrist more accurately determine whether medications are working, whether side effects are emerging, and determine when changes in medications or dosing are in order.

Don't wait until you're asked to become involved. Family members need to be proactive in communicating that they want to participate as a member of the treatment team:

1. **Ask for the name of the person who's responsible for your loved one's care.**
2. **Request an initial meeting with that person.**
3. **Indicate that you have valuable information about your loved one's history of symptoms and treatments, what worked and what didn't, which you're happy to provide.**
4. **Make sure that you come away from your initial meeting with a clear understanding of your loved one's diagnosis, plan of treatment, and prognosis, even if you have to be very firm in making the request to ensure that you do.**
5. **Find out how the professional would like you to communicate with each other on an ongoing basis.**

If the professional is reluctant to provide you with information and hides behind the mask of confidentiality, ask your loved one to sign a release providing his consent to have the doctor communicate with you. Even if your loved one is unwilling to provide consent, there is no breech of confidentiality in your providing information to the doctor (see Chapter 14).

Planning for the Future

One of the most persistent themes we hear from families is their worry about what will happen when they're gone. This is extremely difficult because it means facing one's own mortality and the fear of possibly not living long enough to see your loved one reach the stage of recovery you had hoped for.

As parents age, their energy, abilities, and resources to care for a relative with mental illness may diminish. They may be entering a time of life when they begin developing chronic health problems of their own. Living on fixed incomes, they may also have less funds available to support their loved one with schizophrenia.

If you have a relative with a serious, long-term, and disabling illness of any kind, including schizophrenia, you need to plan for the future. A number of nonprofit organizations assist families in planning for health insurance, powers of attorney, guardianship, healthcare proxies, supplemental needs trusts, housing, and other critical legal and financial issues that need to be addressed. Depending on the family, parents, grandparents, siblings, or children may be the ones involved in future care planning (see Chapter 7).

NAMI has been actively involved for many years in developing Planned Lifetime Assistance Network (PLAN) programs to meet the needs of families with adult children. Currently there are 23 such programs in operation in 18 states. To find out more about these programs and other options, contact the National PLAN Alliance at 518-587-3372 or by e-mail at `npa@nycap.rr.com`.

Chapter 12

Developing Coping Skills

In This Chapter

- Helping your loved one fit in
- Coping with troublesome behaviors
- Fostering independence
- Finding information, support, and advocacy

There's no instruction manual for helping a loved one with schizophrenia live as normal and productive a life as possible. Although books like this one are invaluable, most of the skills necessary to cope with schizophrenia are learned through on-the-job training — for both the family and the person with schizophrenia. It's definitely not easy with a disease as baffling to understand, frightening to witness, and challenging to treat as schizophrenia.

The challenges of integrating a person with schizophrenia into both the family and into the community can be stressful, depressing, and anxiety-provoking for everyone involved. In this chapter, we focus on coping skills that will benefit both caregivers and patients in learning to live the best life possible with schizophrenia.

Helping Your Loved One Live with Others

Schizophrenia's impact often extends far beyond the individual directly affected by the illness. As with many mental illnesses, schizophrenia leads to behaviors that make it difficult for the individual to fit into not only the family, but also the community at large. Because schizophrenia is a poorly understood, and often feared, diagnosis, educating not only yourself and your loved one, but everyone else who comes in contact with your loved one can be a big part of your job.

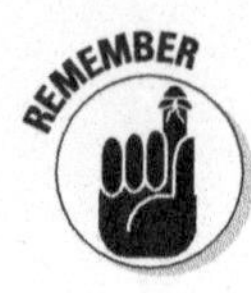

Keep in mind the following:

- **Chronic mental illnesses affect more than one person.** Schizophrenia creates collateral damage and is likely to have implications for the whole family (parents, spouses, children, siblings, grandparents, uncles, aunts, cousins, and so on), as well as friends, acquaintances, co-workers, and classmates. This leads to stress for the whole family.
- **Brain disorders affect every aspect of life.** Any brain disorder can have a profound effect on health, employment, finances, social ties, and relationships.
- **Schizophrenia requires a long-term mindset.** Part of coming to terms with the illness (see Chapter 11) is realizing that schizophrenia isn't a one-time illness; it requires the support of family and friends over the long haul. It also means that your job as teacher, cheerleader, and community liaison for your loved one is never done — new situations requiring new learning skills and new coping mechanisms will continue to arise.
- **The stresses you feel as a caregiver will change over time.** The period before and soon after diagnosis is often the toughest on caregivers.

In this section, we show you ways you can help both your loved one and yourself cope with the stress of living within a community, *any* community — whether it's a family unit or a city — when you're dealing with schizophrenia.

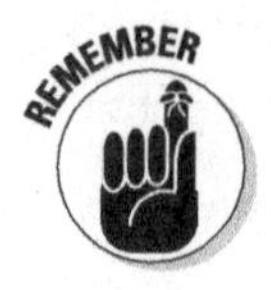

You don't need to reinvent the wheel. People who have been there before you (other consumers, family members, friends, and professionals) have practical advice to share. Don't hesitate to draw upon their experiences to make your own less stressful.

Understanding the unique stress factors of mental illness

Any chronic disorder causes stress, but mental illnesses like schizophrenia come with their special stressors, which require special coping mechanisms:

- **The disease usually has a long-term chronic course.** Schizophrenia can be managed and controlled but not cured, which means that you and your loved one are going to have to deal with schizophrenia for a lifetime — a daunting thought under the best of circumstances.
- **People with the disorder often lack insight into their own illness and may be their own worst enemies.** They may not recognize that they're sick and need help.

- **Your loved one will likely have to take medication for a long time, if not for the rest of his life.** Some people resent this constant reminder of their illness and experiment with changing doses, going on self-proclaimed "drug holidays," or going off medication altogether with grave consequences.
- **More than medication alone is necessary to enhance a person's sense of self-esteem and ability to function.** This means that either you or your loved one will have to find, pay for, and coordinate a range of treatment, basic services, and supports.
- **The ups and downs of the illness make its course and your life unpredictable.** Things can be going along fine, and then they're suddenly derailed. This leads to anxiety and worry about when the next shoe will drop and makes it hard for families to plan ahead, even something as simple as taking a vacation.
- **Crises will occur; although many can be avoided, some cannot.** This inevitably leads to setbacks, frustration and disappointment.
- **The apathy that often accompanies schizophrenia can be aggravating to others.** You need to remember that your loved one isn't simply being lazy or provocative — and keeping this in mind when you're frustrated or at your wit's end can be tough.
- **Any serious illness is likely to take a toll on family life and causes disruptions.** It may necessitate time off from work for doctors' visits or hospitalizations and lost opportunities for participation in leisure and social pursuits.
- **Professionals may care, but they tend to come and go; family is the most constant influence on the individual with schizophrenia, filling in the gaps whenever necessary.**

Improving communication skills

Communicating with people who have schizophrenia is often difficult, for a number of reasons. Here are some of the main barriers you may encounter:

- Your loved one may be fearful of you (because of suspiciousness or paranoid thinking) and, therefore, may not *want* to communicate.
- She may be too sleepy — because of medication side effects — to listen or to speak.
- Your loved one may not *hear* what you're saying because he's distracted by voices or other stimuli in the environment.
- She may not *understand* what you're saying because of anxiety or difficulties processing information.
- Your loved one may not be able to *act* on what you're saying because of lack of motivation or inability to carry through.

Each of these problems may make it hard to get your message across or to have a meaningful conversation. But communication is an essential part of life, and you need to find ways both to communicate directly with your loved and to help him communicate with the larger world.

Here are some techniques that have proven helpful under these circumstances:

- **Remember that timing is everything.** Try to approach your loved one when she's most likely to be willing and able to communicate with you. Try to find a time when she's relaxed, as opposed to upset, anxious, distracted, or angry — especially if you're bringing something up that may be emotionally charged.

  Speaking about tough topics may be easier in the morning (when your loved one is rested and fresh) than it is at night (when she's sleepy). Conversely, if she's having a hard time getting up in the morning, it may be better to talk later in the day. Unsure? Ask your loved one when she would like to talk.

  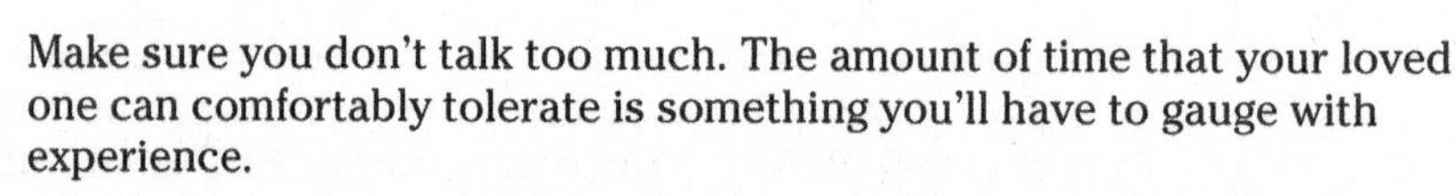

  Make sure you don't talk too much. The amount of time that your loved one can comfortably tolerate is something you'll have to gauge with experience.

- **Respect your loved one's body language.** If he's pacing, tapping his foot, or otherwise appears agitated, put off your conversation for another time. Instead, take a walk, take a drive, have a snack together, or watch TV.

- **Pick your place.** Because your loved one may have a hard time with competing stimulation, pick a quiet place with as few distractions as possible. Is he more comfortable talking at home, riding in the car, or sitting on the grass at a park? Unsure? Ask him.

- **Choose the right medium.** Talking face to face may not always be the best way to discuss difficult topics. Talking on the phone or via e-mail may be easier and less stressful in certain instances.

  Tone is difficult to convey via e-mail, so make sure that you word your messages carefully so that they aren't misinterpreted.

- **Keep in mind that emotions run in two directions.** If you're the one who's upset or emotionally charged, it may **not** be a good time for you to begin a conversation. For example, if you found that your loved one did something that sabotaged his job and you feel furious, wait until you calm down a bit to find out more about what happened and why before starting a heated argument about it.

  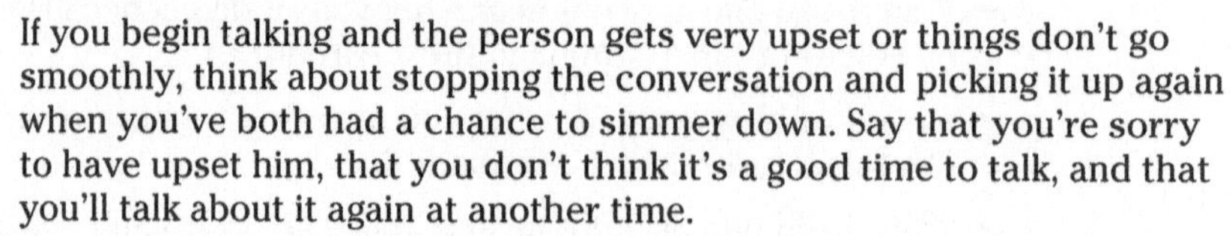

  If you begin talking and the person gets very upset or things don't go smoothly, think about stopping the conversation and picking it up again when you've both had a chance to simmer down. Say that you're sorry to have upset him, that you don't think it's a good time to talk, and that you'll talk about it again at another time.

- **Keep it simple.** Try to be brief, clear, and direct. This is no time to use ten-dollar words. You want to make sure you're getting your point across. Try to keep you discussion simple by expressing or responding to one idea at a time.
- **Don't automatically assume that your loved one understands you.** She may not be getting what you're saying (or may not really be aware of what you're saying) but doesn't want to admit it. If you aren't sure you're getting through, repeat what you said a different way, or ask your loved one to restate what you said in her own words.
- **Be respectful of your loved one.** Whether the individual with schizophrenia is younger or older than you, treat him as an individual worthy of respect. Try not to sound demeaning or overly critical, or to act in a patronizing manner. For example, don't scold your adult daughter in the tone of a voice you would use for a toddler. Don't treat the person as if she were mentally deficient, and don't say things that are rude, abusive, or hurtful. Never make fun of the person's illogical thinking. When someone is upset, he isn't likely to understand humor.

  Because a person with schizophrenia may be very sensitive, if you have something critical to say, be careful not to say it in front of other people who don't need to hear it.

- **Be an enabler (in a good way).** When you think that your loved one wants to say something and is having a tough time expressing it, openly ask if he wants to tell you something. He may just need your help in starting the conversation. One way of doing this is to ask simple questions, modeling what the person may want to say, to see if he responds. You could say, "I think you're disappointed about not getting that job you wanted so badly, aren't you? But maybe it really wasn't a good fit." Just make sure you don't fall into the role of an interrogator or put words in the person's mouth.
- **Be honest but supportive.** If your loved one has done something that you disapprove of (for example, dropping out of a job-training program or deciding to stop taking a necessary medication), you need to be candid about your disappointment but also understanding and supportive. For example, you might say, "I'm sorry that you weren't able to continue attending the program, but I hope you'll feel better about going next week" or "I think that the lithium really helped manage your mood swings, so I hope you'll talk to your doctor about your decision to stop taking it."
- **Keep the lines of communication open.** Remember the importance of maintaining an open relationship with your friend or relative. If you react too critically to what she says, you effectively cut off communication. After a conversation about difficult things, try to keep the communication light. Talk about movies, TV, sports, or anything she's interested in that's free of conflict.

Reducing stress

Stress takes a toll on anyone's physical or mental health, but it can be particularly toxic to a person diagnosed with schizophrenia: Too much stress can worsen symptoms or even precipitate relapse. Although it's impossible to eliminate all stress, reducing stress whenever possible will make your life and your loved one's easier in the long run. Identifying stressors and giving your loved one tools to reduce stress will pay dividends for everyone.

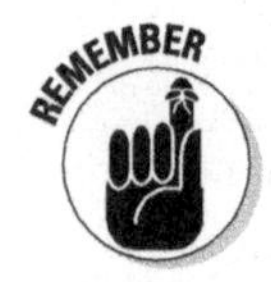

People with schizophrenia are likely to be sensitive, experiencing stress in situations where you might not. They also tend to react to stress in an exaggerated way. For example, even a minor change in your loved one's schedule or environment can be a significant stressor. Anticipatory anxiety, such as having plans to go to dinner with a new friend, may make your loved one feel very nervous and anxious about what to say or what to do. Changing jobs, apartments, or therapists may throw him into a frenzy. Even sustained contact with another person for too many hours in a day may be hard for your loved one to bear. A trauma, such as the loss of a friend or the death of a parent, may be so stressful that it leads to severe depression or psychotic thinking.

Stress also takes its toll on caregivers, who are more likely to be depressed and have physical problems like diabetes and heart disease, than those who aren't caregivers. Caregiving can be physically demanding and emotionally draining for people who are juggling multiple responsibilities — such as holding down a job, caring for children, and then also caring for a spouse with schizophrenia.

Signs of stress aren't always obvious. Here are some indicators that your loved one (or you!) may be experiencing stress overload:

- Problems sleeping (either getting too little sleep or sleeping too much)
- Changed eating patterns (eating too little or too much)
- Irritability
- Anger
- Anxiety
- Sadness
- Fatigue (most of the time, as opposed to just occasionally or just at bedtime)
- Physical problems (like headaches, pains, or gastrointestinal problems)
- Loss of interest in things that are generally enjoyed (such as sex, socializing, and so on)

When one person in a family — or one person among a group of people who live or work together — is stressed, it's likely to have a negative spill-over effect on the people around him. Conversely, relieving stress can have an exponential payoff — for more than one person.

You *can* control and minimize stress. Here are some ways to lessen stress — both for your loved one as well as for yourself:

- **Set priorities.** It's easy for people with schizophrenia to feel overwhelmed. This is particularly true after someone who has had an acute psychotic episode is just getting back to her normal activities, which may suddenly feel as difficult as climbing Mount Everest. Transitions of any kind can be especially stressful — moving to a new apartment, taking on a new job, adding new responsibilities to an old job.

  Some of the symptoms of schizophrenia make it hard to focus, making it especially important for your loved one to identify and order her priorities and stick to them.

  Written lists can be extremely helpful if your loved one has trouble remembering what she needs to do next or prioritizing. Suggest that she make a list of the things that need to be done, rank the items in order of priority, and cross off each task when she completes it. There's something very satisfying about going down a checklist and marking things off! (If your loved one is comfortable with a computer, Web sites like Remember the Milk [`www.rememberthemilk.com`] can be helpful list-making and memory tools.)

  Help your loved one break big tasks into little ones so they don't feel so overwhelming. For example, the first step to going back to school might be to take one class; the first step to getting back to work may be volunteering for a job; the first step to taking a shower may be picking out clothes to wear; and the first step to making a friend may be learning how to smile when you meet someone new.

  Caregivers often feel stressed when they fall into the trap of thinking they can do it all. Chapter 11 provides some tips for avoiding caregiver burnout.

- **Get physical.** Exercise and physical activity help reduce stress. Make sure that you and your loved one are both getting regular exercise. If your loved one has no motivation to exercise, find ways to be encouraging. For example, suggest taking regular walks together or give her a gift of membership in a health club or gym. Even owning a dog can encourage people to get outdoors and get moving.

- **Get a pet.** A number of studies have shown that having a pet can reduce stress — spending time with animals is associated with decreases in heart rate as well as blood pressure. For people with serious mental illnesses, pets also provide the benefit of companionship and help ward off loneliness.

Having a pet entails responsibility so this needs to be factored into the equation. If a dog or cat is too much of a hassle to care for, similar benefits can be achieved by keeping an aquarium with fish. Or maybe your loved one can volunteer at a local animal shelter — he'll get the dual benefits of spending time with animals and easing back into the workforce through volunteering.

- **Take a deep breath.** Meditation, breathing exercises, and yoga can help reduce stress. These activities lower the heart rate, slow down breathing, and lower blood pressure — all of which make you feel calmer and less stressed. Because they aren't treatment per se, they're socially acceptable, come without a stigma, and offer opportunities for meeting new friends.
- **Laugh.** Anything that produces a hearty laugh, like watching old sitcoms on TV (like *I Love Lucy, Seinfeld, Friends,* or *Everyone Loves Raymond*) can help reduce stress. Studies have shown that laughter can reduce certain stress hormones.
- **Find a hobby.** Whether it's playing a sport, following a sports team, knitting alone or in a group, or going to the movies, finding something that interests you and keeps your mind off yourself and your problems is an excellent stress reliever.
- **Try to plan and stick to a routine.** Because people with schizophrenia often have difficulty adjusting to change, setting up a predictable routine so that things are done pretty much the same way and at approximately the same time each day is helpful. This is especially important for eating and sleeping. When changes to the routine are made, they should be done gradually.

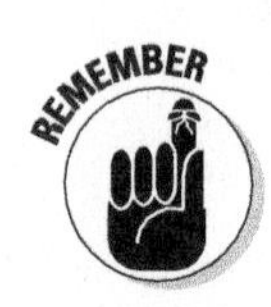

- **Mix it up occasionally.** As comforting as routines may be, everyone seems to benefit from an occasional change. If you find that your loved one is feeling very stressed, think about how you can help her get "unstuck." A mini vacation — like going for a ride in the country on a spring day or spending a day at the beach in the summer — may help reduce stress and restore equilibrium.
- **Allow for a "bad hair day."** Things happen that can throw someone off kilter, and they have nothing to do with the person's illness. A coffee spill on a new suit, a supervisor who came to work angry, or a bus that come late and resulted in a missed therapy appointment. Make allowances for stuff that happens.
- **Treat it.** If other more conservative approaches to managing stress don't seem to work, you may want to consult your loved one's psychiatrist, therapist, or case manager. In fact, in the best of circumstances, they'll recognize it before you do.

Stress often manifests itself as anxiety. If your loved one appears to be uncontrollably anxious, it may be a side-effect of one of the medications he's taking.

If it isn't a medication side effect, the doctor may want to add an anti-anxiety drug to control anxiety. Talk therapies (see Chapter 9) may also be helpful in teaching your loved one techniques to lessen anxiety.

- **Check in periodically.** Like anyone else, people with schizophrenia may not always realize when they're feeling overly stressed. If your loved one lives under your roof, you may periodically ask her how things are going. If she lives elsewhere, call to check in on how she's feeling. On special days when a person may be more stressed (such as Christmas, anniversaries of deaths, birthdays), be preemptive in making sure your loved one has a good plan for how to handle the day. Just talking to another person about the sources of stress may lighten the load.

Setting realistic limits

Whenever two or more people live together, whatever their relationship, there needs to be some discussion, and probably some negotiating, to ensure that one person doesn't overstep another's boundaries. This is especially true when one of the people has schizophrenia, because the symptoms and behaviors associated with the illness often magnify the challenges.

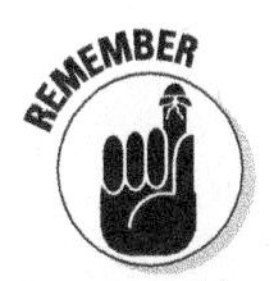

It's better to have a clear-cut set of limits and boundaries in place *before* problems occur than it is to try dealing with issues as they arise. The time to sit down and go over rules is when everyone is in a receptive mood, thinking clearly, and able to comprehend what's being said.

Writing out the rules in a type of "contract" can be helpful. Putting the agreement in writing gives everyone an opportunity to go back and read it when things seem fuzzy.

Setting the rules

When it comes to setting rules, no answers are set in stone — every family's tolerance for certain behaviors will be different. But to avoid constant conflict, and recurrence of the same circumstances over and over, you need to make sure that you, your loved one, and anyone else living in your home are on the same page when it comes to expectations.

The amount of structure needed will depend on how organized or disorganized your loved one's mind is at the time. Also, you may need to renegotiate rules as situations change, particularly during transitions (for example, when he returns from a hospital, jail, or rehab program). If your loved one is already living in the household, you may need to set new limits if there's been a great deal of friction; some rules may need to be relaxed, and others may need to be tightened, to decrease conflict and stress.

When you're coming up with your list of rules, you need to differentiate which ones are tolerable and which ones aren't. Some of the areas to consider on such a list are whether your loved one will:

- See a clinician regularly
- Take medication consistently
- Attend a program
- Apply for entitlements
- Attend school or go to work
- Have to maintain certain hygiene standards
- Dress in a particular way
- Contribute to the rent or other expenses
- Adhere to certain house rules
- Be allowed to smoke in the house or create a fire hazard
- Have access to a car or other means of transportation
- Help with certain household tasks or chores
- Keep certain hours
- Refrain from alcohol and/or drugs on or off premises
- Refrain from dangerous or assaultive behavior

Try not to concentrate exclusively on the *don'ts*. Phrasing things in a positive way, such as, "You will wear a shirt and pants in the house" may be more effective than saying, "No walking around in your underwear."

Setting limits may be helpful even when you're not living with your loved one. For example, are you willing to pay rent indefinitely for your loved one if she's able but unwilling to work? Is your loved one allowed to come to your house and drop in unannounced?

An experienced therapist or case manager can be helpful in zeroing in on areas of difficulty that people typically encounter or on the pitfalls specific to your situation. Talk to your loved one's therapist to avoid potential land mines.

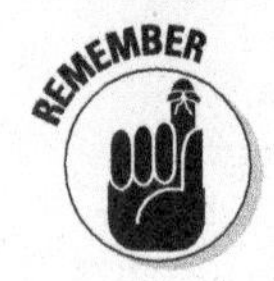

You have rights but also responsibilities in terms of your agreement with your loved one, too. You need to give your loved one a voice in telling you some of *her* expectations, so the agreement isn't a one-sided edict. Including your loved one in the discussion and listing your own responsibilities will help enhance her self-esteem, clarify areas that may be muddy, and increase the odds of sticking to her side of the bargain. Some issues that may arise in your discussions may include the following:

- How much privacy will you give your loved one in terms of access to her bedroom or access to the telephone or e-mail?
- Will you be open to your loved one's friends visiting your home?

- Will you be willing to drive your loved one to work?
- Will you provide extra financial support?
- Are there other ways you can help enhance your loved one's recovery?

As you make this list, you may realize that you need to set some boundaries in relation to your personal involvement. Realistically, what are you able and not able to do? For example, providing support and care to a loved one with schizophrenia may entail cutting back on your own hours at work. How many hours can you afford to lose without adversely affecting yourself or the rest of your family? Providing constant companionship to your relative may entail cutting back on your own friendships. How much are you willing to give up? Will devoting all your time to your loved one undermine the quality of your relationship with other relatives? When you think through these issues, you may need to find ways to offload some responsibilities to other family members, friends, or professionals.

Enforcing the rules

One of the thorniest issues arising in caregiving is the question of what to do when rules are broken. If the goal of the contract is to support your loved one's recovery, you don't want to throw him out on the doorstep except for the most serious offenses. It's important to distinguish between rules that "would be nice" the rules that, when broken, are real deal-breakers with major consequences, such as removal from the house. Minor infractions call for a less-serious response (for example, reminders, reinforcements, or penalties), whereas serious infraction may demand medical and/or legal intervention.

Most families are (or should be) unwilling to tolerate the following behaviors in their homes:

- **Assault:** Your loved one is not allowed to physically harm you, and you're not allowed to physically harm him.
- **Persistent suicidal thoughts or gestures:** If your loved one is talking about suicide or attempting suicide, you need to treat this as an emergency and insist that your loved one call his therapist or a suicide hot line (if the therapist is unreachable). See Chapter 14 for more information.
- **Aggressive or violent behavior toward you or anyone else:** If your loved one is aggressive or violent, you need to report this behavior to his clinician and possibly law enforcement.
- **Abuse of property:** For example, throwing or breaking furniture in the home is not allowed. In order to live in your home, your loved one must respect your property.

- **Engaging in other dangerous, risky, or self-abusive behavior** (for example, refusing to eat, driving erratically, and so on).
- **Breaking the law:** For example, if your loved one is using or selling illicit drugs, he's not allowed to live in your home.

You can negotiate with someone who is relatively stable. But it's probably useless to invoke punishments for breaking rules when someone is psychotic and out of touch with reality. In this case, the rules are completely different (see Chapter 14) and you probably need outside help — doctors, therapists, police — to help resolve the issue.

Consequences only work if they're enforced. Don't threaten consequences that are unenforceable. Thinking of rules and consequences beforehand can prevent you from making idle threats.

Recognizing the role of negative symptoms

Many of the negative symptoms of schizophrenia (see Chapter 3) can lead to behaviors that drive you wild. Understanding obviously psychotic behavior is sometimes easier than it is to understand apathy, apparent laziness, and *avoidance behaviors* (being afraid or unwilling to engage in life) that, even in the good times, often accompany schizophrenia.

Your loved one may appear lazy but just may not have the energy or motivation required to get dressed or leave the house. He may be having problems comprehending the same work that came so easily before the breakdown. You need to carefully balance support and limit-setting — which is often difficult to do.

Try to not mete out punishments during a time of anger or say nasty things impulsively that you can't take back. When rules are broken, try to use the modest approach in taking action — if your loved one purposely breaks a plate, tell her that she can't stay in the kitchen, as opposed to telling her she can't stay in the house. If your loved one isn't taking his medication, tell him that he must speak to his clinician about it instead of saying he needs to be hospitalized. If you aren't sure whether you're being too strict or playing the role of a doormat, talk about it to a friend, relative, or health practitioner to gain some perspective.

Handling unrealistic thinking

Many times, a person with schizophrenia may say things that have no bearing in reality — statements that are so illogical that they leave you dumbfounded as to what to say next. When this happens, your options are to

- Challenge or disagree with something that you know is blatantly unrealistic
- Totally agree and accept something that you know to be untrue
- Dodge the issue in some way

Only the last approach — dodging — is acceptable. Delusional thinking is virtually impossible to challenge or change. It's based on a fixed belief that defies logic (see Chapter 3), and you'll never convince the person about what is real and what isn't. For example, if your loved one thinks that people in red cars are looking for him, nothing you can say can convince him otherwise. In fact, challenging the statement is counterproductive. He's probably frightened (hey, you would be, too, if you thought people were looking for you), and challenging him may simply make him agitated, angry, and more entrenched in his position. You also don't want to reinforce delusional thinking by agreeing with it. In this case, your best bet is either to distract the person and talk about something else or just let it go.

It doesn't hurt to find something to say in a reassuring manner to calm your loved one down and help him feel safe. For example, "The people in the red cars can't see into our house, and we're safe in here right now." Another approach is to focus on the person's *feeling* rather than the content. You can say, "I know you're feeling very anxious, but I think the feeling will pass if I keep you company for a while."

If a person is very fearful that harm is imminent, he may strike out at anyone who is perceived to represent a danger. Be careful, and take any threats seriously. Don't take any chances involving your own safety, or that of your loved one or other family members. No one wants to call the police to calm down a loved one who is out of control, but sometimes it's the more prudent course of action.

Be sure to distinguish between unrealistic thoughts and delusional thinking — the two demand different responses. How do you know the difference? As you get to know your loved one with schizophrenia, you can sense the difference between the two. Delusional thinking is more fixed, impermeable, and isn't likely to change no matter what you say.

When a person is just thinking unrealistically (as opposed to having delusions), you can ask pertinent questions or raise alternative explanations to help her think more clearly. For example, if your loved one thinks that starting a small business is easy and anyone can do it, that's a naïve belief, not a delusion. You can provide her with information about the proportion of small businesses that go under, and she may be stubborn, but she'll probably be open to hearing what you have to say.

Defusing conflicts

Arguments, disagreements, and conflicts are inevitable, even when things are going fairly well. When disagreements arise, you need to give your loved one ample opportunity to speak and tell his side of the story and allow him to hear yours. When people have the opportunity to talk things out calmly and feel that their side is being heard, it often diffuses anger and leads to quicker resolution without making the situation worse.

Never make the mistake of presuming that the other person's point of view isn't valid just because the person has schizophrenia. Listen carefully to hear what your loved one is trying to say and make sure you get it right. You can do this by repeating it back so the other person can hear how his side of the argument sounds to you. This strategy will help the other person recognize that, even if you don't agree, his point is being heard. It can also provide an opportunity to validate his feelings. For example, you can say, "I know you're very angry that I'm not allowing you to use my car, but I can't afford the cost of the gas or additional insurance for another driver right now." This example validates what the person is feeling and also provides an explanation for the basis of the disagreement.

In some instances, consistent disagreements or very intense conflicts over little things may suggest that an individual is having symptoms like anxiety, which should be discussed with a clinician.

Some situations can lead to the potential for an explosive and potentially dangerous situation. Try to recognize the early signs of a conflict and act quickly but calmly to defuse the situation. If your loved one appears to be menacing, try to deescalate the conflict until things calm down or you can get help. Here are some strategies for defusing the situation:

- Don't shout. Speak calmly and softly.
- Don't touch or threaten your loved one. Keep a respectful distance and tone of voice.
- Avoid continuous eye contact, because that can be construed as threatening.
- Don't wave your finger or point at your loved one.
- Try to distract your loved one with something else. If that doesn't work, stick to the topic at hand and don't bring up conflicts from the past.
- Never challenge or dare the person to defy you.
- Minimize critical remarks.

- Comply with any requests that are safe and reasonable.
- If you feel like your own safety is compromised, make that known and do what you have to do to keep yourself safe.

If your loved one has a prior history of self-destructive behavior, you may want to encourage her — while she's well (and rational) — to use an *advance directive* that will provide guidance about how she should be treated when she's ill and irrational (see Chapter 7).

Handling Troublesome Behaviors

Living with someone who has schizophrenia can be extremely disruptive on a number of fronts. You may have to cope with sleepless nights, scuffles with the law, or embarrassing behaviors in front of family, friends, or neighbors, to name just a few issues.

Sleep disturbances

Many people with schizophrenia, as well as those with schizoaffective disorder (see Chapter 3), have sleep issues. Some of these problems may be related to the illness itself; others may be related to medication. Research suggests that these impaired sleep patterns are associated with impaired ability to cope, both socially and vocationally.

Your loved one may sleep *too* much, which may lead you or your family members to believe that she's lazy or not meeting her responsibilities. Conversely, your loved one may have insomnia and pace the floors all night, listening to TV or loud music — interrupting the sleep of you and everyone else in the household.

If your loved one has problems getting asleep or staying asleep, and the problems are only occasional, they may be stress-related. Getting more exercise, keeping regular hours, practicing relaxation techniques, and avoiding caffeine may help.

If your loved one is up all night with manic energy or has reversed night and day, psychotic symptoms may be keeping him awake. If sleeping problems persist more than a few days, tell your loved one's clinician. Changing medication, the dose of medication, or adding a sedative may rectify the problem fairly rapidly.

Bizarre behaviors in public

Some people with schizophrenia may look and behave differently from other people. Often, the faces of people with schizophrenia have a recognizable flat expression that makes it appear as if they aren't experiencing any normal emotions. Over the years, either because of the illness or because of powerful medications, they may also develop peculiar gestures or odd movements.

Many people with schizophrenia also neglect personal hygiene, have poor grooming habits, or have a lack of insight into or concern about how their appearance is perceived by others. Some of these characteristics are tied to negative symptoms of schizophrenia (see Chapter 3).

Some psychosocial rehabilitation programs focus on providing practical instruction to people with schizophrenia on how to better take care of their appearance. This might include teaching a woman how to apply makeup or teaching someone how to dress for an interview or for a date.

Depending on whether the illness is stabilized, your loved one may say or do inappropriate or embarrassing things in public settings — for example, urinating on a lawn when a bathroom isn't accessible or taking something from a store without paying. When these behaviors occur, it's usually a symptom of the illness rather than a reflection of the person's character or personality. Cognitive behavioral therapy can help a person with schizophrenia learn how to behave more normally in common social situations.

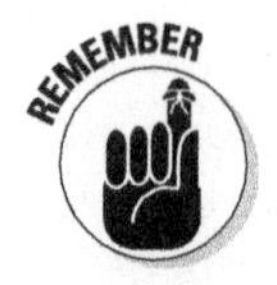

It's important to help define and redefine boundaries. You need to distinguish between public behaviors that are merely embarrassing and those that may be dangerous and illegal. Talk with your loved one beforehand about which behaviors are acceptable, which aren't, and why.

Before attending a potentially stressful social event, you and your loved one may want to role-play the situation so he has clear expectations about what to expect. Talking through the sequential steps that will occur can lessen stress and symptoms. For example, if you're going to a wedding ceremony in a church, you can say that you're taking a 20-minute drive to the church and that the ceremony and mass will last about 45-minutes and that you'll be going home after that.

Give your loved one a means of escape if too much tension builds up. Plan in advance how she can manage her stress without acting up or acting out. For example, in the case of the church wedding, you might tell your loved one that if she's feeling very anxious, she should walk outside to the garden and you'll meet her there as soon as the ceremony is over.

Bizarre behaviors can be mortifying, but the person with schizophrenia often can't help his behavior. In embarrassing situations, you have to remember that you love this person, you want him to be able to enjoy as normal a life as possible, and that most people are going to recognize that there's a problem and not be too harsh in their judgment of you or your loved one. If you think others may not be aware of your loved one's situation, letting them know about your loved one's illness before the event can go a long way toward fostering empathy and understanding.

Fostering Independence

When an adolescent or young adult is struck with schizophrenia, the illness often interferes dramatically with the normal progression into independent adulthood. It may interrupt the person's schooling, interfere with her ability to form social relationships with peers, or limit her opportunities to find and keep a job. Given these barriers, it's easy for a person with schizophrenia to fall back on family and remain dependent on them.

Families, friends, and clinicians need to help people with schizophrenia be as independent as possible in making decisions and controlling the way they live their lives. Helping your loved one find activities that build his self-esteem and give him a sense that he can succeed is invaluable. Limit criticism and heap on praise for things well done — this can encourage your loved one to try new things and master them.

If you find that your loved one is consistently asking others to help do things he can do himself, you may be (unintentionally) fostering his dependence and inadvertently impairing his ability to do things on his own. Sometimes, therapists can help you see these patterns when they're not obvious to you. Even in the best of circumstances, the natural instinct of families is to protect — and often to overprotect. Although you don't want to do a dramatic about-face in your relationship style (which could be upsetting to your loved one), you can encourage him to participate in self-help and peer-support groups to gain self-confidence and acceptance. Increased awareness of your role in fostering your loved one's independence, combined with taking small steps, can result in big changes over time.

Conflicts about who decides how money is spent are common. People with schizophrenia see money as a sign of their autonomy, while families often worry about whether the person will spend responsibly if she doesn't know how to save or budget. Use of allowances, entitlements, or job earnings is a topic that can be discussed with therapists to avoid conflict and promote independence.

Politically correct terminology

People are sensitive to the words used to describe mental illnesses — and for very good reasons. Words like *crazy, mental,* and *nutcase* were and are used to dehumanize and stereotype people with mental disorders.

Plus, sensationalistic and often inaccurate newspaper headlines make it appear as if people with mental disorders are solely responsible for the most heinous of crimes. Until the last decade, the media created such a sense of shame that people were afraid to talk about mental illness. People with these disorders were shunted aside, warehoused in large mental institutions far away from their homes, families, and neighbors.

Although there is growing acceptance of mental illness, discrimination is still rife in employment, housing, and insurance (see Chapter 15). For this reason, anyone touched by mental illness needs to educate others to use the right words, as well as to do the right thing when dealing with people with schizophrenia. With persistence, doing so will lead to a change of attitudes in the next generation.

Here are some of the terms that should not be used:

- **The schizophrenic:** Doctors and other medical personnel have long fallen into the bad habit of referring to people by their disease, such as "the cardiac in Room 4" (to refer to a person having a heart attack). Schizophrenia is the name of a disease, and *schizophrenic* should always be used as an adjective rather than a noun. Referring to someone as *a person with schizophrenia* is less demeaning, as well as more accurate.
- **Crazy, mental, nuts, loony, bananas, or nutcase:** These demeaning terms — and others like them — have no place in anyone's vocabulary. If you hear people using them, let them know that this is wrong and demeaning, and that you have a loved one with schizophrenia who deserves respect.
- **Patient:** People who are under a doctor's care are generally called *patients.* But many people with schizophrenia are offended by this term because it casts them in the role of a patient rather than a person. Alternative terms like *consumer, survivor, client,* and *recipient of care* are preferred by many patients and former patients, but there's no denying that these terms are still somewhat awkward to use and not universally understood by everyone. If you're not sure what term will make someone feel comfortable, ask that person.

Seeking Support for You and Your Loved One with Schizophrenia

When mental illness first strikes, you experience a gamut of feelings — including fear, guilt, confusion, and loss. No family is ever adequately prepared to understand the strange symptoms of the disease that robs people of their personalities; the complex treatments that control symptoms but do not offer cures; or the fragmented and underfinanced service-delivery system that has gaping holes every place you turn.

Family-support groups, consumer-run programs, and peer support programs provide safe havens where people can talk to others who share their pain and problems. These groups have also provided a platform from which people continue to work collectively to change the face of mental-health research, treatment, and service delivery. Through participation in seminars, monthly meetings, speaker series, annual conferences, family-education courses, support groups, and a telephone help line, consumers and families no longer feel alone.

To find a support group in your area, contact the National Alliance on Mental Illness (NAMI) at 800-950-6264 or 703-524-7600. You can also go to `www.nami.org`, and choose State and Local NAMIs from the Find Support drop-down list.

Chapter 13

Housing Choices: Figuring Out Where to Live

In This Chapter

- Deciding whether living at home is an option for your loved one
- Understanding other specialized housing options
- Determining the right fit for your loved one
- Evaluating residential-care programs
- Preventing your loved one from being homeless

Having a stable place to live and call home — whether it's an apartment, a private room in someone's house, or a bed in a supportive residence — is such a profound human need that it's one of the cornerstones to recovery for people with schizophrenia.

Ideally, people with schizophrenia should be able to choose a home based on how it meets their preferences in terms of where, how, and with whom they want to live, something many people take for granted. However, for most people with serious mental illnesses — in most communities across the nation — housing choices are either limited or, more often, nonexistent. Either choices are made for them (by others) or choices are made impossible by virtue of the scarcity of available housing options.

In this chapter, we look at the various housing options open to people with schizophrenia, from living at home to living in a group home, and help you find solutions that will work for everyone involved.

Recognizing the Challenges in Finding Housing

Finding a place to live can be one of the most difficult challenges in life for people with schizophrenia. Most people with disabilities live on limited and/or fixed incomes. Plus, the stigma and discrimination associated with schizophrenia compound the problem of finding housing and earning a living wage — especially if the individual has or has had a co-occurring substance abuse problem, has ever been involved with the law, has had tenant-landlord problems in the past, or needs to be hospitalized for an extended period of time.

When there are no viable alternatives, many people with untreated schizophrenia end up homeless, winding up in hospitals, in jails, in shelters, or on the streets.

In the following sections, we cover some of the challenges in finding housing for people with schizophrenia.

The financial cost

Many people with schizophrenia live on disability or on what they earn at minimum-wage jobs. This means that housing choices are extremely limited, especially if living at home isn't an option.

The availability of affordable housing in the United States is nothing short of a national crisis. For the individual with schizophrenia, there is a huge gap between the cost of housing and disability income. According to one recent report, in 2006, the average income of an individual dependent on Supplemental Security Income (SSI) was $632 per month, while the average cost nationally to rent a one-bedroom or efficiency unit was $715 per month. Given other essential expenses, such as food, transportation, healthcare, and clothing, this puts conventional housing out of the reach of the average person with schizophrenia.

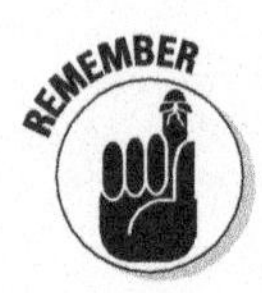

Most sources of funding for housing for people with schizophrenia fund programs rather than people. The exceptions are Section 8 certificates and rent vouchers that are available on a very limited basis from religious or non-profit organizations. In addition, some private health insurance and disability policies may provide benefits for programs that provide residential treatment.

It may fall to parents or other relatives to bridge the gap in housing costs, subsidizing their loved one's SSI with additional money to rent a suitable place. Some families set up special trusts so that their offspring inherits their home upon the death of both parents, to help keep the burden of support off other relatives when they're gone.

The scarcity of subsidized housing

Although some housing is available at below-market rates, the units are so few in number and waiting lists so long that it has become discouraging for people to even apply. For example, there are far too few Section 8 slots available for individuals with schizophrenia who are eligible; the average waiting time is almost three years!

To fill the gap, a number of substandard for-profit facilities exist in various communities, especially in high-cost cities with tight housing markets. Even though the cost of these facilities often taps a significant portion of an individual's disability income, families recount their relatives living in rodent-infested buildings with numerous code violations, including leaks and insufficient heat and hot water.

Because of the lack of options, people often are forced to live where units are available. This may mean compromises in terms of the nature of the neighborhood; accessibility to services; and proximity to family, friends, and other natural supports.

Lack of continuity

A too-common scenario is that a person with schizophrenia moves in and out of his family home (after a squabble or hospitalization) or from one substandard or inappropriate housing situation to another. This lack of continuity necessitates frequent changes in service providers and having to learn to negotiate new neighborhoods, one after another. Yet, people with schizophrenia need stability; any lack of permanency in their living situation can have a negative impact on their psychiatric condition.

Sometimes people with schizophrenia are thrown out of housing settings because they're deemed to no longer need services. Ironically, it may be the stability of their current housing situation that has helped them to stabilize.

Because housing is so scarce and expensive, people with schizophrenia find that shared living situations (or having roommates) is often the only way to make ends meet. It's difficult for *anyone* to negotiate living in close quarters with a complete stranger, let alone someone with schizophrenia. As a result, the privacy of residents living together is often compromised, and tensions arise from living in close quarters with unrelated adults who share few common bonds besides their illness.

The availability of the right amount of support and supervision can make all the difference in an individual's success or failure in community tenure. People with schizophrenia need varying degrees of support and supervision at various times. Resources (such as transportation and medical care) need to be accessible, and mental-health support services need to be able to respond flexibly based on a person's needs.

There's a great deal of controversy about whether housing should be contingent on an individual's willingness to accept services. Many consumers and some professionals see this as coercive and counterproductive to recovery.

Because of the gaps in housing and supports, many people with schizophrenia wind up inappropriately placed in more costly inpatient settings and local jails. A substantial number also join the ranks of the vulnerable homeless, living in shelters or on the streets.

Living at Home

Because of the scarcity of housing, many families pitch in to fill the gap, often at an extremely high cost — both financially and emotionally — to them and to their loved one. Parents or other relatives may offer housing to the individual in their own home or alternatively, support the cost of housing someplace else. Many people open their homes with justified trepidation about the potential conflicts of living under the same roof with their loved one with schizophrenia.

Understandably, living with relatives often precipitates or exacerbates conflicts in the household. This is especially true if the person with schizophrenia is an adult offspring living with one or more parents.

In many cases, parents are older and may have challenging chronic health problems of their own. They may also be facing financial problems: both in terms of declining incomes as they approach or have reached retirement, coupled with savings that have been sharply cut into after years of caregiving for someone with schizophrenia. One 76-year-old woman we know struggles — financially, logistically, and emotionally — to take care of two sisters with schizophrenia on her own. She's unsure how much longer she can continue without compromising her own health.

Moreover, because parents generally don't outlive their offspring, this obviously isn't a long-term solution, and the uncertainty can be unnerving. Parents worry about what will happen when they're gone and what role other siblings will be pressed into playing in the future (see Chapter 11).

In rare instances, living at home works out well and is reciprocal for the person with schizophrenia and her family. No one feels burdened or put out by the arrangement. For example, we know an able-bodied young person with schizophrenia who is a wonderful support to his ailing mother who oversees his mental-health care and provides meals. But this should be a mutual choice, not a default because no other options exist.

Having a written list of rules to abide by can be very beneficial if you plan to live with your relative with schizophrenia. (See Chapter 12 for more on the issues that arise when people with schizophrenia live with others.) Keep in mind that caregivers should have rules to abide by as well. Just because someone's living in your house, for example, doesn't give you carte blanche to go through her things or get angry if he wants to go out with friends on weekends.

If life were a fairy tale, we'd all live happily ever after, but it's not. Sometimes keeping a person with schizophrenia becomes untenable. Any one of the following reasons can lead to a decision that your loved one needs to live elsewhere:

- The individual is threatening and represents a danger to himself or to other members of the family.
- The person has untreated substance abuse problems that require a different type of care and approach than you can provide (such as inpatient detox).
- There are financial, social, and/or medical problems that make it prohibitive (for example, elderly parents dealing with a life-threatening illness).
- The illness is causing so much stress in the family that it's highly disruptive to relationships between spouses or parents and other children.
- The person with schizophrenia is unwilling to accept any treatment and is actively psychotic, leading to chaos in the household.

If you decide that it's impossible for your loved one to live at home, expect to feel guilty, but don't let it overwhelm you — or change your mind in a situation that you know is really impossible. In the long run, this decision will benefit you and your relative. Give yourself time to talk over the decision with other people you respect and who understand the situation.

Specialized Housing Options

If your loved one can't live at home, and isn't able to care for herself without help in her own place, you may need to look at specialized housing. Specialized housing for people with schizophrenia (generally subsidized by government or private-sector organizations) can take one of several forms:

- Housing programs for people with disabilities (including or limited to people with mental disorders)
- Mixed-used housing in the community (with units set aside for people with mental illnesses or other special needs)
- Scattered-site apartments or housing units for people with mental disorders that are fully integrated into the community

Nursing homes aren't just for the elderly; people who need 24-hour skilled nursing care for any reason are eligible for nursing-home care. People with schizophrenia may have health needs in addition to schizophrenia that may make a nursing home a good fit. The downside: It may diminish opportunities for socializing with peers.

When you first start searching for care for a relative who is actively hallucinating or delusional, you may think that long-term hospitalization in a mental-health facility is a logical choice. Although this was true several decades ago, it's rarely an option today.

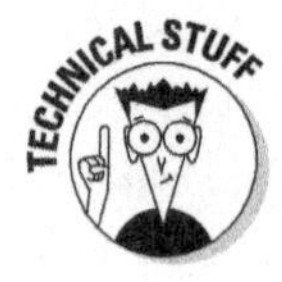

Long-term hospitalization isn't an answer to the housing shortage. In fact, even as a treatment option, it's being used less and less frequently because of changed philosophies of treatment and the rapid escalation in the costs of inpatient care. With the move toward treatment of schizophrenia in the community, state psychiatric hospitals have dramatically reduced their number of inpatient beds and reduced the length of stay of their patients accordingly. For someone to be hospitalized for a long time today, he would need to represent an ongoing danger to himself or others.

There are upsides and downsides to each of these options. Mixed-use or scattered-site housing generally is more integrated into the community as a whole, but specialized housing programs may be more helpful to people with serious mental illnesses. Additionally, such programs may provide greater opportunities for peer support.

Searching for housing

For a person with schizophrenia, finding a place to live is no easy feat. Eligibility and application requirements for affordable housing programs are often complex and difficult to understand. It requires a lot of legwork and networking with other people and organizations to find out what resources, if any, exist in the community. It may also entail signing up on long waiting lists.

Your loved one will likely need your help if he's looking into housing programs. In fact, you may feel like you've taken on a full-time job — a frustrating one, because you'll be dealing with government agencies much of the time — while assisting your loved one in finding housing.

Some of the community resources that may be of assistance in your search include the following:

- **The local mental-health authority,** which may directly sponsor housing units, contract out to other community organizations, or support services in housing operated by others
- **The state mental-health authority or health department,** which may license certain categories of housing within a state (for example, adult homes, board and care homes, or supportive housing programs)
- **The local public housing authority or U.S. Department of Housing and Urban Development (HUD) regional office,** which may be aware of opportunities for low-income housing or HUD-supported programs

- **The National Alliance on Mental Illness (NAMI) and other family organizations,** which may be familiar with resources because of their experience with relatives living in these units or because they've heard about them from others
- **Peers in day programs, social clubs, support groups, and treatment settings,** who may be able to provide some housing leads

If you or your loved one is hospitalized, you need to start planning for his discharge and where he'll live almost from the time he's admitted to the hospital. Given the length of waiting lists for various housing options, you may need both an interim plan as well as a long-term one. The hospital social worker or discharge planner may be able to help you get started.

Making sense of the options

When you're buying a house, you learn to interpret the overly optimistic descriptions used to describe housing. A "fixer upper" is a house that's falling off its foundations; "cozy" means the place is suitable only for one (very short) person. Unfortunately, it's not so easy to decipher the terms used to describe housing for people with mental problems. The same terms (for example, *transitional housing*) may have different meanings and conditions in one state, community, or program than they do in another.

In the following sections, we look at terms commonly used and what they generally (if not always) refer to when searching for housing.

There is no commonly accepted *typology* (classification) of housing terms. They vary from state to state and sometimes from community to community. *Supportive housing,* for example, may have very different meanings in terms of the actual type of supervision provided.

Permanent versus transitional housing

Permanent housing means it's your loved one's for as long as he can pay the rent and uphold the conditions of his lease. The benefit of permanent housing is that it allows the person with schizophrenia to stay in a known setting, to find a place within the community, and to develop a sense of belonging and security. Because change and transition can be disconcerting for someone with schizophrenia, these are real pluses.

Permanent-housing programs may or may not require the resident to take advantage of treatment and support services as a condition of living there.

By definition, *transitional housing* is temporary and available only for a l imited time. Usually, the expectation is that the person will "graduate" to permanent housing. Programs funded by HUD, for example, have a 24-month limit.

Transitional programs are sometimes called *halfway houses,* because they provide care in between an inpatient stay and independent or supportive living in the community.

Transitional housing programs are generally intended for people who require services and support before they're able to live independently, so there's often a requirement that residents take advantage of the services they provide. These may include 24/7 assistance with the activities of daily living, vocational rehabilitation, medication management, social-skills training, provision of cafeteria-style meals, substance-abuse services, and so on.

Transitional housing can take place in a large congregate care setting (such as a community residence) or in a smaller group home that is shared by two or more unrelated adults who may or may not have their own bedrooms.

Supportive housing versus supported housing

Despite the name similarity, supportive housing and supported housing are two different things. In *supportive housing* units, a range of services are provided on-site and people live in close proximity with others who have been diagnosed with mental illnesses. In *supported housing* (also called *scattered-site housing*), services are provided off-site and are usually more limited.

Supportive housing is generally intended for people who require some degree of ongoing on-site support and supervision in order to live in the community. Supported housing may include independent apartments or single-family homes with mobile outreach services.

Both supportive and supported housing tend to offer permanent rather than transitional stays unless there is an egregious breech of house rules.

Certain housing settings are specifically designed for people with co-occurring mental-health and substance-abuse problems. *Wet housing* refers to residences that provide housing for people who still aren't able to pledge abstinence. If this housing weren't available, they would likely be homeless. *Damp housing* is intended for people who are willing to be abstinent in the residence, although they may use drugs or alcohol away from it while they work toward sobriety.

Although supervised housing offers many benefits for people who might otherwise have no other alternatives and may otherwise cycle in and out of hospitals, when units are supervised by staff, many residents feel as if they're institutionalized, having to account for their behavior and whereabouts 24/7. In other words, there can be an overemphasis on control to the extent that respect for the individual falls by the wayside, which can lead to clients leaving in a huff and then not being allowed to return. Make sure you and your relative understand the rules about leaving and returning before she moves in.

Boarding homes and foster-care homes

Boarding homes (where unrelated adults live together in someone's home, sometimes with meals) and *foster-care homes* (where there is more supervision, the amount of which varies from state to state) can be licensed or unlicensed homes where someone in the community houses one or more people with mental disorders, providing them with room and board. Both proprietary boarding homes and foster-care homes can be highly variable in terms of what they offer to a particular person with schizophrenia; many can be purely custodial as opposed to therapeutic.

If you find that rare person who boards people with mental illness out of a genuine love and care for them, do everything in your power to hold on to them! These saints are one in a million. Conversely, if you sense that something's not right in your relative's living situation, try to get him to talk about his life there, and start looking into alternative situations, because you may have to move him out very quickly under emergency circumstances.

One international study suggested that, worldwide, boarding homes are the least desirable type of residential setting in terms of their access to social support, meaningful activity, and work.

Starting the Conversation: Questions to Discuss with Your Loved One

Families, friends, and service providers can play an important part in helping an individual with schizophrenia think about housing options. Some of the questions you need to openly discuss with your loved one include the following:

- **Can your loved one live independently or does he need support and supervision?** For example, is he responsible for taking care of his own needs? Does he show good judgment? Does he know how to handle an emergency?
- **Is your loved one able to access services in the community, or would it be more beneficial to have those services on-site?** Does your loved one require supervision and oversight or would she be able to take advantage of community-based programs on her own?
- **Is it reasonable for the person to live with family, or would it cause too much friction?** Is there enough space? Are you able to handle the burden of another person in the house? Do you think you would be arguing much of the time?

- **How much money does your loved one have available for housing each month (based on entitlements, income, and/or contributions from the family)?** What kind of housing can your loved one realistically afford?
- **What are your loved one's preferences?** People should have some say in the types of settings and locations that most appeal to them, given their choices are consistent with their needs and resources.

Evaluating Residential Care

Sometimes you just know you've found the right living situation for your family member, but more often, you have to choose between several acceptable-but-not-perfect alternatives. When you find a potential housing opportunity, some of the questions you should ask include the following:

- What type of housing is provided?
- How long can an individual reside here?
- What is the philosophy of the operation?
- Who supervises the residence and what type of degree or training does that person have?
- What types of clients are most successful in this setting?
- What is the out-of-pocket monthly cost?
- Are services provided? If so, what types of services? On-site or off-site?
- What are the rules regarding drug and alcohol use?
- What oversight agencies license or accredit the facility?
- How are infractions of rules handled?
- How is relapse handled? Is a room/apartment saved for when the individual is discharged from a hospital?
- Do residents participate in the governance, operation, and/or evaluation of the facility or program? If so, in what way?
- Are there mechanisms in place for interested family members to communicate with staff?

Finally, ask yourself, "What's my gut reaction to this place?" "How would I feel living here?" Never ignore that nagging feeling or intuition that something's just not right.

The need for community acceptance: Understanding and averting homelessness

Everyone thinks there should be housing available for people with mental illness, but no one wants it next door to their house. Historically, when government or advocacy groups have tried to develop specialized housing units to serve the population, the most common response has been "not on my block" or "not in my town," a phenomenon so commonplace that it's nicknamed NIMBY (not in my backyard). As a result, many communities are now grappling with the problem of homelessness among people with serious mental illnesses.

With shrinking budgets at every level of government and the difficulties in establishing supportive housing or subsidized units in regular housing, people with schizophrenia are forced to compete on the open housing market like everyone else, albeit with several strikes against them. Clearly, many of them aren't able to overcome these hurdles: It's estimated that about one-third of people who are homeless have serious mental illnesses — and the majority of them have schizophrenia.

A number of federal programs, sponsored by HUD, are focused on providing affordable housing and support or averting homelessness for people with disabilities. The HUD programs are intended to provide a coordinated strategy for communities to provide a continuum of care, which includes outreach; intake and assessment; emergency shelter; transitional housing; supportive services; permanent supportive housing; permanent housing; and homelessness prevention. The programs include

- **The Sec 811 Supportive Housing Program for People with Disabilities:** This is the sole program providing supportive housing for non-elderly low-income people with disabilities.
- **The Section 8 Housing Choice Voucher (HCV):** This can be used to obtain private rental housing in properties that meet the HCV requirements. Administered by local public housing authorities, there is also a home-ownership option.
- **The McKinney-Vento Homeless Programs:** The components of this legislation include a Supportive Housing Program, a Shelter Plus Care Program, and a Section 8 Moderate Rehabilitation Single Room Occupancy (SRO) Program.

These federal programs are always under siege and threat of cuts when more, rather than less, is what's actually needed. In the private sector, many landlords still continue to discriminate against people with mental illness.

It's important for mental-health advocates to understand that housing is a basic need of people with schizophrenia and to advocate for ways to provide more housing options that offer dignity and support recovery. Some of this entails educating landlords, legislators, service providers, and taxpayers about what may seem obvious — the importance of a place that feels like home to any person's health, mental health, and sense of well-being.

Chapter 14

Coping with Crises

In This Chapter

- Being prepared for psychiatric emergencies
- Recognizing signs of an impending crisis
- Watching for suicide risks
- Knowing what to do if your loved one disappears
- Handling arrests

A psychiatric crisis is a frightening event for everyone — the individual, family and friends, sometimes even the community at large. A psychiatric crisis handled poorly can quickly turn dangerous for the person with schizophrenia or others around him.

Just like the Boy Scouts motto suggests, being prepared is key to coping with any crisis. Having a plan not only allows you to act quickly and appropriately, but also helps minimize stress for everyone involved. In this chapter, we help you prepare for psychiatric emergencies — from psychotic breaks and attempted suicide to disappearances or arrests. We also show you how to recognize signs of possible crisis early and show you how to cope effectively to end the crisis, with a good resolution, as quickly as possible.

Accepting Crises as Part of Schizophrenia

Life may seem to be going along well; your loved one is improving on medication and coping reasonably with life. Then a crisis occurs. You wrack your brain wondering if you should've seen this coming, and feel like you could have done something to prevent it.

But the reality is that schizophrenia is not only a chronic disorder, but also a cyclical disorder, characterized by periods of relative well-being that are interrupted by *relapse* (a severe worsening of symptoms that interferes with a person's functioning). The same type of waxing and waning of symptoms also occurs with other chronic medical disorders, such as arthritis and asthma; even some cancers are seen as chronic diseases that relapse and remit.

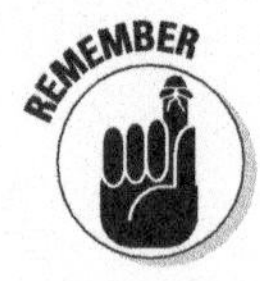

Mental health crises — which can be a sudden worsening of symptoms, or a more gradual change that eventually reaches the point where the person with schizophrenia is out of control and/or can't function — are not uncommon and can't always be prevented, although their frequency and severity can be minimized.

Relapse can occur for a variety of different reasons. The cause of relapse may be apparent at one time and a complete mystery at another. Often, more than one factor contributes to the relapse.

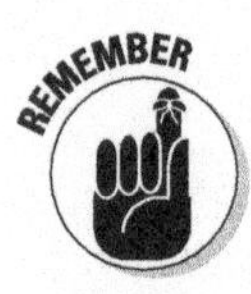

The most common cause of relapse is stopping medication. Either people stop taking medication on their own, or they're advised to stop by a doctor (perhaps because of intolerable side effects). Other potential triggers include the following:

- **Susceptibility to stress in the environment:** Stressful interpersonal or living situations — such as annoying roommates; the threat of eviction or loss of housing; or conflicts with friends, family members, employers, or clinicians — can exacerbate symptoms.
- **Medications failing to work as well as they once did:** The reasons for this situation are still unknown, but it does happen.
- **Laxness in taking medications regularly:** People with schizophrenia may forget a dose here or there, just as people may do when taking a prescribed course of antibiotics. This is especially true when they're feeling better and forget that "feeling good" is probably due to the medication.
- **Complexity of medication schedules:** People with schizophrenia may have to take multiple drugs with different dosing schedules. Following these schedules consistently may be particularly difficult.
- **Unwillingness to adhere to the regimens prescribed by doctors:** It's common for people to experiment, taking more or (usually) less medication than prescribed.
- **Costliness of medications:** New medications that are still under patent are especially expensive. The medications often become unaffordable because of insurance limitations or lack of insurance.

- **Alcohol and/or other drug abuse:** A relapse of a co-occurring substance-abuse problem can precipitate a downward spiral. For example, the person may be unable to stay on medication due to eviction or arrest.
- **Discouragement, depression, or stress:** If someone feels hopeless or overwhelmed, she may neglect many aspects of staying healthy, including taking medication.

Psychiatric crises can also crop up spontaneously, without any identifiable cause, just as part of the disease. When this happens, it's especially frustrating to people with schizophrenia, their relatives, and clinicians who have done everything humanly possible to keep the illness at bay.

The disappointment and frustration associated with relapse is often exasperating for families when the person who is ill doesn't believe or refuses to admit that he is sick. He may instead blame everyone else for what's happening to him. This situation makes it difficult to convince the person that he's sick and needs help. It may also cause friends and family members to question their own behavior, wondering whether they have, in fact, caused or contributed to the crisis.

As a friend or family member of someone with schizophrenia, you have to keep your own emotions on an even keel and not fall prey to the idea that you're somehow responsible for a deteriorating situation. Realizing that relapse is a possibility and recognizing the first signs of it, can help you remind your loved one that he needs to be seen by his doctor.

Anosognosia is the technical term used when an individual has no insight into or awareness of his own illness.

Many people with schizophrenia need to be taught by their clinicians to recognize the warning signs of relapse. In a perfect world, the person in crisis would recognize that she needs help and seek it herself or ask you to intervene. Frankly, this doesn't often happen because, as the illness worsens, awareness and insight — that the illness is causing the disordered behavior — tends to disappear.

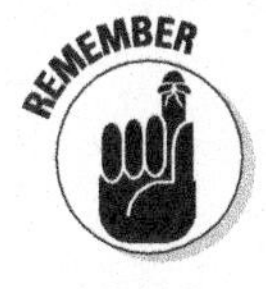

When you recognize that the person with schizophrenia no longer has insight, get help — and don't allow her to persuade you that nothing is wrong.

Being Prepared Before a Crisis Occurs

Many crises can be averted or resolved quickly when you work collaboratively with the person's psychiatrist or other clinician. This is where being prepared ahead of time really pays off. In this section, we help you make sure you're ready to act quickly and effectively in a crisis:

Keeping essential information in a central location

When you're in the middle of a crisis, you don't want to have to search frantically for phone numbers, medical information, insurance cards, and other essential scraps of paper. Instead, keep all the information you need in one convenient location, preferably in a bound notebook near a telephone at home or in your personal address book. It should be readily accessible and easy to find when you need it.

Here's the information you want to have at hand:

- **A list of the names, titles, and phone numbers of your loved one's treatment team so everyone in the household has access to them, including the person with schizophrenia:** This includes the names of the psychiatrist, psychologist, social worker, psychiatric nurse, other clinicians or peer counselor; the name of the person's case manager; and contact information for how each of these professionals can be reached during working hours and off-hours in an emergency.
- **The phone number of the local hospital emergency room and local crisis services**
- **The phone number of a friend or family member who understands and can help**
- **The phone number of the local police department**
- **Your loved one's diagnosis and the approximate date when she was last seen by a clinician**
- **A list of all the medications (psychiatric and any other) the person with schizophrenia is taking, including the names of the drugs, their dosages, and their frequency**
- **A succinct history of the medications your loved one has taken in the past, along with notes about what worked, what didn't, and any adverse reactions**
- **History, if any, of alcohol and/or other drug abuse and its treatment**
- **Any pertinent information about the person's physical health**

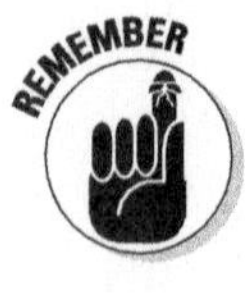

Be sure to update these lists as medications and service providers change.

Although the field of medicine is moving toward electronic medical records to enable consumers (and often their doctors) to have access to their personal health information on the Internet no matter where they are, the reality is that some systems can't "talk" to others, and communication between one provider and another may not be as timely or reliable as it should be.

If possible, purchase a password-protected USB flash drive on which you can store your loved one's electronic medical record. This empowers consumers and families to maintain control of their own information and always have it accessible in an emergency, whether at home or away. At the very least, keep hard copies of all clinician visits, pertinent lab results, and previous hospitalization records.

A *USB flash drive* is a portable hard drive, about the size of your thumb, that plugs into any computer's USB port. You can find these drives in places like the big-name office supply stores or computer stores. A small 1GB drive can be had for less than $20; drives with greater capacity will run you closer to $75 or more (and there are numerous options at prices in between). Look for one with a metal loop attached, so you can put it on your keychain and always have it handy.

Surveying crisis resources before you need them

The best time to learn about crisis resources is before you need them, when your loved one is stable. These resources include mental-health inpatient, outpatient, and crisis programs (alternatives to hospitalization) in the community such as:

- *Mobile outreach teams* (trained teams of professionals who conduct clinical assessments and provide services wherever patients are located, at home or in the community)
- *Crisis response teams* (mental-health professionals who can come to your home in the event of a psychiatric emergency, much like a volunteer ambulance corps might come in the event of an injury or heart attack)
- Assertive Community Treatment (ACT) programs, which use multidisciplinary professional teams to provide comprehensive, round-the-clock services to clients in the comfort of their own homes and in the community
- Hospitals
- Local law enforcement programs intended to divert people from jails

Although all facilities sound wonderful in their brochures or in the phone book, in reality, some may be ill-equipped to handle a person with serious psychiatric issues, may not offer after-hours admitting services, or may not take your insurance — or any insurance at all. When possible, phone or visit these programs in person and speak to the staff to find how they may be able to help during a crisis and to get a feel for the facility or program and whether you would feel comfortable having them provide care for your loved one.

Some of the best sources of up-to-date information on facilities in your area are members of local affiliates of the National Alliance on Mental Illness (NAMI; a national membership organization of families providing education, support, and advocacy), who have vast experience and are willing to share their expertise. Professionals who work with your loved one may also be knowledgeable about community resources.

Also be sure to contact your local public mental health authority (county or city) to find out about the range of crisis services they offer. They're usually listed in the Yellow Pages under government agencies. Depending on where you live, there may be publicly funded mobile outreach services, short-term crisis residential services, consumer-operated safe houses (shelters), and hot lines that can help.

Because crisis stabilization services aren't available everywhere all the time, hospitalization is often a necessity of last resort.

Also, most community hospitals lack a sufficient number of crisis beds resulting in long waits in the emergency room or transfers to other facilities. Knowing what's available at each of your area hospitals can make the difference in the quality of care your loved one gets in a crisis. Consider the following:

- **Make sure the hospital is an in-network provider, participates in your relative's insurance plan, or accepts patients with Medicaid.**
- **Find out if the hospital's behavioral healthcare program is accredited by the Joint Commission (`www.jointcommission.org`).** In that way, you can be assured that the facility meets certain standards. (Although this is desirable, you may not always have a Joint Commission–accredited hospital in your area.)
- **Make sure that the hospital has psychiatric beds.** Some hospitals don't have these beds. If your loved one winds up in such an emergency room, she'll likely be sent elsewhere, wasting time.
- **Ask about the number, demographics, and diagnoses of the psychiatric patients.** If your loved one is in his 80s, you probably wouldn't want him on the same unit as young people with dual diagnoses. On the other hand, if your loved one is an impulsive teenager, you may not want her to be on a mixed-sex ward.
- **Find out who supervises the unit.** Because medication is one of the mainstays of inpatient treatment, ideally the person supervising the unit will be a competent *psychopharmacologist* (an expert in psychiatric medications).
- **Inquire about the visiting policies for patients and whether those hours will make visiting convenient for you.**
- **Find out about the smoking policies if your loved one is addicted to nicotine.**

- **Ask whether your loved one will be able to go outdoors during his stay if it extends more than a few days.**
- **Check with other people who know the hospital about the competence of the physicians who will be taking care of your loved one.**
- **If your loved one doesn't speak English or is of a racial/cultural minority, make sure that the staff is linguistically and culturally sensitive.** Ask whether translators are available when needed.
- **Ask if you can visit the hospital beforehand, to see its facilities.** Don't be surprised if staff isn't welcoming about families visiting a facility beforehand. Typically, they're trying to protect the confidentiality of the patients who are there so your visit may be restricted to certain times or certain areas of the facility.

- **Most important: Find out about the hospital's policies about communicating with families.** Do they see them as part of the problem or part of the solution? Will they allow you to provide information? Will the hospital be willing, with the patient's permission, to share information with you?

Proprietary services on the Internet, like HealthGrades (`www.healthgrades.com`), provide information on individual hospitals and their doctors. Hospitals are rated, with information about their costs, patient volumes, and safety record. You can also find out about doctors, their training, certification, length of time in practice, and whether they've been subject to any disciplinary actions.

Recognizing the Signs That Something Is Wrong

The signs of a beginning recurrence of schizophrenia may or may not be obvious. The onset may be insidious, developing over a long period of time; other times it appears suddenly, seemingly out of the blue. Alerting yourself to the most common early signs that all is not well can help avert a crisis.

Noticing a downward spiral

The signs of an acute psychiatric crisis can't be missed, but symptoms that appear gradually may be easily overlooked or explained away, unless you're aware that they may represent an impending crisis. Many of these signs are also characteristic of the *negative symptoms* of schizophrenia (described in Chapter 3), and it can take an attentive eye to recognize the subtle differences between your loved one's "normal" behavior and an increase in negative symptoms.

Confidentiality policies: Separating fact from fiction

In 1996, the U.S. Congress passed the Health Insurance Portability and Accountability Act (HIPAA), a lengthy and complex law that regulates and protects the sharing of all health (including mental-health) information. Many people don't fully understand the provisions of the law, and some professionals use it as a handy excuse to deny all communication with families. (Additionally, independent of HIPAA, some policies established by mental-health programs are even more restrictive than the federal law.)

The ethical standards of conduct of many mental-health professions (such as psychology, psychiatry, and others) also uphold patient confidentiality in therapeutic relationships. But if a patient is at imminent risk of harming herself or others, clinicians have a duty to inform appropriate individuals, including the family.

In the case of patients with schizophrenia, practitioners need to be sensitive to the ways in which disclosure, with the patient's permission, can actually *benefit* treatment. As a general rule, with explicit permission from the patient (usually in writing), clinicians can share relevant information with the family. If the patient is deemed incompetent, the patient's permission isn't necessary if the family member has legal authority to make medical decisions on behalf of the patient.

Hiding behind the law, some clinicians and hospital employees cite the risk of fines and jail terms if they divulge information to anyone but the patient. In truth, as long as a patient doesn't object, a health practitioner can share information about a patient with family members. Many times, clinicians fail to ask patients their preferences and assume they don't want their families involved (which isn't always the case). Instead, they should discuss the importance of family involvement and support. Even if the patient voices an objection, the doctor isn't prohibited from *listening* to families who can provide vital information about the patient, his illness, and prior treatments.

In some cases, the law is taken to such an extreme that some hospitals are unwilling to put telephone calls through when a relative calls and asks to speak to a patient, not wanting to reveal that the person is hospitalized there. To eliminate any confusion, you might ask your loved one to write a note giving her permission for a doctor to speak to you or for a hospital to release information. (See Chapter 7 for more information on advance directives.)

Regardless of any policy prohibitions against sharing patient-specific information, professionals have an ethical responsibility to share nonconfidential "educational" information — such as information about psychiatric disorders and their treatment, community resources, tips for coping, and information about the availability of NAMI groups and meetings in the community.

Although your loved one may not want a relative — including you — to know all the intimate details of his life, he may want them to know the name of his disorder, its symptoms, its treatment, the expected course, warning signs of relapse, and how they can know if he might be at risk of hurting himself or others. You may need to remind your loved one (and his clinician) that family members and friends can be an important source of support and encouragement on a person's journey to recovery.

Some signs that may indicate a gradual decline include

- Becoming increasingly withdrawn (not interacting or speaking with others)
- Losing interest in eating or eating excessively
- Becoming irresponsible about self-care routines such as washing and dressing
- Spending more and more time asleep or in bed
- Severe mood changes

Spotting the signs of an acute crisis

Symptoms of an acute exacerbation of illness are much more noticeable — and frightening — than the subtle signs that may precede it. These are also the so-called *positive symptoms* of schizophrenia (see Chapter 3).

A person in acute crisis may

- Feel threatened and become hypervigilant
- Hear voices when no one is speaking (known as *hallucinating*)
- Become suspicious and frightened that someone or some group wants to hurt him (known as being *delusional*)
- Become agitated
- Say things that don't make sense
- Pace incessantly, or be unable to sit still

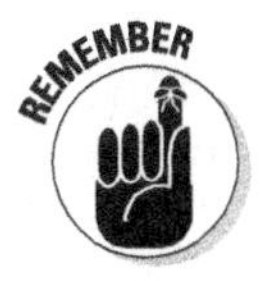

During a crisis, it's easy to let emotions escalate as your fears take hold. However, it's extremely important that you maintain a calm demeanor when speaking to your loved one with schizophrenia. Even if that person is acting belligerent, threatening, or isn't listening to you, it does no good to yell, argue with, or provoke the individual in any way. Instead, your goal should be to diffuse the situation and get help as quickly as possible to protect the patient, yourself, and anyone else who is present. To achieve that, you need to maintain a positive relationship with the person, reassuring him, building his confidence, and letting him know that you're there for him when he feels frightened and out of control.

Calling for Professional Help

If your loved one is in no immediate danger when a crisis begins, the best course of action is to seek immediate medical advice from the person's own psychiatrist or other clinician.

Although only a physician can prescribe medication (except in a few states where psychologists have prescribing privileges), psychiatrists are often overextended and hard to reach, especially if crises occur after hours, on holidays, or on weekends.

Other mental-health professionals often have better luck contacting the psychiatrist than family members or consumers have, or they may be able to render their own help.

Even if you can't reach your loved one's own doctor, typically another doctor will be covering her practice. Other times, you may have to contact a clinic or crisis center where no one is familiar with your family member.

If you're dealing with an unfamiliar clinician, identify your relation to the person with schizophrenia, and be prepared to describe what unusual behaviors or symptoms the person with schizophrenia is experiencing. You'll also need to know the name of the person's doctor, when your loved one was last seen, his diagnosis or diagnoses, and current treatments. (See "Keeping essential information in a central location," earlier in this chapter, for the kind of information to have on hand before a crisis.)

With the information you provide, the clinician will be able to suggest a course of action for you to take. This might include

- Changing medications or changing the dose of one or more medications
- Making an appointment for the person to be seen at a clinic or private office as soon as possible
- Recommending a visit to the emergency room of your local community hospital
- Making arrangements for admission to a psychiatric hospital or a general hospital with psychiatric beds
- Some other course of action based on the patient and family's needs and the available community resources
- Calling the police if the clinician feels the person is dangerous to himself or others

Knowing Whether Hospitalization Is Necessary

Although images from old books and movies may have you very concerned about the possibility of hospitalization for your loved one, rest assured that the scary images of the past no longer represent modern psychiatric facilities. In fact, the images portrayed in old movies (like *The Snake Pit*) actually helped reform them.

Not everyone in crisis needs inpatient hospitalization today; outpatient management may be all your loved one needs. The next sections describe the options of hospitalization and outpatient care.

The decision to hospitalize

When does your loved one need to be hospitalized rather than treated on an outpatient basis? The short answer: when she needs to receive 24-hour care in a more protected and secure environment (which may or may not be locked) than you can provide or when medical treatment requires 24-hour monitoring and observation.

Here are some examples of when hospitalization is necessary:

- When a person needs to be protected (he's dangerous to himself, he's dangerous to others, or his judgment is so impaired that he can't be responsible for himself)
- When the patient would benefit from close observation of symptoms and side effects in a controlled setting (for example, during an acute relapse)
- When the patient needs intensive medical oversight (to rapidly switch medications, to withdraw from illegal drugs, to assess or treat medical complications)
- When the patient would benefit from intensive therapeutic programming (that is, behavioral modification)
- When the family can no longer handle care on their own or they need some respite from providing care and supervision
- When there is an acute drug overdose (whether prescribed, over-the-counter, or illicit drugs)

Even though you think your loved one may be an imminent danger to herself or others, it may be difficult to have her hospitalized involuntarily if she doesn't agree with you and refuses to be evaluated. In many cases, professionals must witness the behavior themselves — but often, they may be willing to accept information you provide.

Involuntary commitment laws are complicated and vary from state to state. Depending on where you live, you or a mental-health professional may need to call the police to transport your loved one to a hospital or file a petition seeking an involuntary psychiatric evaluation. You may be able to contact your local mobile crisis service to bring your loved one to a psychiatric emergency room. To find out about your state commitment law, its standards, and what you need to do in the event of an emergency, contact your local mental-health department or go to www.treatmentadvocacycenter.org/LegalResources/Index.htm.

What to bring with you for hospital admission

Sometimes, hospitals will allow you to arrange for a scheduled admission screening. Other times, you may be required to show up at the emergency room and wait. Either way, these are some of the things you may want to bring with you:

- Insurance cards from Medicaid or any third-party insurers
- A written summary (no more than a couple of pages long) that includes information about your loved one's current medications, a brief list of her current symptoms, a brief history of her medications, what worked, and what didn't
- Information about any health problems your loved one has or had — treated or untreated
- Outpatient provider information (to assure that the treating team has access to prior information about the patient and to facilitate continuity of care after discharge)
- Contact information for the family

Generally, at least two people should accompany the individual to the hospital so one of them can drive and the other can provide support to the person with schizophrenia and assistance to the driver, if necessary.

Alternatives to hospitalization

If your family member isn't a danger to himself or others, outpatient care may be all he needs to get through a crisis — which can help avoid the stigma of a first hospitalization or the demoralization that often results because of a subsequent one. Some of the alternatives that may prevent or avoid hospitalization include

- **More intensely supervised outpatient care:** Checking in with a doctor or case worker more frequently to provide crisis support and monitor or adjust medication.
- **Injectable medication (generally an antipsychotic or sedative medication) administered at a physician's office or in an emergency room**

- **Mobile outreach teams:** See "Surveying crisis resources before you need them," earlier in this chapter.
- **ACT programs:** See "Surveying crisis resources before you need them," earlier in this chapter.
- **Crisis housing:** A short-term residential alternative to hospitalization that offers intensive crisis support.
- **Partial hospitalization:** A program in which patients continue to live at home but spend a certain number of hours in a hospital setting, either during the day or at night.
- **Assisted outpatient treatment (AOT):** Also called *outpatient commitment,* AOT may be an option for people who are consistently unwilling to take medication and, as a result, are unable to live safely in the community. Forty-two states permit the use of this type of court-ordered treatment, although it's used more infrequently than you might think. For more information on AOT, contact your state mental-health authority (see the appendix) or go to `www.psychlaws.org/BriefingPapers/BP4.htm`.

Reducing the Risk of Suicide

The risk of suicide for individuals with schizophrenia is estimated to be 50 times higher than that of the general population. In fact, it is the most common cause of premature death for people with the disorder. (Over 90 percent of Americans who kill themselves have a mental disorder.)

In some cases of suicide among people with schizophrenia, the suicide is considered unintentional — a product of delusional or disturbed thinking. More often, suicide among this group is linked to severe depressive symptoms. That shouldn't be surprising considering all the losses associated with schizophrenia — financial, education, vocational, and social.

If a person with schizophrenia is expressing hopelessness or suicidal thoughts, making suicidal threats, getting rid of her prized belongings, or putting her affairs in order, these behaviors and suicidal thoughts should be taken seriously. No suicidal threat or gesture should ever be ignored; people who talk about or threaten suicide are at high risk for following through.

Although there is no typical suicide victim, some of the factors that increase the risk of suicide include

- Being male
- Having a mental disorder
- Engaging in substance abuse

- Having suffered recent losses
- Being impulsive
- Having attempted suicide in the past or a family history of suicide
- Having access to firearms

If a person is considering suicide, you can take certain precautions to decrease the risk:

- Remove dangerous objects (guns, knives, or other sharp objects).
- Take responsibility for the person's medication supply and only provide a dose at a time.
- Explicitly ask the individual if he is contemplating suicide.
- Give the person the opportunity to talk about her feelings; don't simply dismiss them. Try not to provoke a confrontation.
- Explain that the person is important to you and that his suicide would be a painful loss to you rather than any type of relief.
- Make it clear you want to help and ask the person to promise not to attempt suicide for a certain period of time.
- Explain that depression and suicidal thinking are part of his illness, that schizophrenia is treatable, and that you want to make sure he gets professional help as soon as possible.
- Your loved one may be willing to allow you to make an appointment with a mental-health professional for her. (Generally, a person who has attempted suicide or is considered suicidal can be hospitalized involuntarily.)

If you can't reach a mental-health professional in your community, contact the National Suicide Prevention Hotline at 800-273-8255. The hot line will route your call to the crisis center closest to you that has trained suicide counselors available 24 hours a day, to provide advice to individuals who are suicidal and to their families.

Dealing with Local Law Enforcement

You may think the last thing you need is the local police knowing all your family business. However, when a loved one has schizophrenia, family privacy often goes out the window, and you become much better acquainted with local law enforcement than you ever expected to be.

The best time to get acquainted is before a crisis occurs. Call or visit your local police department and make personal contact before you end up meeting in the middle of a chaotic situation. Explain your loved one's illness and determine, in the event of an emergency, how you should contact law enforcement and what information they'll need. You may be surprised and touched at the compassion law enforcement officers have when they understand the situation you're in.

When to call the police

Some family members have told us that "calling the police on a family member" has been the most difficult thing they've ever had to do. In an emergency, you may have no alternative but to contact the police or call 911 if your loved one with schizophrenia is suicidal, acting threatening to others, has been assaultive, or has a weapon. Be prepared to explain the situation and clearly state that the person has a history of mental illness. Tell the police about the events that precipitated the crisis.

With increased efforts to properly train law-enforcement personnel, they've become more informed about mental illness. Police officers will not generally arrest an individual with schizophrenia unless an actual crime has been committed. Police often provide assistance, in fact, in transporting the person with schizophrenia to a hospital or other facility.

What to do when a person with mental illness is arrested

The phone rings, and it's the local police department. An officer tells you that your loved one with schizophrenia has been arrested for a nuisance crime (perhaps urinating on someone's lawn, touching a stranger, or picking up something from a store counter without paying).

Although people with mental illness are more often victims rather than perpetrators of crime, people with mental illness often get into trouble with the law because of symptoms of their mental disorder — lack of judgment, impulsivity, and inappropriate behavior.

If you get a call saying your loved one has been arrested, do the following:

- **Find out where the person is being held.**
- **If you can, try to prevent the arrest by explaining that your loved one has a mental illness and ask the officer to help you get psychiatric care at an emergency room in lieu of arrest.**

- **If the person has already been arrested, ask the police if they can drop the charges.** If they won't, see if they'll release your loved one if you assure them that she'll appear in court.
- **If your loved one is being arraigned, be sure to attend the arraignment hearing and tell the defense attorney who you are.** Provide specific information about the person's psychiatric illness and treatment needs. See if you can get the charges lowered or dismissed to avert her being jailed.

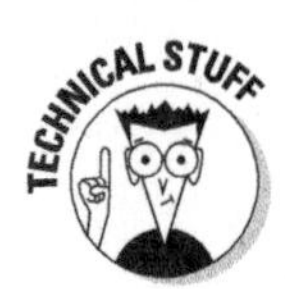

For some nonviolent individuals with mental illness who are not diverted from arrest or pretrial detention, some communities have established *mental-health courts* to allow these defendants to participate in court-supervised treatment designed and implemented by a collaborative team of criminal justice and mental-health professionals. For more about mental health courts, go to `www.ojp.usdoj.gov/BJA/grant/mentalhealth.html`.

- **If your loved one is jailed, assure that she's safe while in custody.** The risk of suicide is very high during the first day or two. State the facts plainly: Explain that your loved one has schizophrenia and you're afraid she might try to kill herself.
- **Engage a defense attorney to work with you and your loved one.**
- **Stay in touch with the mental-health staff at the jail to make sure that your loved one's release is planned in advance.** It's common for people to be released from jails without proper planning. You want to make sure that your loved one is linked to appropriate community mental-health services before her release.

People with schizophrenia should always carry some form of identification with a phone number for a relative or case manager in case of an emergency.

Mentally Ill and Missing

It isn't uncommon for people with schizophrenia to disappear suddenly in an attempt to escape their problems or to search for a better life. This situation is a nightmare for families who realize their loved ones are unable to take care of themselves and fear for their safety. There are steps you can take to find your loved one, however, so don't panic — but take appropriate action as quickly as possible.

Your first step will probably be to call the police, but keep in mind that they won't be able to take any immediate action. After three days, your loved one can be placed on an "endangered adult" list that's compiled by the FBI and sent out over a national alert.

While you're waiting, there's plenty you can do on your own. For example, you can:

- **Contact NAMI.** NAMI provides support and guidance for families of missing persons. You can reach them at 800-950-6264.
- **Develop your own one-page "missing person" flyer, with a picture and description of your relative, and put it everywhere you can think of.** NAMI suggests posting the flyers the following places:
  - Houses of worship
  - College campuses
  - Community health centers
  - Banks
  - Hospitals
  - Public libraries
  - Mass transportation centers
  - Free meal sites
  - The Red Cross
  - The Salvation Army
  - Homeless shelters
  - Social security offices
  - Social service agencies

  A family we worked with was reunited with their relative when his picture was noticed on a bulletin board by an alert nurse in a hospital emergency room.

  With the ease and speed of electronic communications, you can develop such a flyer and rapidly circulate it to everyone you know and to facilities in the community. You may also want to call the local newspaper to see if it would be willing to run a story about your missing relative.

- **Alert friends and relatives that your loved may show up in their area looking for a place to stay.** If you haven't been upfront with friends and relatives about what's happening with your loved one up to this point, now is the time to start.
- **Contact all your loved one's known hangouts and alert regular staff to call you if your loved one comes in.**
- **Make yourself accessible day and night.** Always have a cellphone with you and make sure the number is displayed on your flyers.

Advance Directives: Helping People Decide for Themselves

Healthcare power of attorney is a well-known and often-used tool in general healthcare — it's a written legal document that enables another person you name (known as your *proxy*) to make decisions on your behalf if you're unable to make them independently.

Psychiatric advance directives (PADs) for mental-health decision-making are a specific type of healthcare power of attorney that allows patients who are well (competent) to express how they want to be treated if they become ill again, generally as a result of a recurring mental illness like schizophrenia.

In Canada, PADs are called *Ulysses contracts.*

PADs are based on the idea that someone who was hospitalized in the past, perhaps involuntarily, may have definite preferences about the treatments he wants to have (or not have) next time around. For example, your loved one may realize that medication is helpful even if he's opposed to it when he no longer has insight into his schizophrenia. Conversely, he may not want a certain medication to be used against his will because he found the side effects intolerable.

Generally, your loved one shares his PAD with his psychiatrist or other primary clinician, or another person he trusts to serve as his healthcare agent. Depending on where your loved one lives, the state may or may not *require* him to appoint an agent. Having a PAD in place accomplishes the following:

- It ensures that the healthcare provider — and whoever else your loved one gives copies of the document to — knows his preferences.
- It facilitates an open dialogue between your loved one and his clinician about future care.
- It can prevent potential disagreements between your loved one and concerned family members or physicians around the use of medication.
- It can prevent court battles over involuntary treatment.
- It can help prevent relapse, by encouraging timely treatment before emergencies occur.
- It can specify directions for the care of the person's minor children in the event that he's incapacitated, which can be very comforting to a parent who has schizophrenia.

In the following situations, PADs are *not* followed:

- If the treatment requests in the PAD aren't feasible or acceptable
- If the PAD conflicts with emergency procedures
- If the PAD is outside the law

The National Resource Center on Psychiatric Advance Directives (www.nrc-pad.org) provides information about how to craft a PAD and offers state-specific information and forms. Also, the Bazelon Center for Mental Health Law has a fact sheet on advance directives that provides information and resources (www.bazelon.org/issues/advancedirectives).

Every state has a federally funded protection and advocacy (P&A) system that can advise you about the laws in your own state or refer you to a lawyer who can. To find the contact information for your state P&A, visit the Web site of the National Disability Rights Network (www.napas.org) or call 202-408-9514.

Chapter 15

People Are More Than Patients: Addressing the Needs of the Whole Person

In This Chapter

- Recognizing the fundamental importance of hope
- Facilitating the recovery process
- Meeting the basic needs of people with schizophrenia
- Identifying the roadblocks you'll encounter

People with schizophrenia are, above all else, people. They have hopes, dreams, and human needs like everyone else. When you're in the trenches dealing with the day-to-day challenges of the disorder, remembering this can be difficult.

Every day, people with schizophrenia live in a society that moves fast and often doesn't take their needs into account. Life doesn't stop while people with schizophrenia recover.

Although coping with an illness is vitally important, planning for the rest of the story is equally important. In this chapter, we look at the roadblocks, sometimes seemingly insurmountable, standing between the person with schizophrenia and a fulfilling life, and the realistic goals for normal living that can — and should — be set. Finally, we offer suggestions on how you can help move mountains for your loved one on their journey.

Overcoming Negative Expectations

About 40 years ago, two educational researchers conducted what has become a classic study about the effects of expectations. They found that when teachers expected students to succeed, the students succeeded, and when teachers expected them to fail, the students failed. In other words, what other people *think* you can accomplish can make a huge difference in what you *do* accomplish. The idea that expectations can affect outcomes has become known as the *self-fulfilling prophecy.* We believe that the same theory holds true in the lives of people with schizophrenia.

For many years, people with schizophrenia were *expected* to live a life behind institutional walls, with little hope of recovery and the ability to live a normal life. Fortunately, today's expectations are much more hopeful, although there's still a long way to go.

The expectations that people with schizophrenia set for themselves or that others set for them can dramatically influence whether their lives are "lives well lived." People with schizophrenia, their families, and their friends need to maintain a sense of hope and optimism. This idea isn't Pollyanna-ish — on the contrary, it's realistic! Like heart disease, diabetes, or asthma, schizophrenia should be thought of as a chronic but manageable condition that involves cycles of relapse and recovery. You and your loved one may not have exactly the same life you imagined (no one ever really does), but it can still be a satisfying and productive life!

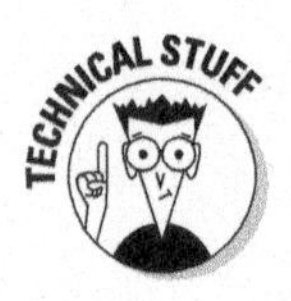

Expectations for people with schizophrenia have undergone a tremendous metamorphosis over the years. In 1896, German psychiatrist Emil Kraepelin used the term *dementia praecox* (early dementia) to describe the symptoms that are now encompassed by the term *schizophrenia.* He and others of his era saw the disorder as one with an inevitable downward and worsening course.

Time and solid research have disproved that idea. Long-term follow-up studies of people with the disorder have proven that schizophrenia is a chronic, but manageable disorder — typically with remissions when symptoms disappear and relapses when symptoms worsen. With early intervention, good treatment, and proper care, periods of wellness are longer, there is less disability, and more people (even most) are able to lead better lives.

If you or someone you know has ever had an elderly relative who received custodial care hidden in a remote state hospital for most of his adult life, never getting better or living a somewhat normal life, get that depressing, hope-crushing picture out of your mind. Mental illnesses are treated differently today.

For more on why schizophrenia was once seen as hopeless, see the nearby sidebar, "The low expectations of the past."

The low expectations of the past

The reason why schizophrenia was once viewed as a grim, and perhaps even hopeless, diagnosis can be explained, in part, by several phenomena:

- **Lack of treatments:** Until the mid-1950s, when the first generation of antipsychotic medications (major tranquilizers, neuroleptics) were introduced, the only way to control the positive symptoms (hallucinations, delusions, agitation, disorganized thinking) of schizophrenia was with sedative drugs such as barbiturates or chloral hydrate. These drugs had to be given at doses that caused sedation, stupor, and sleep before the positive symptoms were controlled. People medicated this way couldn't function and needed to remain in a protected environment.
- The advent of antipsychotic medications to control positive symptoms without making people zombies raised the specter that people with schizophrenia could return to their communities. Fortuitously, *deinstitutionalization* (a social movement oriented to treatment in the least restrictive environment) was taking hold and changed the once-dismal outlook for patients and families. (For more on deinstitutionalization, check out the sidebar "Overcoming the broken promises of deinstitutionalization," in this chapter.)
- **A life of institutionalization:** Because there were no effective treatments for controlling symptoms until the last half-century, people with the disorder had to be hospitalized (mainly for their own protection) for long periods of time, usually far away from their homes, families, and friends. In these asylums, there were no opportunities for the normal stimulation, socialization, and learning that others have living in the community — so people with schizophrenia became impoverished in both thought and behavior and began to look and act "institutionalized," distinct from the symptoms of their illness.
- **The clinician's illusion:** Another reason for negative expectations is the phenomenon known as the *clinician's illusion.* Clinicians (especially psychiatrists) are more likely to see patients with the most severe and intractable forms of schizophrenia rather than milder, more treatable cases. For decades, this situation biased their perceptions about what the disease looks like and how effectively it can be treated. Only when large-scale follow-up studies of entire groups of people with schizophrenia were analyzed did researchers realize that many people with schizophrenia have fairly successful outcomes.

Achieving the Goals of Recovery

An emphasis on recovery has provided renewed hope for people with schizophrenia, as well as their families and friends; it has also changed the expectations of people who provide treatment and care. The concept of *recovery* suggests that individuals shouldn't be reduced to their illness or symptoms alone; instead, they are "whole" individuals who have the same dreams and aspirations as anyone else does. After all, no one, regardless of her condition, wants to be viewed as only a patient — that denies the individual her personhood.

Although recovery may not take place along a straight line, it generally has a positive trajectory (even though there may be some bumps along the way). Recovery shouldn't be relegated to the later stages of schizophrenia — it should be an important concept from the very start of the illness.

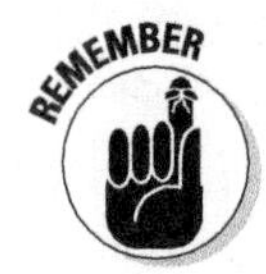

In the same way that people with physical disabilities are empowered when they have equal access (for example, a person in a wheelchair who uses a ramp to mount a curb or an elevator to catch a train), people with mental illnesses require and deserve the basic supports and accommodations they need to achieve the promise of recovery.

One essential element of recovery is the idea that people with schizophrenia should be able to manage and self-direct or self-determine his own care, to the extent possible, making decisions about the range of treatments or supports that are acceptable to him. This control is important for the individual's self-esteem.

The fact that patients vote with their feet, and will only comply with services that are acceptable to them, can positively or negatively impact their treatment plan. For example, if a program isn't welcoming and doesn't treat clients respectfully, they won't attend regularly.

The idea that a person with schizophrenia could recover enough to direct her own care is a fairly recent one. *Recovery* today has a much more positive definition than it did several decades ago, when full recovery and a move back into normal society were rarely possible.

The notion of recovery implies that the person with schizophrenia — without being cured — can still live life fully with the illness: living with as much autonomy as possible despite any residual impairments or disabilities. Recovery is an active and ongoing process that continues over time.

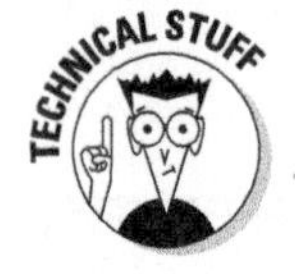

Maybe it's more accurate to use the verb, *recovering,* because it reinforces the ideas that people continue to grow and change incrementally, but continually.

Recovery is multifaceted because schizophrenia affects different domains of functioning in different individuals in different ways. For example:

- Someone's hallucinations and delusions may disappear completely with antipsychotic medication, but that person may still be unable to experience pleasure (in what's called *anhedonia*).
- An individual may no longer be suspicious or have feelings of paranoia, but she may be unable or unmotivated to seek work.
- A person may gradually ease into full-time work but may be unable to completely quell the voices he hears while working.

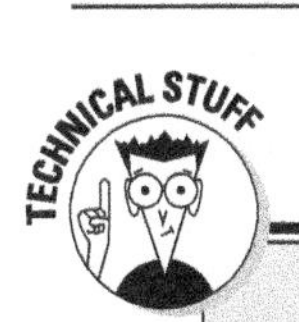

Overcoming the broken promises of deinstitutionalization

Few advances in mental-health treatments were welcomed as enthusiastically as the move to "mainstream" people with mental illness instead of keeping them warehoused in psychiatric hospitals, overmedicated, undertreated, and accorded few of the basic human rights. Popular movies and books like *The Snake Pit* portrayed mental institutions as horrific places, and the move to community care was the result of good intentions.

Having good intentions, however, doesn't always result in positive solutions. As primitive, ineffective, and sometimes inhumane as treatment was in the era of asylums, patients in these institutions were at least assured three square meals a day, clothes on their back, a roof over their heads, and a modicum of safety. Unfortunately, that isn't true today. With all the advances that have been made in scientific knowledge and improved treatments, and the growth of patient and family advocacy, there are still formidable barriers to decent care for people with serious mental illnesses like schizophrenia in the United States. In many cases, taking people out of institutions and putting them on the street has done a tremendous disservice to them, leaving many much worse off than they were before.

In essence, the movement toward deinstitutionalization in the United States ended up as a broken promise. Changes in federal legislation prohibited Medicaid reimbursement for inpatient stays in state mental hospitals. So in an effort to cut costs to state governments, patients were released from these institutions to communities that were often less than welcoming. The full array of community-based treatments and basic supports (especially affordable housing) never materialized for those who were most in need. Even today, too many people with schizophrenia still cycle in and out of local jails; live in substandard housing, in shelters, or under bridges; wait hours in crowded hospital emergency rooms only to be sent back to their families or the streets without treatment; and swell the ranks of the nation's homeless population. (It's estimated that about one-third of the homeless population suffer from severe mental disorders — the majority of them with schizophrenia — including many who are dually diagnosed with mental illness and substance-use disorders.)

One of the scariest end results of deinstitutionalization is the ability of people with mental illness to simply disappear into the streets and alleys of our nation's cities, leaving behind panic-stricken, desperate families with no way to contact them. If your loved one disappears, contact your local police department immediately, as well as the police departments in areas where you think your loved one might turn up. If she remains missing more than three days, the information you provide will be handed over to the FBI, and your relative will be considered an "endangered adult." Many families have had success in locating a missing relative after preparing a flyer with a picture and identifying information and posting it in shelters, hospital emergency rooms, and other places where their relative might go for help.

Despite these grim facts, there's much to be hopeful about in the aftermath of deinstitutionalization. With the right support systems, people with schizophrenia are much freer today to work at the jobs of their choice, live where they please, and live much like everyone else. The key to living a satisfying life is to identify goals, plan for them, and work toward them step by step. There will be bumps and detours along the way, but at least the ability to pursue the goals your loved one chooses for himself are there in a way they never were for those with schizophrenia several decades ago.

Being realistic about immediate "cures"

Medicine in general looks for "cures" as the definition of successful treatment. Although this approach may work in the case of surgery or a broken limb, chronic diseases — including schizophrenia — aren't cured in one simple step. All the snake-oil salesmen's claim for miraculous cures through use of a newly discovered herb oil have failed to deliver a permanent "cure" as well. It's more realistic in chronic diseases to see the stabilization that results from treatment as a positive recovery.

You and your loved one should think of recovery as a *process* with parallel paths and multiple goals rather than a single path with one endpoint.

Most important, the concept of recovery acknowledges the rights of all people, including those with disabilities, to have rewarding friendships, meaningful employment, and enjoyable leisure-time pursuits. It empowers them to set life goals and to move toward them instead of waiting for "total cure" or even remission of symptoms before engaging in life.

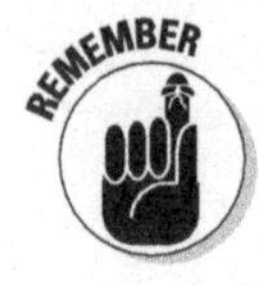

You need to convey to your loved one your confidence in her ability to help herself. When family members understand the notion of recovery, they're less frustrated about rough patches — they see them as part of the illness as opposed to a failure of their loved one or themselves, which helps them cope more constructively.

Breaking Through the Roadblocks

Because the burden of mental illness can be financially and emotionally overwhelming, people with schizophrenia and their families need to rely on community support. It takes a village. Yet, some already-gaping holes in the so-called safety net are getting noticeably larger rather than smaller. A number of recent national surveys have described the roadblocks to recovery; we summarize them for you in the following sections.

Experiencing long delays in getting treatment

Because people typically tend to minimize or be unaware of early symptoms of schizophrenia until the disease is undeniable, there's a lengthy gap between the time symptoms first appear and when they're treated (see Chapter 4 for more on the course of schizophrenia). People with schizophrenia experience delays averaging 8½ years before they get treated — despite research suggesting that early recognition and intervention improves outcomes and minimizes disability. (It's estimated that two-thirds of people with mental disorders remain untreated!) These alarming statistics point to the need for improved mental-health literacy that extends to families, family doctors, teachers, employers, and the general public.

Also, quality mental healthcare is unaffordable for many individuals and families. Despite advocacy efforts to implement mental-health parity legislation at the federal level and in many states, disparities between physical and mental-health coverage remain in the form of co-payments and coverage (see Chapter 7 for more on ways to finance care). State Medicaid and managed-care formularies often restrict access to more costly but effective psychiatric medications.

To ensure that your loved one gets treatment as early as possible, trust your instincts. You know your loved one better than anyone else. If you think something is wrong with him (perhaps after reading this book or learning some of the warning signs of schizophrenia), be direct and suggest that he see a mental-health professional for an evaluation. Gently explain to him that the symptoms he's experiencing (and you're noticing) are often associated with a treatable mental disorder and that you're concerned enough that you want him to check it out.

Don't be surprised if he doesn't think there's a problem and dismisses your concerns — it may take some time for him to come to terms with his symptoms and accept help. Unless the situation is an emergency, be patient. Just because *you* finally realize something is wrong doesn't mean he's on the same page. (See Chapter 6 for concrete suggestions on how to deal with lack of insight.)

Finding your inner activist

If you want to work to create change in the treatment of mental illness, or understand more about the systemic problems with mental-health care, check out the following:

- ***Achieving the Promise: Transforming Mental Health Care in America:*** You can get this 2003 report online at www.mentalhealthcommission.gov/reports/reports.htm or order a copy by calling 800-789-2647 and asking for item number SMA 03-3832, *Final Report for the President's New Freedom Commission on Mental Health.*
- ***Schizophrenia: Public Attitudes, Personal Needs:*** This report, published by the National Alliance on Mental Illness (NAMI) in June 2008, is available online at www.nami.org/schizophreniasurvey.
- ***The Insanity Defense: How America's Failure to the Treat the Seriously Mentally Ill Endangers its Citizens,* by E. Fuller Torrey (W. W. Norton)**
- ***Crazy,* by Pete Earley (G. P. Putnam and Sons)**

On the other hand, don't wait more than a week or two. Wait for a calm moment when he's open to listening and raise the issue again. Don't let yourself be deluded into thinking that if you just ignore things, they'll get better. In most cases, untreated mental disorders just get worse. If your loved one does have schizophrenia, you want to get on top of it sooner rather than later, to improve the outcomes.

When your loved one agrees to see someone, offer to do the legwork to find a clinician or suggest how he can go about it (see Chapter 5). If your loved one is insured, he needs to check with his insurer (or you can do so on his behalf) to find out about the mental-health provisions of the healthcare policy. If he isn't insured, find out whether your community offers free or low-cost services. (See Chapter 7 for advice on paying for care.)

Having no place to go in a crisis

According to a recent survey by the American College of Emergency Physicians, nearly 80 percent of emergency rooms report that waits for psychiatric patients in crisis average four hours or more; another 10 percent said waits typically exceed a day. Imagine sitting in a waiting room for four hours or more with someone who is agitated, upset, and actively psychotic and being told to wait before you can even speak to a doctor!

The number of psychiatric hospital beds in most communities is insufficient to meet the need. Since 2000, there has been a 12 percent decline in the availability of community beds for individuals whose treatment needs can't be met in outpatient programs. In 2008, the Treatment Advocacy Center reported a shortage of 100,000 psychiatric beds across the United States. The escalating costs of healthcare, an acute shortage of psychiatrists, and a scarcity of community-based alternatives to hospitals have coalesced to create a crisis in mental healthcare.

Once considered places of last resort for individuals with serious mental illnesses who were at risk of harming themselves or others, even state hospitals are no longer open to many people who need them. With states transferring financial burdens to the federal government, many state hospitals have reduced the numbers of their beds and now have lengthy waiting lists. As a consequence, with no hospitals or crisis alternatives available in their communities, people may be sent to hospitals far away from their homes and families or left to fend for themselves on the streets. This situation is particularly acute for young children and teens with schizophrenia.

To ensure that you and your loved one aren't left in a lurch during a crisis, prepare ahead. Check out resources in your community before you need them. Contact your city or county mental-health department and ask for information about crisis services — and keep it in a place where you can easily find it when you need it (see Chapter 14). Check with the state mental-health authority to become familiar with the laws for involuntary commitment and assisted outpatient commitment, in case they're needed.

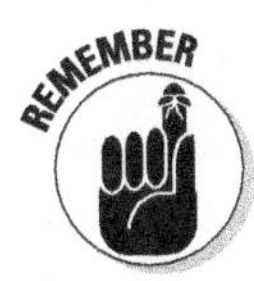

When you first interview psychiatrists, find out how they could help you in the event of a psychiatric emergency. Do they have admitting privileges at a local hospital or contacts with a crisis-response team?

If your loved one is living in a supervised or semi-supervised setting that is adequately staffed, or if you're able to sustain him at home, it may turn out that the crisis is relatively brief, and you may be able to ride out the crisis while he receives outpatient care. Many times, an acute crisis can be stabilized fairly quickly with rapid medication management and a bit more support from you, her psychiatrist, and other members of your team. Finally, both you and your loved one need to do all that you can by being alert to the earliest signs of relapse (see Chapter 18) and staying on medication that's working.

Looking at mental illness as a crime

According to the U.S. Department of Justice, mental illness is three to four times more prevalent among individuals in the criminal-justice system than it is in the general population. Forty-four percent of people with serious mental illnesses are arrested at some point in their lives. This is because people with untreated mental illness often get picked up for petty charges and misdemeanors that are due to their illness — sometimes by compassionate police officers who fear for the safety of these individuals on the streets. Police are twice as likely to arrest people who have mental illnesses, although most of them need treatment and services.

Jail diversion programs such as specialized *mental-health courts* (developed jointly by mental-health and criminal-justice providers) can provide more appropriate and less costly services. (See Chapter 14 for more about mental health courts.)

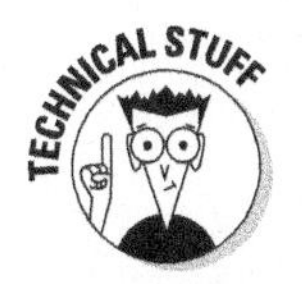

The Los Angeles County Jail has been called the largest mental-health treatment facility in the world, spending more than $10 million per year on psychiatric medications alone. Nationally, there are more people with mental illness in state prisons than there are in state psychiatric centers.

If your loved one is arrested, you'll have to move into action mode and intervene quickly. Following the steps outlined in Chapter 14, try to prevent the arrest by explaining that your relative has been diagnosed with schizophrenia — a brain disorder — and needs mental healthcare. In communities, where there are no formal jail-diversion programs, suggest that the officer divert your loved one to a psychiatric emergency room for evaluation instead of making an arrest.

Make sure that your loved one always carries some form of identification card, either with your name as an emergency contact or that of her case manager, so the police will know who they can contact in the event of an emergency.

Being over-represented among the downtrodden

Unfortunately, there's a strong association between schizophrenia, poverty, and homelessness. The large majority of people with schizophrenia have a hard time making ends meet and are often forced to live on the fringes of society. Mental disorders are the leading cause of disability among adults — and if you can't work in this country, you tend to wind up among the very poor.

Approximately one-third of individuals with mental disorders live below the poverty line. Nearly three out of four live on less than $20,000 a year; one in five lives on less than $500 a year. Plus, bureaucratic barriers make applying and appealing unfair denials for Supplemental Security Income (SSI), Social Security Disability Insurance (SSDI), and food stamps challenging for people with mental disabilities. And they may fear losing their benefits if they become employed at competitive wages.

With the stock of safe, affordable housing eroding, individuals with schizophrenia are often last in line for public housing in their communities. Thus, finding a decent place to live can be extremely frustrating. (Chapter 13 describes some of the limited options.) As a result, nearly three out of five individuals rely on their family or friends for financial support; half depend on them for housing. People with disabilities deserve safe and stable housing and opportunities to work and become self-supporting.

If your loved one has no money, she'll have a hard time paying for treatment of *any* kind. To help her, make sure that she has applied for all the benefit programs to which she is entitled, such as SSI, SSDI, Medicaid, food stamps, VA benefits, and so on. The Social Security Administration (SSA) offers an online Disability Planner (`www.ssa.gov/dibplan/index.htm`) explaining how to apply and qualify for these programs (see Chapter 7 for more information).

The eligibility requirements for public benefits are confusing, and filling out applications and providing supporting documentation can also be a daunting task. Your loved one will likely need your assistance in filling out forms and keeping all relevant information organized and in one place. In fact, you may want to seek outside advice from an expert, someone who understands the intricacies of these programs, perhaps a social worker or case manager.

If your loved one has troubling managing money, SSA and the VA have representative payee programs that allow another person (a relative, a professional, or a program) to oversee and assume responsibility for helping the individual to budget her money.

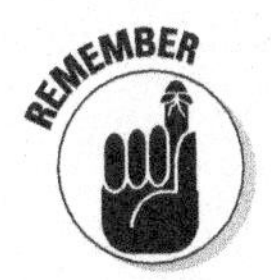

Working provides more than a paycheck to someone with schizophrenia. To feel productive, is vital to recovery. There may not be a straight line from A to B, but various vocational rehabilitation programs (see Chapter 7 and Chapter 14) can help your loved one define achievable steps to employment.

Receiving substandard healthcare

Disparities in healthcare are so great that people with schizophrenia die 25 years earlier than their peers. One out of four people with a mental-health disorder, substance-abuse disorder, or co-occurring mental-health and substance-abuse disorders has no health insurance at all, which sets the stage for problems in getting timely healthcare. Many people with schizophrenia never see any other physician besides their psychiatrists, who, unfortunately, are likely to focus only on their mental disorder as opposed to their overall health.

Yet, people with schizophrenia are more prone than the general population to get diabetes, heart disease, and other conditions (sometimes due to the side effects of antipsychotic medications), all of them chronic physical conditions that could be better managed with appropriate treatment. General medical needs are too often overlooked, ignored, or simply not addressed by primary-care doctors (if the person with schizophrenia even has a primary-care doctor). Nearly half of people with schizophrenia report that doctors take their medical needs less seriously upon hearing their psychiatric diagnosis.

Make sure that your loved one continues to be seen by a primary-care doctor the way you're seen — for yearly exams and other basic and preventive care. If your loved one is taking one of the newer atypical antipsychotic medications (see Chapter 8), you need to encourage her to monitor her weight and be seen by an endocrinologist to lessen the risk of diabetes.

In addition, you want to encourage your loved one to get regular exercise. Aside from its obvious health benefits, exercise can help lessen symptoms of anxiety and depression. Joining a gym or attending an adult-education class focused on wellness can help your loved one improve her self-esteem and find new friends.

Dealing with a complex treatment system

Even when services exist, people with schizophrenia often find it difficult to access appropriate care. They may not know where to turn or may get bounced back and forth between providers. For example, even though co-occurring mental-health and substance-abuse problems are commonplace rather than an exception, a substance-abuse program may not accept people with schizophrenia, and mental-health programs may not admit people with substance-abuse disorders. Instead of what has been termed "ping-pong therapy," people need an integrated approach to their disorders that addresses both conditions simultaneously.

Also, people may have to depend on costly and sometimes difficult-to-access public transportation or travel long distances to keep appointments with therapists. Like general medical care, navigating the maze is difficult under ordinary circumstances, but it's especially difficult if you aren't feeling at the top of your game. Think of the discomfort of riding in a train, feeling suspicious about the person sitting beside you, and having to remember which stop to get off at. When and if a person finally arrives there, rushed and often underpaid providers may be insensitive to sensitive clients and further undermine their already low self-esteem by failing to listen to them or involve them in treatment decisions.

When people have no insight, their families often encounter inordinate difficulties convincing mental-health programs that they need help until their relatives have been overtly dangerous to themselves or others. Many providers hide under the cloak of the Health Insurance Portability and Accountability Act (HIPAA), not only refusing to talk but also refusing to listen. (For more on HIPAA, turn to Chapter 14.)

Most of these problems are driven by the way services are funded and organized, leaving individuals and families burdened to find ways to bridge the gaps and make care more continuous. There are too few ACT teams (see Chapter 5) to provide aggressive outreach and follow-up, and the numbers of people on existing caseloads are often far too high. It's estimated that these programs only reach one in five persons who need them.

To find programs that can provide your loved one with an integrated approach to care, contact your state or local mental-health authority to find out about case-management or ACT programs in your community. Having a person or team who can oversee care helps assure continuity across different programs and providers. Additionally, that individual can serve as your loved one's advocate in making sure that services are accessible and that his needs are being addressed in a respectful manner.

Experiencing gaps between what we know and what we do

Clearly the medical profession's knowledge about schizophrenia and its treatment has been expanding at an exponential pace. Especially in the areas of both pharmacologic and psychosocial treatments, multiple articles and updated treatment guidelines have been published. These have been generated by research scientists, government-convened groups (like the National Institute of Mental Health) and professional organizations (like the American Psychiatric Association), all with the aim of updating clinicians with evidence-based findings that they can use to improve treatment outcomes.

Unfortunately, old habits (including treatment beliefs) die hard, and new information and knowledge about treatment hasn't trickled down to the people who provide care as readily the researchers would like. Thus, many treatments and services that *should* be in place and that have clear scientific backup aren't being used by all healthcare providers.

Books like this one and articles in daily newspapers and online (at sites such as `www.schizophrenia.com`) play an important role in reporting research findings to audiences who need to know about them. Don't hesitate to ask your loved one's clinician about whether your loved one could benefit from the advances you've read about.

You need to be a vocal advocate for your loved one, especially if she can't advocate for herself. This requires constant vigilance (although you don't want to make your loved one doesn't feel like you're hovering over her) so you understand her needs, as well as continuing education so you can keep up with the rapid pace of discovery. Read all you can whenever you can. Attend lectures and local, statewide, and national conferences sponsored by NAMI.

Facing pervasive stigma and discrimination

Myths and misperceptions still get in the way of full community acceptance of people with schizophrenia (see Chapter 16). Public awareness and understanding is still limited. In a recent NAMI survey, only one out of four people surveyed were familiar with schizophrenia. For example, people still associate schizophrenia with split personalities and serial murderers they see on TV; they don't realize that people with schizophrenia are ten times more likely to be *victims* of violence than the general population.

Due to stigma, people are embarrassed to tell others that they have the illness or that someone in their family is affected. This leads to feelings of shame, humiliation, and isolation that prevent people from seeking treatment when they need it and makes it more difficult to cope. A study of mental illness in the United Kingdom found that one out of eight people wouldn't want to live next to someone with a mental illness. Even treatment providers fall into the trap of forgetting to see their patients as people first, rather than faceless victims of a disease.

Discrimination and stigma restricts the choices that people can make. If your loved one has been diagnosed or you know someone with schizophrenia, become a stigma-buster and help educate others. The latter part of this chapter provides some suggestions of concrete actions you can take within your own community. In addition, NAMI has a StigmaBuster network, comprised of volunteers who help spot inaccurate media portrayals of mental illness and bring them to the attention of those responsible for perpetuating these inaccuracies on TV, in film, and in print. (To get involved, go to `www.nami.org`, and under "Take Action," click on "Fight Stigma.") Also, the federal SAMHSA Resource Center to Promote Acceptance, Dignity and Social Inclusion Associated with Mental Health (`www.stopstigma.samhsa.gov`) offers information and resources to help you understand stigma and its destructive effects on people with schizophrenia.

You can also do simple things to help reduce stigma for your loved one and others. Avoid the use of offensive terms like *crazy*, *loony*, *wacko*, or *nuts*. Use people-first language (see Chapter 12). Starting with yourself and your loved one, make it your personal mission to educate everyone around you that schizophrenia is a serious but treatable, no-fault, equal-opportunity, brain disorder.

Not having enough friends

People with schizophrenia need warmth and companionship like everyone else. If someone told you that he had a chronic health problem like cancer, you would react by offering him compassion and support. This usually isn't the case when friends, employers, and even some families find out about someone having schizophrenia. Disclosing the illness too often creates distance from once-friends, leading to an overwhelming sense of loneliness. For this reason, only about half of those surveyed by NAMI said they would tell someone if they were diagnosed with the disorder. Imagine living with that secret and being unable to share it with more than a few people, if any.

Ongoing companionship and support from family, friends, and the community are essential ingredients to recovery. Consumer-, peer-, and family-run programs can be instrumental in helping people learn to live and cope with schizophrenia — and also in recognizing that they aren't alone (see Chapter 9).

To help your loved one get the support he needs, encourage him to join self-help and peer support groups in your community (see Chapter 8). And make sure you're also getting the support you need as a caregiver by joining NAMI and actively engaging in your own life.

A Call to Action

You may feel so overwhelmed by your own situation at that moment that you feel like you can barely stay afloat. But by working collectively, and doing what you can when you can, you can change the face of treatments, services, and supports for people with schizophrenia. Take heart in knowing that NAMI and many other national organizations and concerned citizens take this task seriously. There is a citizen army working on your behalf!

There will be a time when you'll be able to rise up and have the energy to advocate for yourself, your loved one, and others. You'll be able to give back what you've gotten from others.

Here are some of the basic rules of individual advocacy:

- **Be voracious in your quest for knowledge and information.** Get your facts straight by harnessing and taking advantage of all the information available through people, books, and the Internet to increase your knowledge about schizophrenia and the resources available in your community.
- **Join NAMI and other consumer and family advocacy groups at the national, state, and local levels.** Members of these organizations are like an underground railroad of people who know how to work the system. They know the programs and the players and, most important, they understand what you're going through.
- **Make your voice heard.** Ask questions. If you have concerns about treatment or care, or a policy or legal problem affecting you or a relative, start at the bottom and move up the ladder. Let people know from the outset that you're informed, interested, and part of a larger group — you aren't part of the problem, you're part of the solution!
- **Whenever you communicate or advocate, put your best foot forward.** Stay calm even if you're angry, hurt, or disappointed. Be persistent yet firm — and listen. Use praise, diplomacy, and humor to get your way.

- **Don't sweat the small stuff.** Keep things in perspective, keep your eye on the big picture, and never give up.
- **Take care of yourself and live your life.** Undeniably, no one would wish for any type of mental or physical disorder, including schizophrenia, but you can't allow it to bring anyone's life to a halt — including your own. There are too many reasons for hope.

Whether you're only able to attend a NAMI meeting, write a letter to your local legislator, volunteer at a program, leave NAMI brochures in a doctor's waiting room, or make a phone call of support to another family member, with a little help and advocacy from everyday people like you, people with schizophrenia will be able to achieve the goals all of us share: living a meaningful existence with a sense of purpose, joy, and promise for the future.

Part V
The Part of Tens

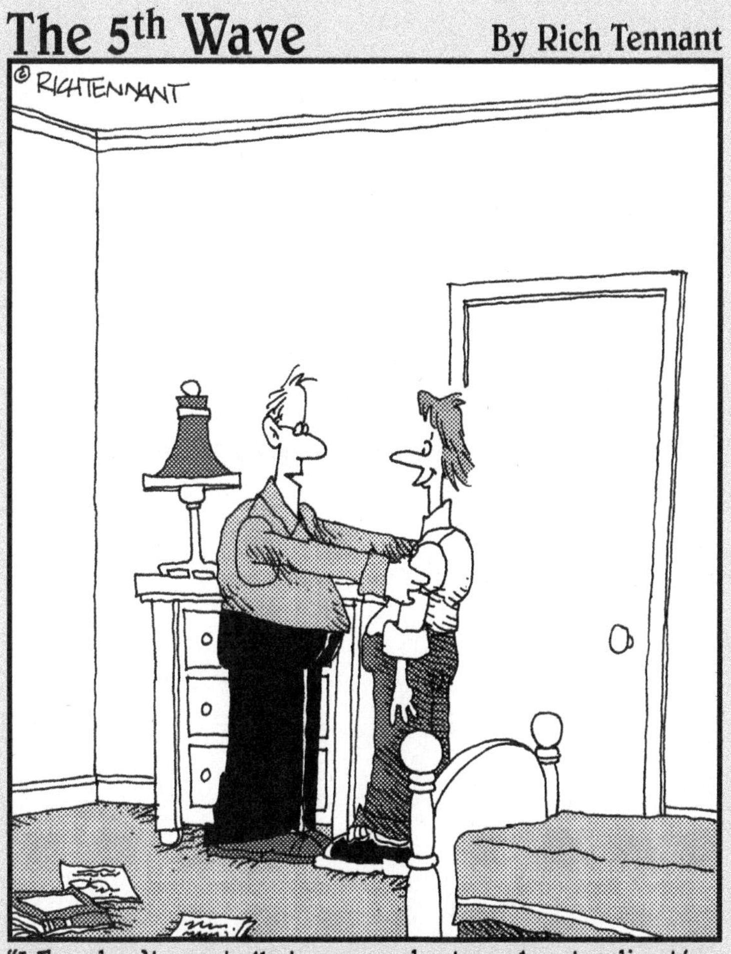

"Why don't we talk to your doctor about adjusting your medication, and then see about building that underground railroad to all your friends' homes."

In this part . . .

Every *For Dummies* book concludes with a Part of Tens that imparts the wisdom of the ages in short-list form. In our Part of Tens, we highlight ten myths and misperceptions about schizophrenia, ten tips for helping family and friends cope, and ten ways to avoid relapse.

Chapter 16

Ten Myths about Schizophrenia You Can Forget

In This Chapter

- Differentiating between what schizophrenia is and isn't
- Understanding the nature of people with schizophrenia
- Exploding the myths and misperceptions about the disorder and its treatment

Schizophrenia is one of the most feared, misunderstood, and stigmatized disorders because myths and misperceptions abound about the diagnosis, its symptoms, and its treatment. Although there still is no cure, schizophrenia is an eminently treatable and manageable, no-fault disorder of the brain.

In this chapter, we dispel some of the myths that get in the way of effective treatment and that impede public acceptance and understanding of people with the disorder.

Myth #1: Schizophrenia Isn't a Brain Disorder

Many people think that someone with schizophrenia is simply "acting crazy" and could behave normally if she wanted to. Nothing could be further from the truth.

Experts generally agree that schizophrenia is a no-fault neurobiological illness involving chemical imbalances in the brain and/or brain abnormalities that affect people in different ways. Symptoms of the disorder can include changes in feelings, perceptions, thinking, and behavior that are *rooted in biology.* Want proof? The growing body of evidence includes

- Measures of brain electrophysiology (as measured by EEG-type equipment) showing differences in people with schizophrenia
- MRIs of the brain structure showing enlarged ventricles and white matter damage in people with schizophrenia
- Functional MRIs showing malfunction in the frontal lobes as well as certain other areas of the brain in people with schizophrenia

What's still missing at this time is the ability to identify the *specific* chemical imbalance or brain abnormality that occurs in any individual diagnosed with schizophrenia. (This would be the equivalent of a lab test like the one that confirms a diagnosis of strep throat.)

It's quite possible that symptoms of schizophrenia are manifest in different ways for different people — just like one person can suffer a heart attack and experience chest pain, and another person suffering a heart attack may have pain in his arm or jaw, but not in his chest. In fact, scientists may eventually find that, like cancer or diabetes, there's more than one type of schizophrenia.

Myth #2: A Person with Schizophrenia Has a "Split Personality"

Schizophrenia is not a *split personality.*

Because the word *schizophrenia* is derived from the combined Greek terms *schizein* (meaning "to split") and *phren* (referring to the mind), people have long come to the erroneous conclusion that schizophrenia means "split personality."

For more than a century, stories about people with split or multiple personalities appeared in different forms throughout popular culture, capturing the imagination not only of authors and screenwriters but also of their audiences:

- Most students have read Robert Louis Stevenson's tale of *The Strange Case of Dr. Jekyll and Mr. Hyde,* in which both good and evil personalities are embodied in a single man.
- Supposedly based on a true story, *The Three Faces of Eve* was an Academy Award–winning movie portrayal of the life of Chris Costner-Sizemore, who was diagnosed with multiple personalities by her psychiatrists in the 1950s after witnessing two deaths and a terrible accident as a child. (Later, the psychiatrists involved in the case are said to have recanted the diagnosis.)

- More recently, the movie *Me, Myself & Irene,* starring Jim Carrey, told the fictional story of a state trooper who develops a split personality after his wife takes up with an African-American dwarf.

Although these stories and others like them are fascinating and entertaining, they've only increased the public's confusion when it comes to schizophrenia. In fact, almost two-thirds of people surveyed by the Harris Organization in the late 1990s still believed that schizophrenia was associated with a split personality. In a more recent online survey examining the mental-health literacy of university students, nearly two-thirds of them thought that a "split personality" was one of the main symptoms of schizophrenia.

The closest Diagnostic and Statistical Manual (DSM) of Mental Disorders diagnosis resembling the stereotypic split or multiple personality is *dissociative identity disorder,* a relatively rare and controversial diagnosis, the symptoms of which are distinct from those of schizophrenia. Making the diagnosis requires that at least two personalities routinely take control of the individual's behavior with memory loss that goes beyond normal forgetfulness. (This cannot be due to substance abuse or medical causes.)

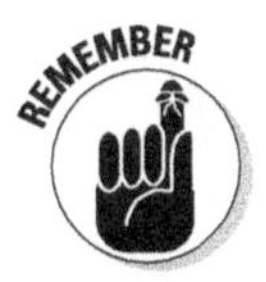

People with schizophrenia have only one personality, but they have problems distinguishing what is real from what is not. So, if there is any split associated with schizophrenia, it is the disconnect between (a) an individual's thoughts, behaviors, and emotions, and (b) what we call reality.

Myth #3: Schizophrenia Is Caused by Bad Parenting

Schizophrenia is a biological disease of the brain, with genetic underpinnings, and its causation has nothing to do with parenting styles.

For many years, even mental-health professionals were trained to believe that bad parenting, particularly by mothers, was the root cause of schizophrenia — so that became the conventional wisdom.

Imagine how it felt to be on the frontline with a family member you love suffering from schizophrenia, only to be told that you're the cause of your relative's illness — either because you were too cold, too rejecting, or too permissive, or because you gave mixed messages! The guilt, shame, and sense of remorse that resulted created enormous gulfs between doctors and families, and between patients and their families.

With advances in research and new imaging techniques that have opened virtual windows into the living brain, doctors have learned that schizophrenia is caused by an underlying neurobiological susceptibility (probably predetermined by multiple genes) that is exacerbated by certain prenatal, environmental, or social triggers.

Now most professionals view family members as partners in care as opposed to seeing them as part of the problem. Therapies focus on the patient rather than the "pathology" of the family. Family interventions are aimed at educating families about the disorder, its symptoms, and treatment; helping them learn necessary communication and coping skills; and providing them with support for their demanding and complex roles as caregivers.

Schizophrenia does run in families: Having a family history of schizophrenia places offspring at a greater risk for the disorder (see Chapter 2). But this association is genetic and has nothing do to with parenting styles. If you encounter a dinosaur doctor who still clings to the idea that families cause schizophrenia, run the other way!

Myth #4: Schizophrenia Is Untreatable

Although schizophrenia can't be cured, it can be treated and managed.

Less than 50 years ago, receiving a diagnosis of schizophrenia was akin to being diagnosed with a terminal illness. Families would resign themselves to the fact that their loved ones would live out their lives in state institutions, far removed from their family members, friends, neighbors, and communities, with little hope for improvement. People with mental illness were shackled for their own safety and protection, and locked behind bars for the protection of society.

With the advent of antipsychotic medications in the 1950s, it became clear that most people with schizophrenia could be successfully treated in the community and would be able to live in less-restrictive settings. Now when someone is acutely ill, she's typically hospitalized for a relatively short time (a number of weeks) until her acute symptoms are stabilized. Alternatively, treatment of an acute episode can sometimes take place on an outpatient basis.

Although scientists still haven't found a "cure" for schizophrenia, psychotropic medications and psychosocial supports are highly effective in addressing positive symptoms (see Chapter 3 for more on the positive symptoms of schizophrenia). The vast majority of people diagnosed with schizophrenia improve significantly with currently available treatments, and research holds the promise that people whose illnesses are now deemed "treatment-resistant" will be able to be helped in the future. Scientists are also working on recognizing the earliest signs of schizophrenia among those at high-risk, to prevent the disorder and to intervene early to minimize its disabling effects.

Significant gaps still exist in the availability of evidence-based treatments to reduce the negative symptoms of schizophrenia (see Chapter 3) and to get rid of the cognitive deficits associated with the disorder, but ongoing research is targeted in these directions. Most experts believe that, with proper treatment, at least one-quarter of those diagnosed with schizophrenia totally recover, another quarter improve considerably, and another quarter show some modest improvement.

Myth #5: All People with Schizophrenia Are Violent

Unfortunately, the media often sensationalizes stories about people with mental illness who are involved in acts of violence because it makes for catchy headlines, feeding into people's fears and misunderstandings about the disorder.

Although people with schizophrenia can be unpredictable, they're more often victims of violent crime than perpetrators of it. This is because they often appear to be frightened and confused, making them look like easy prey for criminals.

When individuals with schizophrenia *do* commit crimes, they're usually petty misdemeanors that are an outgrowth of their poverty and despair. For example, a homeless person with schizophrenia might urinate on someone's lawn because he has no access to a public restroom or may be charged with petty theft for stealing food when he has no money and is hungry.

When serious crimes do occur that involve people with schizophrenia, it's because their illness is untreated or is aggravated by drug or alcohol abuse. Acutely psychotic patients may have outbursts of aggression: Untreated psychosis — as well as the presence of substance abuse — increases the chances of an individual becoming violent or aggressive in response to voices they hear, feelings of being persecuted or followed by enemies, or feelings of loss of control over impulses. Psychotropic medications reduce the risk of violence as does substance-abuse treatment.

Myth #6: People with Schizophrenia Are Just Lazy

People with schizophrenia aren't lazy per se. However, they may *appear* that way due to symptoms of the illness, as well as the side effects of medications used to treat it.

People with schizophrenia often seem to lack motivation, energy, or "get up and go." They find it difficult to adhere to a regular schedule; instead, they sleep too much, sleep too little, or keep irregular hours. They may show no interest in getting a job or spending their time productively — preferring to stay in bed or watch TV for endless hours. These behaviors may convey the impression that they are just lazy and unwilling to do anything for themselves.

Understandably, people get very frustrated when they see a loved one taking it easy while they struggle to make ends meet. When they try to motivate the person, they may be met with a flat "I don't care" attitude. In addition, people with schizophrenia may show little interest or concern for other people, even those they love, and have difficulty making or keeping friends, or sustaining relationships with relatives.

For a long time, these "negative" symptoms were seen as side effects of psychotropic medication. This is true to some extent — but a constellation of negative symptoms is associated with the illness, including low energy, lack of interest in other people and things, and the inability to form social relationships and/or a lack of caring about social relationships.

When you understand that these symptoms are due to changes in brain chemistry and functioning, you realize how pointless it is to harangue your loved one with schizophrenia. It isn't a matter of a flawed character or a lack of will — nor is it something she can just "snap out of" on her own. However, with proper medication and other supports, negative symptoms are often manageable (although they *are* more resistant to treatment than positive symptoms like delusions and hallucinations).

Myth #7: People with Schizophrenia Are Loners Who Don't Want to Have Friends

Although people with schizophrenia typically have limited, narrow social networks, most of them would *love* to have friends and families of their own.

In many ways, schizophrenia is an alienating illness. When people are ill, they may have peculiar mannerisms, poor hygiene, and odd behaviors, all of which may make them unattractive or frightening to other people. They may be suspicious, fearing that others are talking about them, don't like them, or are out to hurt them. Additionally, they lack the social skills necessary to establish new friendships and maintain old ones — they may be less apt to understand social cues one on one, or to respond appropriately in larger social settings.

Schizophrenia is often associated with high rates of poverty and unemployment, too, both of which further undermine a person's sense of self-esteem and confidence. After all, one of the first things someone asks you when you meet is, "What do you do?" Many people with schizophrenia only see themselves functioning in the role of a patient, idling away their time and passively accepting care from treatment providers and support from family members. After paying their bills, they may have no money available for social or leisure pursuits. Stigma and discrimination make it all the more difficult for them to candidly explain their illness and its impact on their lives.

Yet, when asked, patients with schizophrenia often express a profound sense of loneliness and alienation and yearn for companionship. It's only human to want to feel loved and needed. Struck by the illness in the prime of their lives, they may have lost contact with their close friends from high school or college who moved on socially, vocationally, or geographically without them.

Even after recovery, they may be skeptical about renewing relationships with people who knew them then, feeling embarrassed to explain the time they lost due to illness and/or disability. For reasons that are obvious, they may be ambivalent about relationships with other people who have mental illnesses or with those without them. They feel like they simply don't fit in.

As a result of these losses, people with schizophrenia tend to over-rely on family to fill the void in their lives. It's not uncommon for adults with schizophrenia to remain in their parents' homes or depend on them for most of their social interactions. They may even be hesitant to participate in gatherings outside the nuclear family, such as holiday family get-togethers, because of the fear of being uncomfortable and misunderstood.

Peer support groups, therapy groups, clubhouse programs, volunteer jobs, social clubs, drop-in centers, and supported employment and rehabilitation programs can enable people with schizophrenia to gradually develop ties that make them feel more connected and better understood.

Myth #8: People with Schizophrenia Are Stupid

There's no association between schizophrenia and diminished intelligence. People diagnosed with schizophrenia have the same wide range of abilities as the "normal" population does. Yet there are reasons why people may assume otherwise.

Years ago, people with schizophrenia and those with developmental disabilities (once called "mental retardation") were often kept together in the same asylums, so it's easy to see how this misperception evolved.

Because the average age of onset of schizophrenia typically overlaps with the time when young people are pursuing their education and careers, a person who is "doing nothing" — not attending school, not working — may be assumed to be of low intelligence, not smart enough to work or go to school.

Plus, the symptoms of schizophrenia and the medications used to control them can lead to specific cognitive deficits such as impaired memory, inability to respond quickly, difficulty paying attention, and problems organizing and sequencing information. Many of these functional deficits can be minimized through cognitive remediation programs.

Myth #9: When People with Schizophrenia Start to Feel Better, They Can Stop Taking Medication

They're probably feeling better because they're taking medication, and stopping it on their own will increase the risk of relapse.

Schizophrenia is a chronic and relapsing illness that requires medication to be taken for the long-term. Just as someone with diabetes shouldn't stop taking insulin or someone with high blood pressure shouldn't stop taking blood-pressure medication, a person with schizophrenia shouldn't stop taking her antipsychotic medication unless she's advised to do so by her doctor and is carefully monitored.

Studies show that when people stop taking their medication, they're likely to have a relapse within the first year. The major reason people stop their medication often has to do with adverse side effects that feel unpleasant or uncomfortable. These can often be addressed by changing the dosage, adjusting how the medication is taken, switching to another drug, or adding another medication.

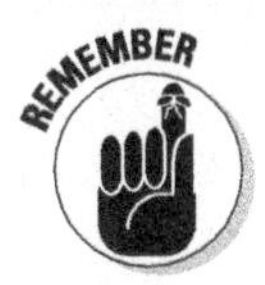

When someone is prescribed medication for a chronic illness, he may worry that he'll need to take it for the rest of his life. In the case of schizophrenia, this isn't always the case, but going off meds should only be done under medical supervision.

Myth #10: You Should Never Tell Anyone That Your Loved One Has Schizophrenia

With increased public understanding of mental disorders, families need to carefully weigh the pros and cons of disclosure.

For many years, people were terribly ashamed of loved ones who were diagnosed with schizophrenia. They never spoke about "eccentric" Uncle Joe who stayed upstairs in his room talking to himself or about Grandma Ethel who was sent away to a state hospital for most of her adult life. To have schizophrenia in your family was stigmatizing and reflected badly on other relatives. It was something that was only discussed behind closed doors.

Now that schizophrenia is accepted as a no-fault neurobiological illness, affected individuals and their families are more apt to be honest in telling friends, neighbors, and potential employers about the illness. That said, you still need to be aware of the potential risks because stigma still exists!

Peer and family support groups give people the chance to learn from each other how to better cope; they also provide some comfort — it helps to know that you're not alone. And legislation such as the Americans with Disabilities Act has afforded protection to people who need accommodations in the workplace.

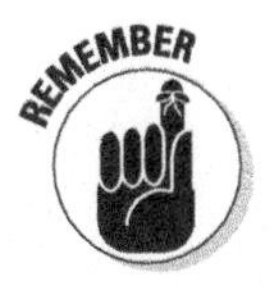

This doesn't mean that you should indiscriminately tell everyone you know about your loved one's illness. Determine for yourself how much to tell and when (see Chapter 11), recognizing that mental-health literacy and a spirit of openness goes a long way toward enhancing public awareness and minimizing stigma and misunderstanding. When the people around you know and understand your loved one's disorder, they can provide you with compassion, support, and understanding when you need it most.

Chapter 17

Ten Tips for Helping Families and Friends Cope and Come Out on Top

In This Chapter

- Building a team
- Partnering with professionals
- Educating yourself
- Supporting your loved one
- Taking care of yourself and the rest of your family
- Remaining hopeful and giving back

Never underestimate the value of family and friends in the life of a person with schizophrenia. The support you give and the advocacy you provide can make a huge difference in the quality of your loved one's life. In this chapter, we list ten ways that families and friends can ease the challenges of living with schizophrenia.

Select Your Team and Choose a Captain

To help someone with schizophrenia, it takes a team of experienced and caring people who are willing to work collaboratively with you and your loved one to:

- Diagnose the disorder.
- Plan and manage a comprehensive plan of treatment including medication, psychosocial rehabilitation, and supports.
- Help the individual achieve independence and move toward recovery. (Contrary to myth, a substantial percentage of people with schizophrenia are able to lead productive lives in their communities.)

Every team needs a leader. If your loved one is showing warning signs and symptoms of schizophrenia (see Chapter 3), seeing a psychiatrist who is well versed in treating schizophrenia is crucial. That person will be able to make the diagnosis and place your loved one on an appropriate medication regimen as soon as possible.

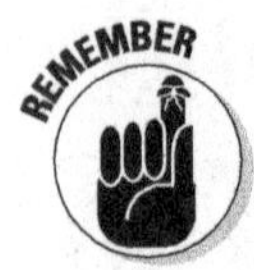

The earlier the illness is treated, the better the odds of recovery and the less chance for the illness to result in disability.

Finding a psychiatrist who specializes in treating schizophrenia isn't as easy as it sounds. The vast majority of psychiatrists (as well as other mental-health professionals) in any community are more likely to treat people for less chronic and/or less serious disorders. But your loved one will receive the best care if he's treated by people who work with individuals with schizophrenia all the time.

Like other hard-to-find medical specialists, the best way to find a psychiatrist is to ask other families or professionals (including your loved one's internist) if they can recommend someone. Your local affiliate of the National Alliance for the Mentally Ill (NAMI) — a family group providing information, advocacy and support — can put you in touch with other families who can share their experiences with you and vet any names that you have; you can find your local NAMI affiliate by going to www.nami.org/Template.cfm?Section=Your_Local_NAMI&Template=/CustomSource/AffiliateFinder.cfm (or by going to www.nami.org, clicking "Find Support," and clicking "State and Local NAMIs"). You also may want to contact the department of psychiatry of a local medical school for the name of an expert in your area.

A successful first visit is vitally important because it can determine whether your family member is onboard with — or alienated from — her doctor and her treatment plan. Interview a potential doctor by phone before making the first appointment, just to get a sense of whether the person will be a good match for your loved one. Sometimes, it's just a matter of making sure the person has the right style.

You also need to find out about the public and private mental-health programs in your community that offer an array of programs and other professionals — such as case managers, social workers, psychologists, psychiatric nurses, occupational therapists, and so on — who will comprise the rest of your team.

Your local NAMI group, the local chapter of Mental Health America (go to www.nmha.org/go/searchMHA to find your local chapter), and your city/county mental-health authority can provide you with information on mental-health programs in your community.

Understand Your Loved One's Diagnosis and Plan of Treatment

Decades ago, some people with schizophrenia were analyzed on couches for years on end as psychoanalysts looked for the root causes of their illness. Most times, parents (especially mothers) were wrongly blamed for causing schizophrenia.

With advances in medicine and technology, physicians, scientists, and much of the general public now know that schizophrenia is a no-fault brain disorder that is a result of both genetic and environmental factors. Medication has become the mainstay for treatment — along with cognitive-behavioral, remediative, supportive, rehabilitative therapies, and self-help and psychoeducational approaches.

Families no longer have to feel ashamed or worried that they did something to cause their loved one's illness, or that they're somehow part of the problem. In fact, families are part of the solution, because they can provide invaluable support and practical assistance to their loved one with schizophrenia.

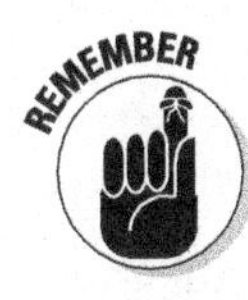

When you and your loved one meet with mental-health professionals, you're consumers who have the right to ask direct questions and get clear answers. The relationship is no different than the one you have with an internist. You'd never expect to leave the doctor's office without some explanation of what he's treating and how. Always make it clear that you're interested and involved in your loved one's care and that you have valuable information to contribute.

One complication that often interferes with family involvement in treatment is the federal Health Insurance Portability and Accountability Act (HIPAA), designed to guarantee patient privacy and confidentiality. If you find a doctor who hides behind HIPAA and is unwilling to discuss the nature of your relative's illness and its treatment with you, find another. You're not asking for personal details about your relative, but you are owed a clear understanding of the diagnosis and course of treatment. And, of course, you can always *provide* information! If your loved one is willing, she can sign a release explicitly allowing direct communication between you and her doctor. (see Chapter 14 for more information about HIPAA).

Even if your relative is reluctant to allow you to participate in her treatment now, her thoughts may change over time so don't give up!

Become the Archivist of Your Loved One's History

Because schizophrenia is a chronic illness, recognize early on that your loved one is likely to be seen by many different mental-health professionals and receive a variety of different treatments over the course of his illness. We all know how hard it is to remember the details of what happened years or even several months ago. For better or for worse, you're likely to forget some of your loved one's treatments over time.

Resist the temptation to write all the information you acquire on little scraps of paper that will get left in pockets, go through the wash, and get lost over time. Buy a hardbound journal or notebook so you can document your loved one's major symptoms, diagnoses, hospitalizations, medications (including doses, which medicines worked best and which didn't, side effects, and adverse effects, if any), and the staff who were involved in treatment.

Like other providers, mental-health personnel come and go. Close friends and family members are generally there for the long haul, so you can serve as the historian who documents and communicates which medications or other treatments worked or didn't work in the past, and why. You provide the continuity over time and can best explain the events that preceded hospitalizations and the approaches that helped foster recovery.

In your little journal or book, also be sure to keep a list of the names, titles, phone numbers, and emergency contact information for your loved one's doctors and other professionals intimately involved in her care.

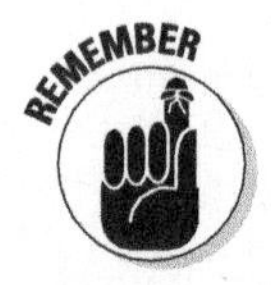

Mental-health emergencies can occur any hour of the day and any day of the week. If you plan ahead and keep information at your fingertips, you'll be able to handle things more smoothly.

Feel Free to Get a Second Opinion

Don't be skittish about seeking out second opinions if you have any concerns about your loved one's care, if there doesn't seem to be any improvement over time, or if you have a nagging gut feeling telling you something isn't right. You'd get a second opinion if you were undergoing a surgical procedure or if a medical treatment wasn't going well; don't feel funny about doing the same when dealing with a mental illness.

As a common courtesy, let your current doctor know you'd like a second opinion; it's always a good idea to leave the door open in case you decide to return to him. If the doctor is defensive about your getting another opinion, run in the other direction. Most competent professionals are happy to be able to collaborate with a colleague over a tough case (see Chapter 4).

If your loved one is part of a mental-health program and you have complaints or concerns, first speak directly to the person involved in her care before you raise the issue with a supervisor. Be open and give the individual a chance to respond. If you aren't satisfied with the response, direct your concerns to a supervisor.

Remember: No one knows your relative better than you do.

Oversee Medication Adherence

It can be hard to understand why someone would refuse to take medication that — to your eyes — obviously helps him. There are a multitude of reasons why patients don't adhere to prescribed regimens of psychotropic drugs. These include:

- Uncomfortable side effects
- Complex dosing schedules
- Confusion and memory problems that interfere with the ability to independently manage medications
- High costs
- Lack of understanding of the importance of staying on medication
- Denial of the illness

Medication is the key to treating schizophrenia. If your loved one isn't stabilized with medication, she's likely to remain out of touch with reality. To the extent that your loved one allows you to do so, become a medication enabler. Encourage her to talk to the doctor about:

- Simplifying dosing schedules
- Changing medications that have bothersome side effects
- Finding out about insurance, patient assistance programs, and entitlement programs that can help pay for medications

Helping your loved one set up and fill a divided pill container encourages her independence in taking the medication as it's prescribed.

Become an Expert

Receiving a diagnosis of any serious illness for the first time is life-altering. The emotional impact of being told that someone you love has schizophrenia cannot be underestimated. After you've had time to regain your equilibrium, you need to ramp up your knowledge and understanding of every aspect of the illness and its treatment.

You're taking the first step in your quest for knowledge by reading this book! Depending on your appetite or needs at the moment, read it in its entirety or in parts. Then read everything else you can and take advantage of all the resources available on the Internet, in the library, and from mental-health organizations (see the appendix). You won't have as much expertise as some of the professionals you'll meet (if you do, find another doctor!), but you'll gain enough wisdom to ask tough questions that need to be asked and deserve to be answered.

Familiarize yourself with the latest evidence-based guidelines and practices, which are available on the Internet at the National Guidelines Clearinghouse (`www.guideline.gov`).

Read memoirs of people who have lived with the illness so you can understand it from the perspective of those who have experienced its symptoms first-hand and of family members like yourself who have struggled and found ways to successfully cope and move forward. A few such memoirs we recommend are

- ***The Center Cannot Hold: My Journey through Madness,*** by Elyn R. Saks
- ***Crazy: A Father's Search through America's Mental Health Madness,*** by Pete Earley
- ***The Day the Voices Stopped: A Memoir of Madness and Hope,*** by Ken Steele and Claire Berman
- ***Divided Minds: Twin Sisters and Their Journey through Schizophrenia,*** by Pamela Spiro Wagner and Carolyn S. Spiro, MD
- ***Hope's Boy: A Memoir,*** by Andrew Bridge
- ***Imagining Robert: My Brother, Madness, and Survival: A Memoir,*** by Jay Neugeboren
- ***Mad House: Growing Up in the Shadows of Mentally Ill Siblings,*** by Clea Simon
- ***The Outsider: A Journey into My Father's Struggle with Madness,*** by Nathaniel Lachenmeyer
- ***The Quiet Room: A Journey out of the Torment of Madness,*** by Lori Schiller and Amanda Bennett

Enroll in a family psychoeducation course — free NAMI Family-to-Family courses, led by trained volunteers, are available in many communities. Attend lectures and courses offered by local organizations and educational institutions.

Don't Neglect Yourself and the Rest of Your Family

Friends and family can easily get lost in the day-to-day responsibilities entailed in helping their loved one with schizophrenia. Don't neglect yourself and the rest of your family. The surest recipe for burnout is to focus only on the person with schizophrenia to the exclusion of everyone else.

Make time in your day for:

- Sitting down for regular meals with your family
- Getting enough exercise
- Spending time with your friends
- Relaxing
- Continuing to do things you like to do

If you're in a relationship, don't forget your partner. Make time to do things together like going to the movies or visiting with friends. Often, relationships between husbands and wives suffer when a child has a severe mental illness because of conflicts over caregiving and the lack of quality time spent together as a couple. Recognize that you can be of tremendous support to one another.

If you have children in your household, don't neglect them or leave them feeling unappreciated. It may be hard for them to understand why so much time is being devoted to one member of the family. But if you make an effort to focus on each child's interests and activities, your kids will be more understanding when you have to spend some time helping your loved one with schizophrenia.

Reach out to other families and support groups. They can be invaluable in helping you realize that you aren't alone and that other people are struggling with similar issues in their families and making positive headway. Just as important, other families will truly understand your feelings and be able to share the wealth of knowledge, experience, and resources they've learned about. Need a doctor who has experience with Clozapine? Someone in the group is likely to know. Need a good CBT therapist? Ask the group for a list of three. Family members who have been there will be able to provide practical advice on how to react if your relative won't leave the house or denies that she's sick.

Familiarize Yourself with the Signs of Relapse

Not all the time, but often, relapse can be prevented. When your loved one initially became sick, what were his symptoms? When he had a recurrence, did he have the same sleep disturbance? Help your loved one spot problems on his own and take the right steps to get back on track. Talk calmly and openly about his symptoms so he feels comfortable doing the same.

Pride yourself on becoming a keen, but unobtrusive, observer so you can recognize the subtle signs that suggest the illness is recurring (particularly if your loved one is unable to do so on her own). Prompt attention often can help avert relapse and hospitalization.

Families find that the signs of relapse are the same, or very similar, for their loved one each time it occurs. These signs may include withdrawing from people, changes in eating or sleeping habits, severe mood changes, or changes in self-care and hygiene habits.

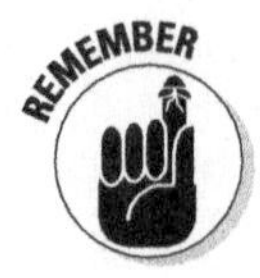

Even with good intentions, close oversight, and rapid treatment intervention, you may be unable to prevent your loved one from getting sick again or needing to be hospitalized. If that occurs, change your focus to how you can help him recover — and don't blame yourself!

Remain Ever Hopeful — With Good Reason

For a multitude of reasons, this is a time of great optimism in the field of mental health and mental illness. With recent research breakthroughs in genetics and neurobiology, there's never been a more hopeful time for people with schizophrenia and their families as we learn more about prevention, treatment, and rehabilitation.

In March 2008, the U.S. House of Representatives and the U.S. Senate approved mental-health parity bills that would help narrow the gap in insurance benefits between health and mental-health coverage and make treatment more affordable to many who have been left to fend for themselves. The proliferation of peer and family advocacy groups has gone a long way in educating the public and raising awareness of schizophrenia as a brain disorder that, although still not curable, is very treatable and manageable.

Families must maintain their sense of hope and optimism and convey it to their relatives. Your loved one may not live the same life you or she had expected, but she can live a "life well-lived," one with a sense of purpose and dignity. You can take pride in her accomplishments and in your role in providing support. Try to minimize criticism and conflict; instead compliment success and find areas of agreement. Allow her to take some risks and make decisions on her own.

Many families and friends of people with schizophrenia find that the close reciprocal relationships they develop with their loved ones are extremely rewarding, as opposed to burdensome. They appreciate the opportunity to provide friendship and concrete assistance to help their loved ones overcome the loneliness and social isolation so often associated with the illness. In return, they find that their loved ones are there for them when they need them, too. When one young man's father became very ill, it was the son with schizophrenia who drove and accompanied his mother to the hospital each day to be at his father's bedside.

And as difficult as it may be when you're in the thick of it, try to maintain a sense of perspective. As bad as things seem, it's likely that today's crisis will eventually pass and become a fading memory (although, of course, you'll have documented it in your journal — see "Become the Archivist of Your Loved One's History," earlier in this chapter).

Give Back

Sometimes it's hard to ever imagine having the time to give back to others or having the expertise to become a trainer rather than a disciple. Your journey as a caregiver will create new opportunities for you to contribute not only to your loved one, but to your community and to society. Many family members and friends of people with schizophrenia find rewarding roles as volunteers, case managers, and group facilitators working with individuals with serious mental illness.

When things are more stable with your loved one and you're up to the task, become an advocate for enhanced mental-health literacy in every segment of your community. As an individual or as part of a group, go out to schools, libraries, civic groups, and businesses to teach people about mental illness and dispel the myths.

Tell everyone you know about NAMI and spread the word that severe mental illnesses are no-fault neurobiological illnesses of the brain. Distribute NAMI brochures so they are available at every office, clinic, hospital, and library. Even many professionals aren't aware of NAMI.

Early recognition, diagnosis, and treatment can minimize disability and lessen family burden. People need to understand these disorders before they hit home. Engage legislators, public officials, and the media in a dialogue. The more patients and their families are willing to speak out and be candid about mental illness, the easier it will be for everyone to understand that schizophrenia is an illness that can strike any family.

Join the fight for mental-health parity and encourage support for psychiatric research at state and national levels. Participate as a healthy volunteer in a research project or encourage others to participate in clinical trials of new treatments. Most families and professionals recognize that research is the best hope for the future.

Chapter 18

Ten Ways to Avoid Relapse

In This Chapter

- Recognizing the signs of relapse
- Avoiding hospitalization
- Staying on track with treatment

When the symptoms of schizophrenia subside, keeping them under control and seeing that your loved one lives as normal and gratifying a life as possible becomes a high priority. In this chapter, we give you tools to help you achieve that goal, in the form of ten tips that may decrease the chance of relapse.

Staying on Meds

The best way for a person with schizophrenia to avoid relapse is to continue taking her medication as prescribed. Research shows that medication adherence reduces the risk of relapse and hospitalization.

Make sure your loved one sticks to a regular schedule, taking his medication at approximately the same time each day. If possible, he should link the time he takes the medicine to some regular event (for example, when he gets up in the morning, goes to sleep at night, or at mealtimes) or to some visual cue (for example, leaving his medication on the shelf where he keeps his toothpaste so he remembers to take it each morning.)

Anyone who takes multiple pills is apt to forget whether they've taken them. Instead of taking each pill from the vial that the medication came in, your loved one can spend a few minutes at the beginning of each week to set up a divided pill case. She may need your help to do this (either initially or on an ongoing basis), so don't be afraid to offer. Setting up the case at the beginning of each week will allow your loved one to see whether she's taken a particular dose.

Complex dosing schedules can make it hard for a person with schizophrenia to adhere to his medication regimen. If a doctor has prescribed one pill four times a day and another three times a day, find out if there is a way that the schedule can be simplified so that it's easier to remember. Sometimes when medication is first prescribed, it's prescribed more times over the course of a day, but afterward it can be taken fewer times per day.

Unless they're very bothersome or dangerous, mild side effects aren't a good reason for discontinuing medication. If the side effects of medication are bothersome, you or your loved one should report them to her doctor so he can change the medication or the dosage. If you or your loved one feels like the medication is no longer working or not working as well as you hoped it would, find out whether the doctor is willing to make adjustments, change the medication, or add another.

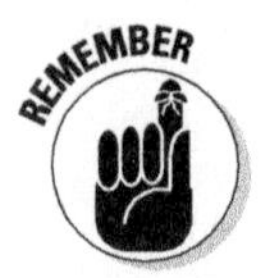

If your loved one feels that taking medication is embarrassing or degrading, remind him that hospitalization and relapse are far worse.

Sometimes people stop taking medication because they're feeling better, losing sight of the fact that they're feeling better precisely *because* they're taking it. This would be similar to women stopping birth control pills because they hadn't gotten pregnant that month, or people with diabetes stopping their insulin when their blood sugar levels were restored to normal. If your loved one says she doesn't need her medication anymore, because she's feeling better, talk to her about why stopping can be risky.

If your loved one's medication needs to be refilled from a mail-order pharmacy and he's running low, or if his prescription is running out and he's not going to see his doctor soon, call his doctor's office and let them know your loved one is worried about running out of medication. The doctor may prescribe a small quantity to tide him over until his next appointment or until the mail order arrives.

Don't wait until your loved one is close to running out of pills to refill her prescription. You never know whether the pharmacy will be closed on a weekend or the mail-order pharmacy will require more time to mail the prescription. Make sure your loved one stays on top of ordering her medications and saving the money she needs to pay for them.

Even co-pays can be costly. If the cost of medication is a barrier, take advantage of a patient prescription assistance program (see Chapter 8).

Considering Depot Medication

Ouch! No one likes the thought of an injection. But if your loved one has already had multiple relapse episodes while taking medication by mouth, it's possible that by using *depot medication* (a medication that's injected so the person doesn't have to take pills daily) these episodes may be avoided in the future. Depot medication is usually administered only once or twice a month.

Generally, these medications are the same kinds that are given by mouth, but they're given in a form that's retained in the body and slowly released into the person's system. This may prevent relapse for two reasons:

- It eliminates the possibility that your loved one will miss his daily doses of medication and guarantees a steady dose at regular intervals.
- Medication taken by mouth is absorbed and directly circulated through the liver, where it's metabolized; medication given by injection is absorbed directly into the body and avoids initial circulation to the liver. This may lead to a more effective use of the medication.

Recently, second-generation antipsychotic medications in depot form have become available (added to the first-generation depot medications, which have been available for some time; see Chapter 8). If while receiving a depot antipsychotic medication, your loved one is showing increased symptoms, it's possible, under medical supervision, to augment the medication by using an oral form of the medication, to raise the dose between injections.

An injection only once or twice a month may be an acceptable trade-off for having to take (and remember to take) medication at least once and sometimes multiple times a day. Not having to take medication every day may allow a person with schizophrenia to feel like she's leading a more "normal" lifestyle without constant reminders of her illness.

Recognizing Warning Signs

If your loved one has been diagnosed with schizophrenia, you and that person need to be aware of potential warning signs that might signal a worsening or recurrence of the disorder.

Early recognition, adjustments in medications, modifications in your loved one's environment, some extra support, or a combination of these things may help avoid relapse. The sooner this happens, the better the odds of warding off a full-blown episode.

Here some of the signs and behaviors you (and your loved one) should be on the lookout for:

- Believing unusual things, like that the television or radio are talking to her, or that the smoke alarms or digital clocks in public places are taking pictures of her
- Saying things over and over that don't make sense
- Hearing voices in his head
- Seeing things she knows aren't really there
- Feeling as if everyone is against him or out to get him
- A sudden or gradual decrease or increase in her ability to think, focus, make decisions, and understand things
- Thinking he's so great that he's world-famous or can do supernatural things
- Having a hard time controlling her behavior
- Having periods of time go by when he doesn't know what has happened or how the time has passed
- Having an unusually hard time keeping her mind on what she's doing
- Retreating from social relationships that were once rewarding
- Becoming afraid of common things like going outdoors or indoors, or of being seen in certain places
- Feeling like something bad is going to happen and being afraid of everything
- Being very shaky, nervous, continually upset, and irritable
- Being unable to sit still
- Doing things over and over again — finding it very hard to stop doing things like washing his hands, counting everything, or collecting things he doesn't need
- Doing strange or risky things, like wearing winter clothes in the summer and summer clothes in the winter, or driving too fast or acting like a daredevil

Although any one of these signs taken alone isn't necessarily a sign of relapse, they're things worth talking about with your loved one's clinician before they worsen.

Because everyone has off moments now and then, you need to learn how to distinguish between an *occasional* lapse (having a very anxious day and getting over it) and a *consistent* pattern or trend that might signal relapse (such as regularly being too anxious to leave the house to go to school or work).

The following are generally considered signs of a true psychiatric emergency (see Chapter 14):

- Feeling like life is hopeless and worthless
- Thinking about dying, having thoughts of suicide, or planning to kill herself
- Taking risks that are endangering his life and/or the lives of others
- Feeling like she wants to cut herself or hurt herself in another physical way
- Feeling the temptation to destroy property or commit a crime

If your loved one has any one of these symptoms, you need to contact a mental-health professional, crisis center, or suicide hot line immediately.

Note: The information in this section was adapted, in part, from *Recovering Your Mental Health: A Self-Help Guide,* a publication of the Center for Mental Health Services (CMHS), which is a part of the Substance Abuse and Mental Health Services Administration (SAMHSA).

Being Alert to and Avoiding Changes in Eating or Sleeping Patterns

Most times, an acute episode doesn't come on like gangbusters out of the blue. Instead, when you look back, you realize that there were subtle signs for days, weeks, or months that something was amiss. One of the most common signs is a distinct change in eating or sleeping patterns. That doesn't mean one night of having trouble sleeping or one day of feeling hyper-vigilant — it means a pattern that is different from normal.

Changes in sleep patterns can include

- Not being able to fall asleep at night
- Not being able to wake up in the morning
- Sleeping too many hours
- Getting only interrupted, fitful sleep during the night
- Having excess energy and little need for sleep

Changes in eating patterns can include

- Loss of appetite
- Excessive appetite

Your loved one should try to maintain a regular sleep schedule by going to bed the same time every night. Sometimes this is hard to do, but he can try to establish a bedtime ritual, repeating the same things each evening to help him sleep (for example, reading or listening to relaxing music for an hour before sleep). Sometimes taking a warm shower or bath, or putting lavender on the pillow, can help a person sleep more easily. Someone with schizophrenia should avoid doing shift work (for example, working nights or working day and night for a day or more) or traveling across multiple time zones, which can be disruptive to the *circadian rhythms* (also called a person's biological clock, they control the sleep-wake cycle).

Your loved one should try to eat balanced meals and keep track of her weight so she knows that she hasn't lost or gained too much weight.

Sometimes, changes in sleep or eating patterns can be signs of relapse, but they also can be side effects of various medications. Suggest that your loved one let her doctor know about these changes so he can help figure out why they're happening and whether they're any cause for concern.

Recognizing Your Loved One's Unique Warning Signs

Very often patients and/or families will recognize that certain behaviors or symptoms occur prior to an acute episode. Getting a feel for your loved one's unique signs is important, so you know which behaviors shouldn't be ignored. For example, one patient we knew started to withdraw to her room and sleep incessantly whenever she was on the verge of relapse. At first, she didn't recognize what was happening — until her sister brought it to her attention. Now, she's vigilant to this cue and consults with her psychiatrist who helps her avert more serious problems.

You and your loved one also need to recognize the specific triggers that may lead to relapse. For example, one young man with a diagnosis of schizophrenia had several failed relationships with female friends that led to breakups. Twice, they precipitated hospitalizations. He learned to approach relationships more cautiously and, in therapy, he found ways to lessen the stress he felt from such losses.

Decreasing Alcohol Use and Avoiding Street Drugs

Although most people don't think of alcohol as a drug, it is one. The reaction that your loved one has to alcohol will be determined by how much she drinks, as well as what other medications she has in her body.

Alcohol is considered a depressant, and when taken in large enough doses, it can put a person to sleep or even lead to death. Before your loved one was taking antipsychotic, antidepressant, or anti-anxiety medications, he may have been able to drink, for example, two glasses of wine, with almost no effect. However, because medications interact with each other, the effect of two glasses of wine when your loved one is taking other medications may be the equivalent of drinking *four* glasses. Your loved one can very easily become impaired on an amount of alcohol that previously wouldn't have affected him in that way.

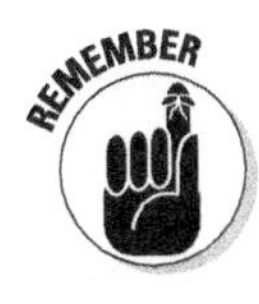

The safest approach is to not drink alcohol at all, but drinking a very small amount — such as half a glass of wine or a can of beer — isn't likely to have a severe adverse effect. However, keep in mind that it may not be possible for your loved one to drink a small amount and keep herself from going on and consuming larger amounts.

Some people with schizophrenia sometimes try to self-medicate by consuming large amounts of alcohol in an effort to control their symptoms. Talk to your loved one about this if you suspect it may be going on, and let him know that it's dangerous. Alcohol does not have an antipsychotic effect, and it can actually make symptoms worse. Let him know that alcohol has side effects and toxic effects. For example, alcohol causes damage to the liver when taken in large amounts over a longer period of time. However, taking alcohol with other medications that may also cause liver damage, may lead to liver toxicity earlier than would be expected from using alcohol alone.

Even over-the-counter medications from a drugstore can be dangerous in certain situations. For example, medications that are used to control allergies, or to help with sleep cause drowsiness; combined with medications someone is already taking, they may lead to excessive sleepiness or even coma.

Drugs of abuse, or so-called *street drugs* (like marijuana, heroin, or cocaine), should be avoided entirely. There's now clear evidence that marijuana in someone predisposed to schizophrenia can facilitate the onset of psychosis. Cocaine in itself is known to produce psychotic episodes, and in someone who already has psychotic symptoms (such as those seen in schizophrenia), this can lead to an acute and disastrous situation. Heroin, which is extremely addicting, can lead to a situation in which the individual not only needs to be treated for schizophrenia, but also requires a detoxification and rehabilitation program to be treated for the drug addiction simultaneously.

Compounding schizophrenia with drug abuse leads to poorer outcomes. So-called *co-occurring* (dual diagnosis) treatment programs are often hard to find in many communities, but people with co-occurring disorders must receive integrated treatment.

Building an Open and Trusting Relationship with Your Loved One

Although many people with schizophrenia don't like to admit it, people close to them (family members, friends, and professionals) may be able to spot the first signs of a problem long before *they* do. For this reason, you need to develop a trusting, supportive relationship with your loved one and encourage her to maintain a regular relationship with a therapist, psychiatrist, and/or case manager — people who can help her stay in touch with her own feelings about how she's doing, and who can point out any problems they see.

Be an active listener and a good observer. If your loved one expresses strange or uncomfortable feelings to you, hear her out and repeat to her what you heard (for example, "I'm hearing you say that you're feeling . . .). Then say, "I know you feel that way, but you really are safe here" or "Let's see if the doctor can help you think about another medication with less troublesome side effects." Try to offer helpful options without being judgmental or dismissing her feelings. The only time you may need to be more heavy-handed in suggesting that she seek medical attention is if you observe behaviors that are harmful to herself or others.

Admittedly, watching someone decline is very difficult, and you're often powerless to change things yourself. All you can do is be there, provide support and guidance, and help your loved one move toward making the right decisions.

Reducing and Minimizing Stress

Stress alone doesn't cause schizophrenia, but it can exacerbate symptoms and increase the chance of relapse.

Your loved one shouldn't be too hard on himself — and you shouldn't be too hard on him either. If he's just coming out of the hospital or is just entering the workplace, help him devise a way to take small steps to reach his goals. For example, doing volunteer work can help him adjust to routines before he returns to competitive employment. If he's returning to a position he previously held, part-time work is a nice way to ease his way back into the routines of the workplace. You might suggest whether this is something he can negotiate with his supervisor or the director of human resources. If he were coming out of the hospital after a major illness or after surgery, he wouldn't expect to return full-time right away; the same is true with schizophrenia.

Your loved one may also need to lower her own expectations or those being placed on her by others. For example, if she was recently diagnosed with schizophrenia, she might need to get her illness under control before she can return to school. In the scheme of things, missing a semester or even a year or two from college isn't a big deal. It's common for people to take leaves of absence for all sorts of reasons. If your loved one has already graduated from college and is thinking about graduate school, she may decide that graduate study is too stressful right now and take some time off to work. This may require your loved one to educate the people around her (including you) and directly tell them that she wants to make every effort to reduce the stress associated with certain types of activities.

You can help in this regard, too — for example, if your sibling has schizophrenia, and your parents have always wanted her to be a doctor, you may be able to sit down with your folks and let them know that, right now, your sister is going to work as a lab assistant or radiation technician, but maybe she'll decide to go to medical school down the road. Let them know that this is a good decision for someone who needs to minimize stress.

When you've been ill, social situations can also be stressful. It may be hard for your loved one to face his old friends or colleagues or to feel good about himself at cocktail parties where he meets new people. Tell him to take one step at a time. Suggest that he meet with one friend for a limited period of time — perhaps coffee or lunch — before he meets with groups or spends an entire day with one individual. He may even feel like he needs to spend some time alone dealing with his feelings or talking them over with a therapist before he takes the dive into the social world.

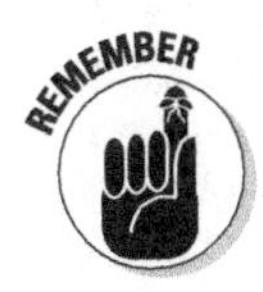

It'll take time before he'll feel back to his "old self." In the meantime, he needs to be comfortable doing less. Suggest that he take one day at a time and gauge how he's feeling before he takes on more — or too much.

Life often throws curveballs, even when you're already having problems. A person with schizophrenia can receive a devastating diagnosis of a life-threatening illness, be left by a spouse, lose custody of a child, be fired from a job, or lose a close family member. One family member expressed it philosophically by saying, "Life still goes on," regardless of whether someone has schizophrenia. Needless to say, these are extraordinary stressors that, in some cases, may be more stressful for someone with a mental disorder. Added stress generally calls for extra support and help — for whomever, whatever the circumstances. So if your loved one is hit with an exceptionally stressful event, make sure you're there to help him however you can, and pay attention for signs of relapse as well.

Planning Ahead

Sometimes, no matter what a person with schizophrenia does or doesn't do — or no matter how supportive his friends and family have been — relapse can't be avoided. For this reason, it's vital to plan ahead for the possibility of relapse.

Keep a list of the medications your loved one is taking, a short history of previous episodes and how they were treated, and the names and phone numbers of key people and contacts you will need in an emergency. This may include

- A crisis hot line or mobile crisis service you or your loved one can call in an emergency
- Your loved one's psychiatrist and case manager
- Your loved one's health insurer (write down her policy number or ID number as well)
- The name of the hospital your loved one would like to be in, if hospitalization is required.

Before a crisis occurs, talk to your loved one about the best way to handle a crisis, and put the plan in writing. (You both hope you'll never have to use it, but think of it like taking an umbrella with you on a cloudy day.) Reviewing past crises can give you a better idea of what works and what doesn't.

Another aspect of planning ahead is making sure your loved one's wishes are known and put in writing, before he's incapacitated in any way, so that his wishes can be carried out. Having *advance psychiatric directives* and allowing someone your loved one trusts to have healthcare power of attorney for him will allow him to make his decisions and preferences known while he's thinking clearly.

The Bazelon Center for Mental Health Law (`www.bazelon.org/issues/advancedirectives`) and the National Resource Center on Advance Psychiatric Directives (`www.nrc-pad.org`) are excellent resources for information, forms, and more specific advice for creating advance psychiatric directives.

Hanging in There

It can be disappointing, aggravating, and stressful to watch your loved one adhere to her medication and *still* hear voices or see things that aren't there. Don't dismay. There are behavioral ways to cope with treatment-resistant symptoms (see Chapter 12), and new medications and behavioral techniques are always in the pipeline. For example, some research suggests that humming reduces auditory hallucinations.

Research offers the hope that new treatments will address symptoms and problems that may now seem beyond your loved one's control and the reach of mental-health treatment. You need to convey this sense of hopefulness to your loved one!

Appendix

Resources

Finding out everything you possibly can about schizophrenia is vitally important when the disease affects you or someone you love. The more you know, the better you'll be able to cope and to seek out effective treatments and services. In this appendix, we fill you in on Web sites and books that we think will be most helpful in your journey.

Resources that are marked with a Tip icon are simply too important to be overlooked.

Web Sites

The Web can be an incredibly rich source of information, available 24/7 for people who want to learn about schizophrenia and locate help and support in their communities. But sometimes wading through the sea of information and finding the truth can be difficult. In this section, we fill you in on the most useful sites out there, so you can go straight for the ones you can trust.

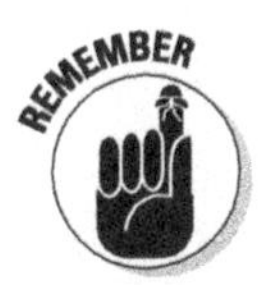

Web sites often change their addresses and/or content. This section is based on information that was accurate at the time this book was written.

For information on schizophrenia

The following national advocacy organizations can provide information as well as offer practical help in solving problems and finding support:

- **The Campaign for Mental Health Reform:** www.mhreform.org
- **Judge David L. Bazelon Center for Mental Health Law:** www.bazelon.org (phone: 202-467-5730)
- **Mental Health America:** www.mentalhealthamerica.net (phone: 800-969-6642 or 703-684-7722)
- **NARSAD:** www.narsad.org (phone: 800-829-8289)

- **National Alliance on Mental Illness:** www.nami.org (phone: 800-950-6264)
- **National Federation of Families for Children's Mental Health:** www.ffcmh.org (phone: 240-403-1901)

Government agencies can also be helpful. Check out the following:

- **Center for Substance Abuse Prevention:** http://prevention.samhsa.gov (phone: 800-729-6686)
- **Center for Substance Abuse Treatment:** http://csat.samhsa.gov (phone: 800-662-4357 or 240-276-2750)
- **Centers for Medicare and Medicaid Services:** www.cms.hhs.gov

- **ClinicalTrials.gov:** www.clinicaltrials.gov
- **Medline Plus:** www.nlm.nih.gov/medlineplus/schizophrenia.html
- **National Center for Complementary and Alternative Medicine:** www.nccam.nih.gov
- **National Guideline Clearinghouse:** www.guidelines.gov

- **National Health Information Center:** www.healthfinder.gov
- **National Institute of Mental Health:** www.nimh.nih.gov (phone: 866-615-6464 or 301-443-4513)
- **National Institute on Alcohol Abuse and Alcoholism:** www.niaaa.nih.gov
- **National Institute on Drug Abuse:** www.nida.nih.gov (phone: 301-443-1124)
- **National Institutes of Health:** http://health.nih.gov (phone: 301-496-4000)

- **National Mental Health Information Center:** http://mentalhealth.samhsa.gov (phone: 800-789-2647)

- **President's New Freedom Commission on Mental Health:** www.mentalhealthcommission.gov
- **PubMed:** www.ncbi.nlm.nih.gov/pubmed
- **Social Security Administration:** www.ssa.gov (phone: 800-772-1213)
- **Substance Abuse and Mental Health Services Administration:** www.samhsa.gov (phone: 877-726-4727)
- **U.S. Department of Housing and Urban Development:** www.hud.gov (phone: 202-708-1112)
- **U.S. Department of Veterans Affairs Mental Health:** www.mentalhealth.va.gov

Also check out the following:

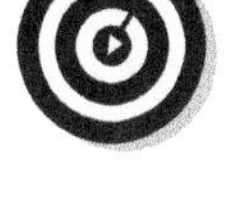

- **Boston University Center for Psychiatric Rehabilitation:** www.bu.edu/cpr (phone: 617-353-3549)
- **Criminal Justice/Mental Health Consensus Project:** www.consensusproject.org
- **Homelessness Resource Center:** www.nrchmi.samhsa.gov
- **Internet Mental Health:** www.mentalhealth.com
- **The Merck Manuals Online Medical Library Home Edition for Patients and Caregivers:** www.merck.com/mmhe/sec07.html
- **National Alliance for Caregiving:** www.caregiving.org
- **National Alliance for Research on Schizophrenia and Depression:** www.narsad.org
- **National Association of State Mental Health Program Directors (NASMHPD):** www.nasmhpd.org/mental_health_resources.cfm
- **National Family Caregivers Association:** www.nfcacares.org
- **National GAINS Center:** http://gainscenter.samhsa.gov
- **National Research and Training Center on Psychiatric Disability:** www.cmhsrp.uic.edu/nrtc

Brochures for the asking

Looking for brochures you can pass on to family, friends, employers, or co-workers to increase their understanding of schizophrenia? Check these out:

- ***Let's Talk Facts about Schizophrenia,*** published by the American Psychiatric Association: http://healthyminds.org/factsheets/LTF-Schizophrenia.pdf
- ***Recovering Your Mental Health: A Self-Help Guide,*** published by the U.S. Department of Health and Human Services, the Substance Abuse and Mental Health Services Administration, and the Center for Mental Health Services: http://mentalhealth.samhsa.gov/publications/allpubs/SMA-3504/default.asp
- ***Schizophrenia,*** published by the National Institute of Mental Health: www.nimh.nih.gov/health/publications/schizophrenia/complete-publication.shtml
- ***Schizophrenia in Children,*** published by the American Academy of Child & Adolescent Psychiatry: www.aacap.org/cs/root/facts_for_families/schizophrenia_in_children
- ***Understanding Schizophrenia,*** published by the National Alliance for Research on Schizophrenia and Depression: www.narsad.org/dc/pdf/brochure.schizophrenia.pdf

- **National Resource Center on Psychiatric Advance Directives:** www.nrc-pad.org
- **National Suicide Prevention Lifeline:** www.suicidepreventionlifeline.org (phone: 800-273-8255)
- **Partnership for Workplace Mental Health:** www.workplacementalhealth.org

- **Schizophrenia Digest:** www.schizophreniadigest.com
- **Schizophrenia.com:** www.schizophrenia.com
- **SchizophreniaConnection.com**: www.healthcentral.com/schizophrenia
- **The Stanley Medical Research Institute:** www.stanleyresearch.org
- **Treatment Advocacy Center:** www.treatmentadvocacycenter.org

For locating clinicians or care in your community

Where do you start when you want to find the best healthcare providers in your area? The following are good sources of information for finding the help you need:

- **American Academy of Child & Adolescent Psychiatry:** www.aacap.org (phone: 202-966-7300)
- **American Association for Geriatric Psychiatry:** www.aagpgpa.org (phone: 301-654-7850)
- **American Medical Association Doctor Finder:** http://webapps.ama-assn.org/doctorfinder
- **American Psychiatric Association:** www.psych.org (phone: 888-357-7924 or 703-907-7300)
- **American Psychological Association:** www.apa.org (phone: 800-374-2721 or 202-336-5500)
- **National Association of Cognitive-Behavioral Therapists:** www.nacbt.org (phone: 800-853-1135 or 304-723-3982)
- **National Association of Social Workers:** www.helpstartshere.org/common/Search/Default.asp (phone: 202-408-8600)
- **National Council on Community Behavioral Healthcare:** www.thenationalcouncil.org (phone: 301-984-6200)

- **SAMHSA's Mental Health Services Locator:** http://mentalhealth.samhsa.gov/databases
- **U.S. Psychiatric Rehabilitation Association:** www.uspra.org (phone: 410-789-7054)

For information on medications and medication-assistance programs

Need to know more about medication choices and how to pay for them? Check out the following resources:

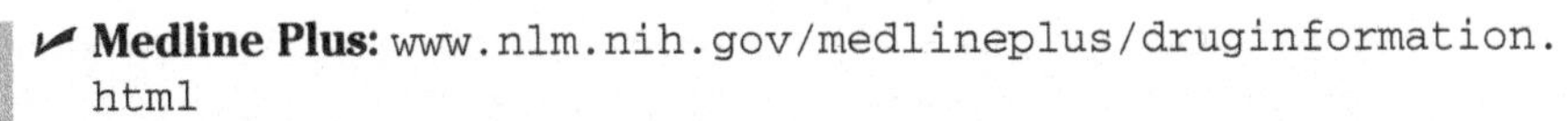

- **Medline Plus:** www.nlm.nih.gov/medlineplus/druginformation.html
- **Mental Health Part D:** www.mentalhealthpartd.org/01_Home.php
- **SafeMedication.com:** www.safemedication.com
- **U.S. Food and Drug Administration Index to Drug-Specific Information:** www.fda.gov/cder/drug/DrugSafety/DrugIndex.htm

The following sites catalog free and low-cost medication programs:

- **NeedyMeds:** www.needymeds.com
- **Partnership for Prescription Assistance:** www.pparx.org
- **RxAssist:** www.rxassist.org

For self-help and family or peer support

Sometimes you need resources for self-help rather than professional organizations. The following will point you in the right direction:

- **Active Minds on Campus:** www.activemindsoncampus.org (phone: 202-332-9595)
- **Consumer Organization and Networking Technical Assistance Center:** www.contac.org (phone: 888-825-8234)
- **Mental Health America:** www.mentalhealthamerica.net/go/find_support_group (phone: 800-723-8255)

- **National Alliance on Mental Illness:** www.nami.org/Template.cfm?Section=Your_Local_NAMI&Template=/CustomSource/AffiliateFinder.cfm (phone: 703-524-7600)
- **National Coalition of Mental Health Consumer/Survivor Organizations:** www.ncmhcso.org (phone: 877-246-9058)
- **NAMI Consumer Star Center:** www.consumerstar.org (phone: 866-537-7827)
- **National Consumer Supporter Technical Assistance Center:** www.ncstac.org (phone: 800-969-6642)

- **National Empowerment Center:** www.power2u.org (phone: 800-769-3728 or 978-685-1494)
- **National Mental Health Consumers' Self-Help Clearinghouse:** www.mhselfhelp.org (phone: 800-553-4539 or 215-751-1810)
- **Recovery, Inc.:** www.recovery-inc.com (phone: 866-221-0302 or 312-337-5661)
- **Schizophrenics Anonymous:** www.sanonymous.com (phone: 800-482-9534, ext.103)

Books

Although *Schizophrenia For Dummies* provides all the information you really need to know, it isn't the only book out there. The following books also provide good information that may be helpful to you. Some of them are more narrowly focused, and others provide more in-depth information to expand your knowledge:

- ***100 Questions & Answers about Schizophrenia,*** by Lynn E. DeLisi, MD (Jones and Bartlett)
- ***Breakthroughs in Antipsychotic Medications: A Guide for Consumers, Families and Clinicians,*** by Peter J. Weiden, MD; Patricia L. Scheifler, MSW; Ronald J. Diamon, MD; and Ruth Ross, MA (W.W. Norton)

- ***Clinical Handbook of Schizophrenia,*** edited by Kim T. Mueser and Dilip V. Jeste (Guilford)
- ***The Complete Family Guide to Schizophrenia: Helping Your Loved One Get the Most out of Life,*** by Kim Mueser, PhD, and Susan Gingerich, MSW (Guilford)
- ***Diagnosis: Schizophrenia,*** by Rachel Miller and Susan E. Mason (Columbia University)
- ***How to Live with a Mentally Ill Person: A Handbook of Day-to-Day Strategies,*** by Christine Adamec (Wiley)
- ***I Am Not Sick, I Don't Need Help! Helping the Seriously Mentally Ill Accept Treatment,*** by Xavier Amador and Anna-Lisa Johanson (Vida Press)
- ***If Your Adolescent Has Schizophrenia: An Essential Resource for Parents,*** by Raquel E. Gur, MD, and Ann Braden Johnson, PhD (Oxford University)

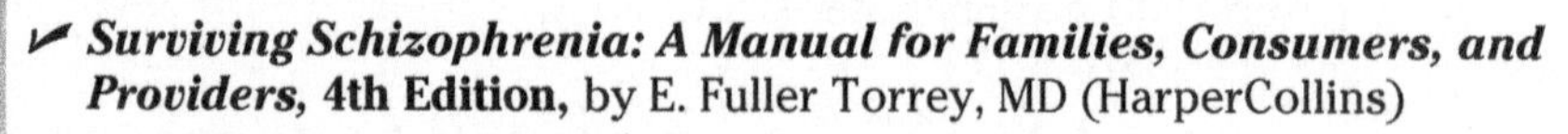

- ***Surviving Schizophrenia: A Manual for Families, Consumers, and Providers,* 4th Edition,** by E. Fuller Torrey, MD (HarperCollins)
- ***When Someone You Love Has a Mental Illness,*** by Rebecca Woolis, MFCC (Penguin)

Index

• Numerics •

• A •

• D •

• E •

• M •

• N •

• O •

• P •

• Q •

• R •

• S •

• T •

• U •

• V •

• W •

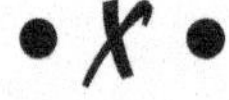

• Z •

INTERNET & DIGITAL MEDIA

AdWords For Dummies
978-0-470-15252-2

Blogging For Dummies, 2nd Edition
978-0-470-23017-6

Digital Photography All-in-One Desk Reference For Dummies, 3rd Edition
978-0-470-03743-0

Digital Photography For Dummies, 5th Edition
978-0-7645-9802-9

Digital SLR Cameras & Photography For Dummies, 2nd Edition
978-0-470-14927-0

eBay Business All-in-One Desk Reference For Dummies
978-0-7645-8438-1

eBay For Dummies, 5th Edition*
978-0-470-04529-9

eBay Listings That Sell For Dummies
978-0-471-78912-3

Facebook For Dummies
978-0-470-26273-3

The Internet For Dummies, 11th Edition
978-0-470-12174-0

Investing Online For Dummies, 5th Edition
978-0-7645-8456-5

iPod & iTunes For Dummies, 5th Edition
978-0-470-17474-6

MySpace For Dummies
978-0-470-09529-4

Podcasting For Dummies
978-0-471-74898-4

Search Engine Optimization For Dummies, 2nd Edition
978-0-471-97998-2

Second Life For Dummies
978-0-470-18025-9

Starting an eBay Business For Dummies, 3rd Edition†
978-0-470-14924-9

GRAPHICS, DESIGN & WEB DEVELOPMENT

Adobe Creative Suite 3 Design Premium All-in-One Desk Reference For Dummies
978-0-470-11724-8

Adobe Web Suite CS3 All-in-One Desk Reference For Dummies
978-0-470-12099-6

AutoCAD 2008 For Dummies
978-0-470-11650-0

Building a Web Site For Dummies, 3rd Edition
978-0-470-14928-7

Creating Web Pages All-in-One Desk Reference For Dummies, 3rd Edition
978-0-470-09629-1

Creating Web Pages For Dummies, 8th Edition
978-0-470-08030-6

Dreamweaver CS3 For Dummies
978-0-470-11490-2

Flash CS3 For Dummies
978-0-470-12100-9

Google SketchUp For Dummies
978-0-470-13744-4

InDesign CS3 For Dummies
978-0-470-11865-8

Photoshop CS3 All-in-One Desk Reference For Dummies
978-0-470-11195-6

Photoshop CS3 For Dummies
978-0-470-11193-2

Photoshop Elements 5 For Dummies
978-0-470-09810-3

SolidWorks For Dummies
978-0-7645-9555-4

Visio 2007 For Dummies
978-0-470-08983-5

Web Design For Dummies, 2nd Edition
978-0-471-78117-2

Web Sites Do-It-Yourself For Dummies
978-0-470-16903-2

Web Stores Do-It-Yourself For Dummies
978-0-470-17443-2

LANGUAGES, RELIGION & SPIRITUALITY

Arabic For Dummies
978-0-471-77270-5

Chinese For Dummies, Audio Set
978-0-470-12766-7

French For Dummies
978-0-7645-5193-2

German For Dummies
978-0-7645-5195-6

Hebrew For Dummies
978-0-7645-5489-6

Ingles Para Dummies
978-0-7645-5427-8

Italian For Dummies, Audio Set
978-0-470-09586-7

Italian Verbs For Dummies
978-0-471-77389-4

Japanese For Dummies
978-0-7645-5429-2

Latin For Dummies
978-0-7645-5431-5

Portuguese For Dummies
978-0-471-78738-9

Russian For Dummies
978-0-471-78001-4

Spanish Phrases For Dummies
978-0-7645-7204-3

Spanish For Dummies
978-0-7645-5194-9

Spanish For Dummies, Audio Set
978-0-470-09585-0

The Bible For Dummies
978-0-7645-5296-0

Catholicism For Dummies
978-0-7645-5391-2

The Historical Jesus For Dummies
978-0-470-16785-4

Islam For Dummies
978-0-7645-5503-9

Spirituality For Dummies, 2nd Edition
978-0-470-19142-2

NETWORKING AND PROGRAMMING

ASP.NET 3.5 For Dummies
978-0-470-19592-5

C# 2008 For Dummies
978-0-470-19109-5

Hacking For Dummies, 2nd Edition
978-0-470-05235-8

Home Networking For Dummies, 4th Edition
978-0-470-11806-1

Java For Dummies, 4th Edition
978-0-470-08716-9

Microsoft® SQL Server™ 2008 All-in-One Desk Reference For Dummies
978-0-470-17954-3

Networking All-in-One Desk Reference For Dummies, 2nd Edition
978-0-7645-9939-2

Networking For Dummies, 8th Edition
978-0-470-05620-2

SharePoint 2007 For Dummies
978-0-470-09941-4

Wireless Home Networking For Dummies, 2nd Edition
978-0-471-74940-0

Do More with Dummies Products for the Rest of Us!

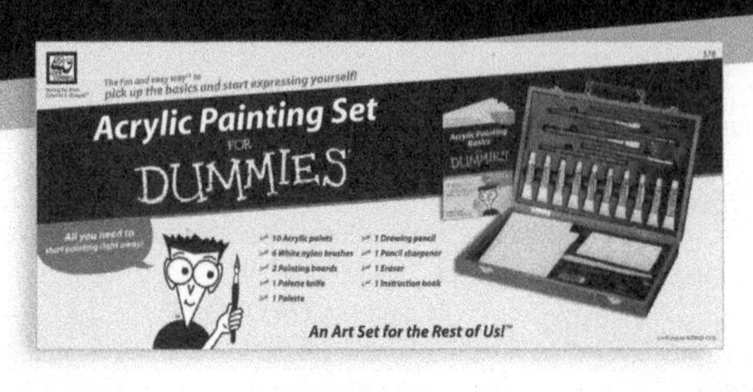

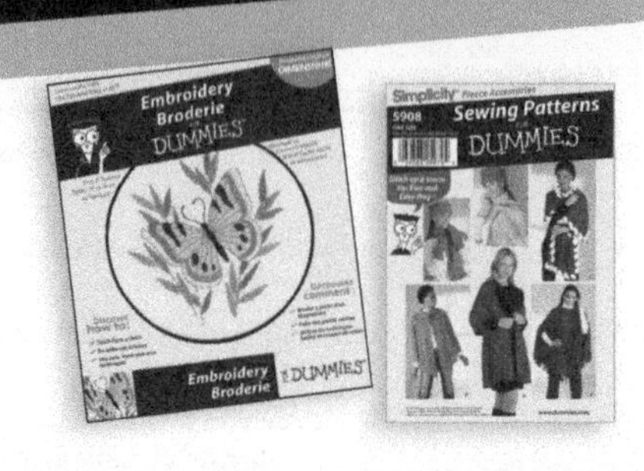

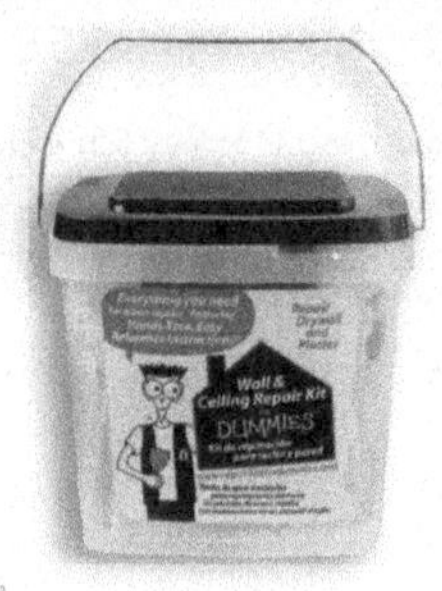

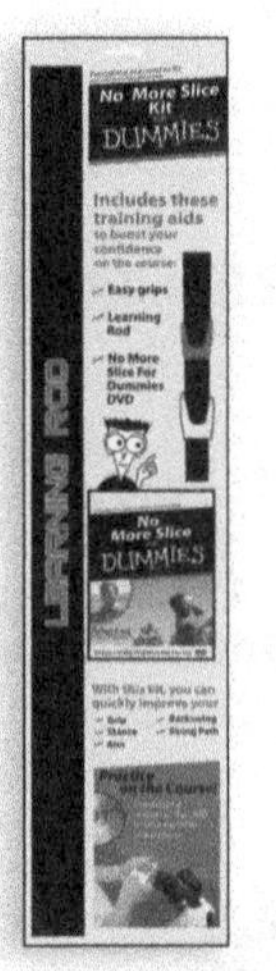

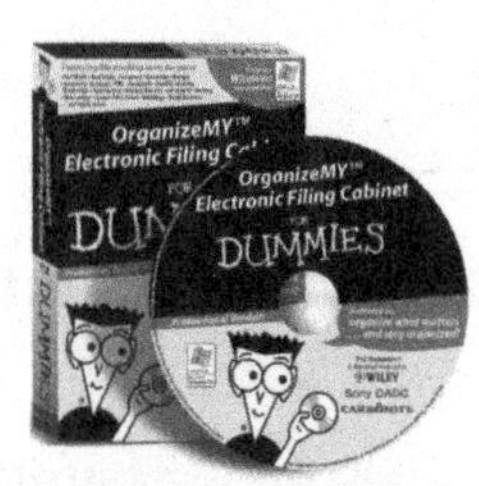

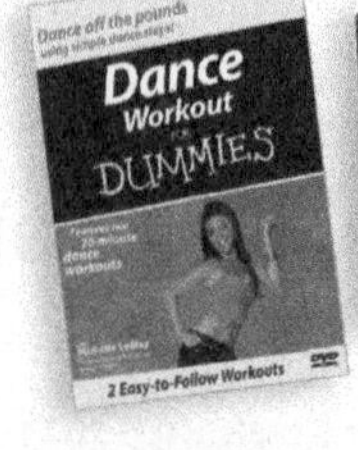

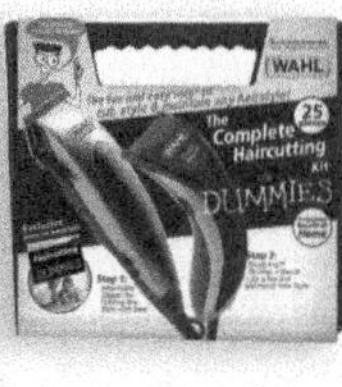

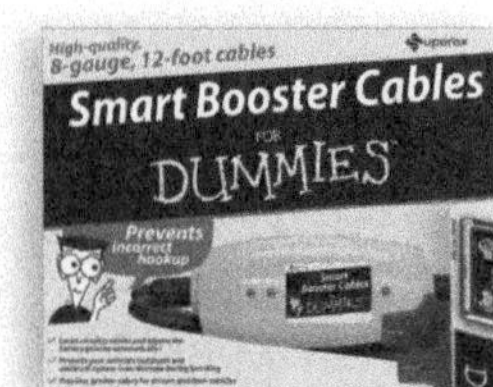

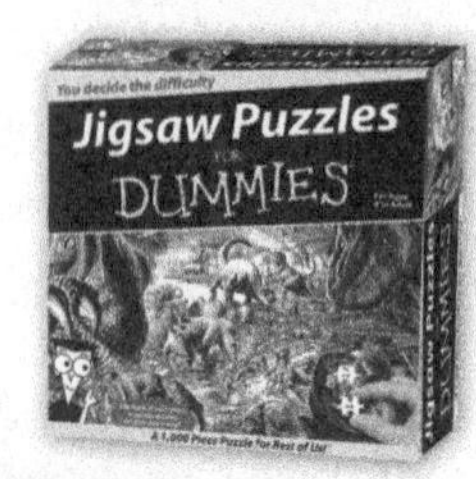

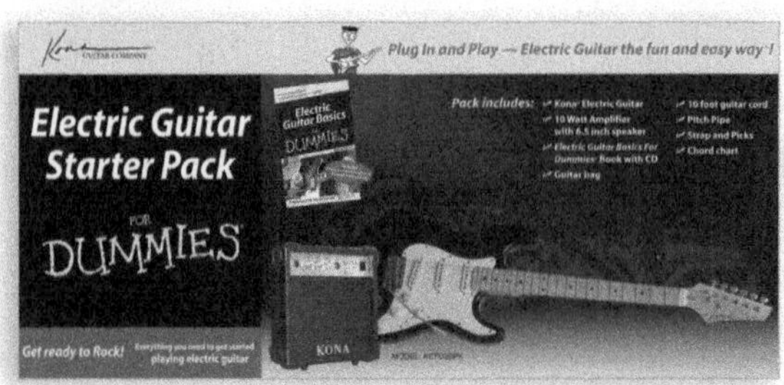

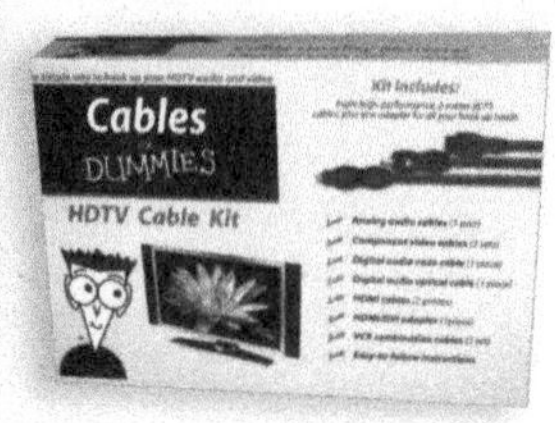

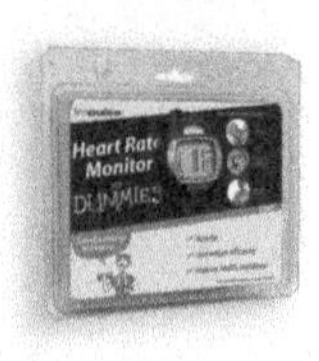

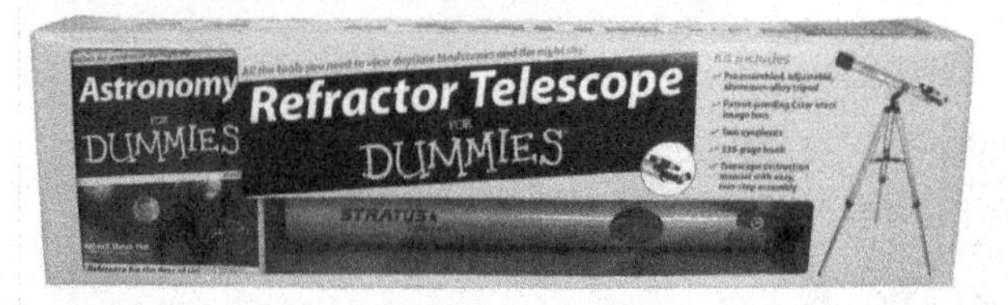

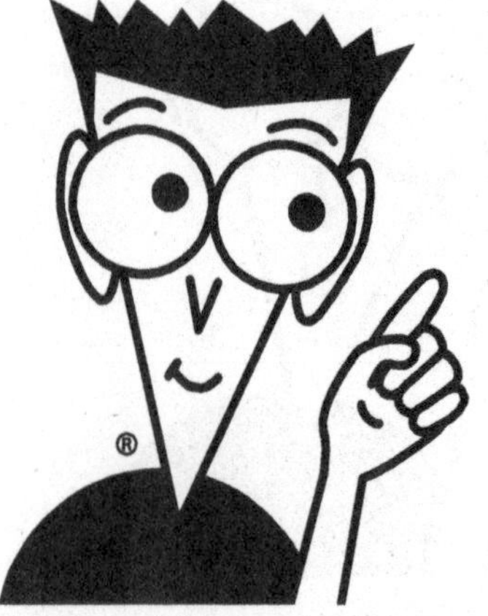

DVDs • Music • Games • DIY
Consumer Electronics • Software • Crafts
Hobbies • Cookware • and more!

WILEY

Check out the Dummies Product Shop at www.dummies.com for more information!